Diagnostic, Prognostic and Predictive Biological Markers in Bladder Cancer—Illumination of a Vision

Diagnostic, Prognostic and Predictive Biological Markers in Bladder Cancer—Illumination of a Vision

Special Issue Editors

Thorsten Ecke
Thomas Otto

MDPI • Basel • Beijing • Wuhan • Barcelona • Belgrade

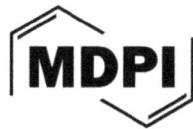

Special Issue Editors

Thorsten Ecke
Department of Urology
HELIOS Hospital Bad Saarow
Germany

Thomas Otto
Urologische Klinik
Städtische Kliniken Neuss-Lukaskrankenhaus-GmbH
Germany

Editorial Office
MDPI
St. Alban-Anlage 66
4052 Basel, Switzerland

This is a reprint of articles from the Special Issue published online in the open access journal *International Journal of Molecular Sciences* (ISSN 1422-0067) from 2017 to 2018 (available at: https://www.mdpi.com/journal/ijms/special_issues/bladder_cancer)

For citation purposes, cite each article independently as indicated on the article page online and as indicated below:

LastName, A.A.; LastName, B.B.; LastName, C.C. Article Title. *Journal Name* **Year**, *Article Number*, Page Range.

ISBN 978-3-03897-634-9 (Pbk)
ISBN 978-3-03897-635-6 (PDF)

Cover image courtesy of Aleksandra Ecke and Alicja Ecke.

© 2019 by the authors. Articles in this book are Open Access and distributed under the Creative Commons Attribution (CC BY) license, which allows users to download, copy and build upon published articles, as long as the author and publisher are properly credited, which ensures maximum dissemination and a wider impact of our publications.

The book as a whole is distributed by MDPI under the terms and conditions of the Creative Commons license CC BY-NC-ND.

Contents

About the Special Issue Editors vii

Preface to "Diagnostic, Prognostic and Predictive Biological Markers in Bladder Cancer—Illumination of a Vision" ix

Thorsten H. Ecke and Thomas Otto
Illumination of a Vision—How Arthur Rimbaud Will Give Us Motivation to Find New Input into Bladder Cancer Biomarker Research
Reprinted from: *Int. J. Mol. Sci.* **2017**, *18*, 2463, doi:10.3390/ijms18112463 1

Thorsten H. Ecke, Sarah Weiß, Carsten Stephan, Steffen Hallmann, Christian Arndt, Dimitri Barski, Thomas Otto and Holger Gerullis
UBC® Rapid Test—A Urinary Point-of-Care (POC) Assay for Diagnosis of Bladder Cancer with a focus on Non-Muscle Invasive High-Grade Tumors: Results of a Multicenter-Study
Reprinted from: *Int. J. Mol. Sci.* **2018**, *19*, 3841, doi:10.3390/ijms19123841 6

Markus Eckstein, Ralph Markus Wirtz, Matthias Gross-Weege, Johannes Breyer, Wolfgang Otto, Robert Stoehr, Danijel Sikic, Bastian Keck, Sebastian Eidt, Maximilian Burger, Christian Bolenz, Katja Nitschke, Stefan Proubsky, Arndt Hartmann and Philipp Erben
mRNA-Expression of *KRT5* and *KRT20* Defines Distinct Prognostic Subgroups of Muscle-Invasive Urothelial Bladder Cancer Correlating with Histological Variants
Reprinted from: *Int. J. Mol. Sci.* **2018**, *19*, 3396, doi:10.3390/ijms19113396 18

Mirja Geelvink, Armin Babmorad, Angela Maurer, Robert Stöhr, Tobias Grimm, Christian Bach, Ruth Knuechel, Michael Rose and Nadine T. Gaisa
Diagnostic and Prognostic Implications of FGFR3^{high}/Ki67^{high} Papillary Bladder Cancers
Reprinted from: *Int. J. Mol. Sci.* **2018**, *19*, 2548, doi:10.3390/ijms19092548 31

Anja Rabien, Nadine Ratert, Anica Högner, Andreas Erbersdobler, Klaus Jung, Thorsten H. Ecke and Ergin Kilic
Diagnostic and Prognostic Potential of MicroRNA Maturation Regulators Drosha, AGO1 and AGO2 in Urothelial Carcinomas of the Bladder
Reprinted from: *Int. J. Mol. Sci.* **2018**, *19*, 1622, doi:10.3390/ijms19061622 45

Jan Gleichenhagen, Christian Arndt, Swaantje Casjens, Carmen Meinig, Holger Gerullis, Irina Raiko, Thomas Brüning, Thorsten Ecke and Georg Johnen
Evaluation of a New Survivin ELISA and UBC® Rapid for the Detection of Bladder Cancer in Urine
Reprinted from: *Int. J. Mol. Sci.* **2018**, *19*, 226, doi:10.3390/ijms19010226 57

Toshikazu Tanaka, Tohru Yoneyama, Daisuke Noro, Kengo Imanishi, Yuta Kojima, Shingo Hatakeyama, Yuki Tobisawa, Kazuyuki Mori, Hayato Yamamoto, Atsushi Imai, Takahiro Yoneyama, Yasuhiro Hashimoto, Takuya Koie, Masakazu Tanaka, Shin-Ichiro Nishimura, Shizuka Kurauchi, Ippei Takahashi and Chikara Ohyama
Aberrant *N*-Glycosylation Profile of Serum Immunoglobulins is a Diagnostic Biomarker of Urothelial Carcinomas
Reprinted from: *Int. J. Mol. Sci.* **2017**, *18*, 2632, doi:10.3390/ijms18122632 70

Makito Miyake, Yoshihiro Tatsumi, Daisuke Gotoh, Sayuri Ohnishi, Takuya Owari,
Kota Iida, Kenta Ohnishi, Shunta Hori, Yosuke Morizawa, Yoshitaka Itami,
Yasushi Nakai, Takeshi Inoue, Satoshi Anai, Kazumasa Torimoto, Katsuya Aoki,
Keiji Shimada, Noboru Konishi, Nobumichi Tanaka and Kiyohide Fujimoto
Regulatory T Cells and Tumor-Associated Macrophages in the Tumor Microenvironment in
Non-Muscle Invasive Bladder Cancer Treated with Intravesical Bacille Calmette-Guérin:
A Long-Term Follow-Up Study of a Japanese Cohort
Reprinted from: *Int. J. Mol. Sci.* **2017**, *18*, 2186, doi:10.3390/ijms18102186 83

Hiroshi Fukushima, Kosuke Takemura, Hiroaki Suzuki and Fumitaka Koga
Impact of Sarcopenia as a Prognostic Biomarker of Bladder Cancer
Reprinted from: *Int. J. Mol. Sci.* **2018**, *19*, 2999, doi:10.3390/ijms19102999 95

Yu-Ru Liu, Carlos J. Ortiz-Bonilla and Yi-Fen Lee
Extracellular Vesicles in Bladder Cancer: Biomarkers and Beyond
Reprinted from: *Int. J. Mol. Sci.* **2018**, *19*, 2822, doi:10.3390/ijms19092822 111

Fumitaka Koga, Kosuke Takemura and Hiroshi Fukushima
Biomarkers for Predicting Clinical Outcomes of Chemoradiation-Based Bladder Preservation
Therapy for Muscle-Invasive Bladder Cancer
Reprinted from: *Int. J. Mol. Sci.* **2018**, *19*, 2777, doi:10.3390/ijms19092777 129

Melissa P. Tan, Gerhardt Attard and Robert A. Huddart
Circulating Tumour DNA in Muscle-Invasive Bladder Cancer
Reprinted from: *Int. J. Mol. Sci.* **2018**, *19*, 2568, doi:10.3390/ijms19092568 143

Iris Lodewijk, Marta Dueñas, Carolina Rubio, Ester Munera-Maravilla, Cristina Segovia,
Alejandra Bernardini, Alicia Teijeira, Jesús M. Paramio and Cristian Suárez-Cabrera
Liquid Biopsy Biomarkers in Bladder Cancer: A Current Need for Patient Diagnosis
and Monitoring
Reprinted from: *Int. J. Mol. Sci.* **2018**, *19*, 2514, doi:10.3390/ijms19092514 157

About the Special Issue Editors

Thorsten Ecke gained his medical degree from Humboldt-University Berlin—Charité (Germany) in 2000 after medical studies in Berlin and Turku (Finland). In 2005, he qualified in urology. In 2012, he became Head of the Prostate Center at Helios Hospital Bad Saarow (Germany). Since 2013 he has been teaching as an Associate Professor at Universitätmedizin Berlin Charité (Germany). He is the author and co-author of more than 70 articles. His areas of clinical and scientific expertise include uro-oncology, tumor markers, urinary-based markers, molecular biology, men's health, and the development of new diagnostic tools.

Thomas Otto gained his medical degree from the University of Essen (Germany) in 1983, and went on to work in the Department of General and Vascular Surgery at the Evangelisches Krankenhaus Mülheim/Ruhr. Between 1987 and 2004, he worked at the University of Essen in the Department of Urology, in addition to undertaking postdoctoral research in the Department of Cell Biology and Molecular Oncology. In 1996, he became an Associate Professor, and in 2001 a Professor of Urology. In 1993, Professor Dr. Otto qualified in urology, and qualified in urological surgery in 2004. In 2004, Professor Dr. Otto became the Head of the Department of Urology at the Städtische Kliniken Lukaskrankenhaus in Neuss. Since 2005, he has also been Head of the Institute of Tissue Engineering at the Städtische Kliniken Lukaskrankenhaus. He is the author and co-author of more than 400 articles. Professor Dr. Otto's areas of clinical expertise include oncology, pediatric urology, urinary incontinence, men's health, and tissue engineering. He is an expert in GMP (good manufacturing practice) and European pharmaceutical law. He has received several awards, including the German Association of Urology's Maximilian Nitze Award, the C.E. Alken Award, the European Association for Urology's (EAU) Scientific Newsflash Award, and the UNESCO Award in Bioethics.

Preface to "Diagnostic, Prognostic and Predictive Biological Markers in Bladder Cancer—Illumination of a Vision"

When medical scientists have the opportunity to meet artists, this mixture will bring new energy to each of them. This happen very often when scientists/medical practitioners love art—which all of them should do. On the other side, it could happen if artists come in contact with medical practitioners—mostly a need, rather than a desire. Let us find some parallels between bladder cancer research and French poetry: Arthur Rimbaud was a pioneer in modern poetry and showed a clear way for all poets following him. Pioneers in medicine are also showing a clear way for their followers. Especially, diagnosis for bladder cancer is a very progressive field in medicine, though there are still two very old diagnostic standards: haematuria and cystoscopy. All of what follows has to be measured with these standards. Due to different pathways in bladder cancer and the heterogeneity of this disease, there are many possible ways to go into its mechanisms. Finally, science could find new ways to help patients with instruments for early diagnostics and with predictive and prognostic markers finding new and personalized strategies for therapy.

The Editors thank all of the submitting Authors for their efforts and time spent on each manuscript. We hope that this Special Issue will prove useful to research work in bladder cancer in future. We hope that many researchers will use any kind of art to improve their professional success and to ameliorate diagnostics and therapy in bladder cancer!

Thorsten Ecke, Thomas Otto
Special Issue Editors

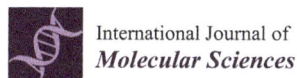

Editorial

Illumination of a Vision—How Arthur Rimbaud Will Give Us Motivation to Find New Input into Bladder Cancer Biomarker Research

Thorsten H. Ecke [1],* and Thomas Otto [2]

1 Department of Urology, HELIOS Hospital Bad Saarow, 15526 Bad Saarow, Germany
2 Department of Urology, Lukaskrankenhaus Neuss, 41464 Neuss, Germany; thomas_otto@lukasneuss.de
* Correspondence: thorsten.ecke@helios-kliniken.de; Tel.: +49-33631-72267; Fax: +49-33631-73136

Received: 9 November 2017; Accepted: 16 November 2017; Published: 19 November 2017

Bladder cancer (BC) accounts for approximately 430,000 new cases and 165,000 deaths each year worldwide [1,2]. Around 30% of bladder cancer patients suffered from muscle- invasive bladder cancer (MIBC) at the time of first diagnosis [3]. The incidence of urinary bladder cancer has increased in the last decades. Bladder cancer has a high rate of recurrence and a significant number of non-invasive tumours will progress to muscle-invasive disease. Due to the heterogeneity of the tumour, new markers for tumour progression are clearly needed as clinical parameters, such as tumour grade and stage are not accurate in predicting the biological behaviour and thus guiding the choice of treatment, especially in high risk cases [4–6].

It seems that urinary-based assays could detect the presence of bladder cancer, because the malignancy is in direct contact with urine. Malignant cells are shed into the urine, and it is likely that urine will contain carcinogens producing the malignancy. But the illusion or vision—again Rimbaud—that one single molecular marker can detect all kinds of bladder cancer accurately is probably not correct [7]. Clinical evidence and molecular studies suggest that there are two pathways in human bladder carcinogenesis: the pTa pathway and the carcinoma in situ (CIS) pathway [8]. pTa tumours are mostly low-grade and often recur, but rarely progress to lamina propria-invasive (pT1) and muscle-invasive tumours (pT2–T4), whereas CIS are always high-grade and are thought to be the most common precursor of invasive tumours. Interestingly markers detecting tumours at low-grade pathway as FGFR3 for example have only a 7% overlapping mutation rate comparing to markers detecting tumours at high-grade pathway as TP53 [9,10]. A urinary-based assay that can diagnose bladder cancer whilst confined to the urothelium or carcinoma in situ could fulfil the criterion to differ between both. This model has also been confirmed by other publications in the past [9,11,12].

Not focus on one marker is the goal, we need to study a combination of several different tumor markers to guide the interval between cystoscopies, and to direct biopsy of clinically meaningful "occult" disease that could not be detected by regular histopathological reports [13]. New markers should be based on their characteristics as well as the particular risk profile of the studied patients. This could lead to greater sensitivity than either marker alone, but worsens overall specificity.

Some promising bladder cancer markers have even a better accuracy than prostate-specific antigen has for prostate cancer screening [14,15]. It will depend by the willingness of physicians and patients whether one of the bladder tumor markers will find more influence in the clinical treatment and the changing of the diagnosis of bladder cancer in future.

Further determination of recurrence and progression marker will contribute to establish better treatments for the individual patient. Molecular staging of urological tumors will allow selecting cases that will require systemic treatment [16,17]. Regarding new therapies, it is also important to know more about cancer progression pathways which allows the evaluation of medical therapies against these specific tumor targets. In order to obtain such objectives, it is necessary to integrate basic and clinical research teams. Such teams would require integration of clinical follow-up information of cancer patients with optimal tumor and serum banks. However, the most important task is to integrate under the same objectives basic and clinical research.

On the other side it should be a need in all further studies about bladder cancer markers to have a very clear classification of the studies into phases I to IV; this had already been recommended by Lokeshwar et al. in 2005 [18]. In that meaning phase I are always feasibility studies showing development and evaluation of clinical prevalence for assays, phase II are including all evaluation studies for clinical utility, phase III are confirmation studies, and phase IV are application studies for validation and technology transfer. Having this in mind we will account these recommendations in the presented studies in our special issue.

Clinical needs in the uro-oncology are related to diagnosis, prognosis and treatment. Uro-oncology is diverse since genitourinary tumors differ histologically in their origin and various clinical behaviour [19].

Another important fact is that bladder cancer is one of the most expensive malignancies in the Western countries, the cost of a bladder cancer patient from diagnosis to death was calculated between $96,000 and $187,000 in 2001 [20,21]. Therefore bladder cancer markers are needed in future to reduce cost intensive and also painful examinations like cystoscopies, and define risk groups to know in advance which treatment is the best for the patient.

This special issue has been introduced with the aim of offering the possibility to publish new research results from old and new pioneers in the field of bladder cancer basic research. While editing this special issue we have learned that an enormous enthusiasm is necessary to go on in bladder cancer research. In our eyes bladder cancer is on one hand a very heterogenous malignancy that's why it makes so difficult to focus on the one and only bladder cancer marker in bladder cancer diagnostic and follow-up. On the other hand bladder cancer has a high importance to find prognostic and predictive factors due to its high incidence and its enormous costs as one of the most expensive malignancies in the world. Finding and development of new bladder cancer markers is still a very dynamic field. Because of the mass of all these markers it is impossible to report all. This special issue is trying to highlight the role of bladder cancer markers in diagnosis and the most important biomarkers studied and reported recently. In this special issue a highlight to some of the most important markers was made. Further determination of recurrence and progression marker will contribute to establish better treatments for the individual patient. Molecular staging of urological tumors will allow selecting cases that will require systemic treatment. It is necessary and important to integrate under the same objectives basic and clinical research.

If scientists/medicines and artists come in contact, the mixture will bring new energy into each of them. This will happen very often, when scientists/medicines love art—what all of them should do. On the other side it could happen if artists come in contact with medicines—what mostly is a need, not a will. Let us find out, what are parallels between bladder cancer research and French poetry: Arthur Rimbaud (Figure 1) was a pioneer in modern poetry and showed a clear way for all poets following him. Pioneers in medicine are also showing a clear way for their followers, especially diagnosis for bladder cancer is a very progressive field in medicine, though there are still two very old diagnostic standards—haematuria and cystoscopy. All what follows has to be measured with that standards. Due to different pathways in bladder cancer and the heterogeneity of this disease there are many possibilities to go into its mechanisms. White is not only white—black is not only black—Arthur Rimbaud would say "L'Étoile a pleuré rose ... " (English: "The star wept rose ... "). At the end he suffers from a malignancy. At the end science could perform new ways (Figure 2: Author T.E. walking on Rimbaud's routes close to Charleville in France) to help patients with instruments for early diagnostics and with predictive and prognostic markers finding new and personalized strategies for therapy.

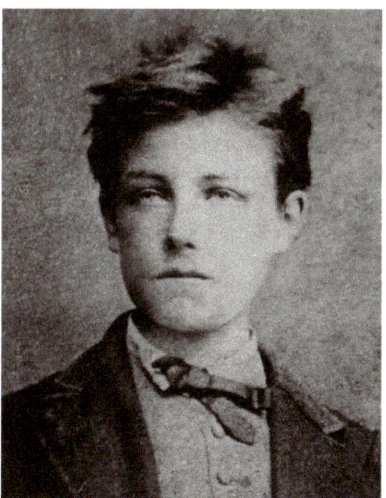

Figure 1. Arthur Rimbaud (1872)—photography by Étienne Carjat.

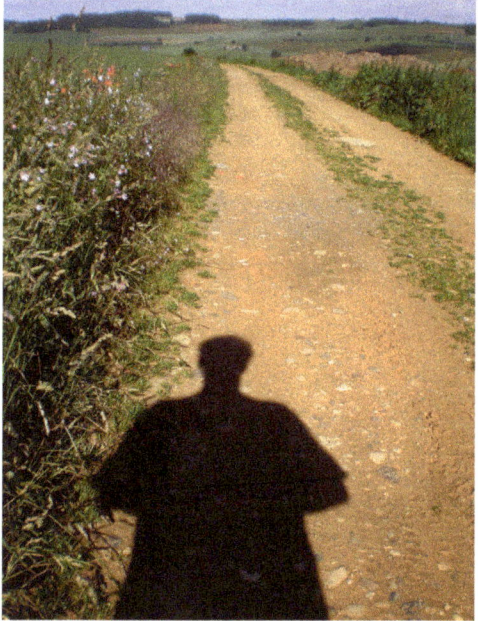

Figure 2. Author Thorsten H. Ecke walking on Rimbaud's routes close to Charleville in France.

The editors thank all submitting authors for their efforts and time spent for each manuscript. The lead editor would like to thank all editors for the time spent in reviewing, assigning reviews, and commenting on submitted manuscripts. As editorial team, we hope that this special issue will prove useful to research work in bladder cancer in future. Hopefully many researchers will use any kind of art to improve their professional success to ameliorate diagnostics and therapy in bladder cancer.

Conflicts of Interest: The authors declare no conflict of interest.

References

1. Sylvester, R.J.; van der Meijden, A.P.; Oosterlinck, W.; Witjes, J.A.; Bouffioux, C.; Denis, L.; Newling, D.W.; Kurth, K. Predicting recurrence and progression in individual patients with stage Ta T1 bladder cancer using EORTC risk tables: A combined analysis of 2596 patients from seven EORTC trials. *Eur. Urol.* **2006**, *49*, 466–477. [CrossRef] [PubMed]
2. Knowles, M.A.; Hurst, C.D. Molecular biology of bladder cancer: New insights into pathogenesis and clinical diversity. *Nat. Rev. Cancer* **2015**, *15*, 25–41. [CrossRef] [PubMed]
3. Witjes, J.A.; Comperat, E.; Cowan, N.C.; de Santis, M.; Gakis, G.; Lebret, T.; Ribal, M.J.; van der Heijden, A.G.; Sherif, A. European Association of Urology. EAU guidelines on muscle-invasive and metastatic bladder cancer: Summary of the 2013 guidelines. *Eur. Urol.* **2014**, *65*, 778–792. [CrossRef] [PubMed]
4. Theodorescu, D.; Wittke, S.; Ross, M.M.; Walden, M.; Conaway, M.; Just, I.; Mischak, H.; Frierson, H.F. Discovery and validation of new protein biomarkers for urothelial cancer: A prospective analysis. *Lancet Oncol.* **2006**, *7*, 230–240. [CrossRef]
5. Sanchez-Carbayo, M.; Cordon-Cardo, C. Molecular alterations associated with bladder cancer progression. *Semin. Oncol.* **2007**, *34*, 75–84. [CrossRef] [PubMed]
6. Mhawech-Fauceglia, P.; Cheney, R.T.; Schwaller, J. Genetic alterations in urothelial bladder carcinoma: An updated review. *Cancer* **2006**, *106*, 1205–1216. [CrossRef] [PubMed]
7. Knowles, M.A. Molecular subtypes of bladder cancer: Jekyll and Hyde or chalk and cheese? *Carcinogenesis* **2006**, *27*, 361–373. [CrossRef] [PubMed]
8. Spruck, C.H., 3rd; Ohneseit, P.F.; Gonzalez-Zulueta, M.; Esrig, D.; Miyao, N.; Tsai, Y.C.; Lerner, S.P.; Schmütte, C.; Yang, A.S.; Cote, R.; et al. Two molecular pathways to transitional cell carcinoma of the bladder. *Cancer Res.* **1994**, *54*, 784–788. [PubMed]
9. Van Rhijn, B.W.; van der Kwast, T.H.; Vis, A.N.; Kirkels, W.J.; Boevé, E.R.; Jöbsis, A.C.; Zwarthoff, E.C. FGFR3 and P53 characterize alternative genetic pathways in the pathogenesis of urothelial cell carcinoma. *Cancer Res.* **2004**, *64*, 1911–1914. [CrossRef] [PubMed]
10. Van Rhijn, B.W.; van der Kwast, T.H.; Liu, L.; Fleshner, N.E.; Bostrom, P.J.; Vis, A.N.; Alkhateeb, S.S.; Bangma, C.H.; Jewett, M.A.; Zwarthoff, E.C.; et al. The FGFR3 mutation is related to favorable pT1 bladder cancer. *J. Urol.* **2012**, *187*, 310–314. [PubMed]
11. Bakkar, A.A.; Wallerand, H.; Radvanyi, F.; Lahaye, J.B.; Pissard, S.; Lecerf, L.; Kouyoumdjian, J.C.; Abbou, C.C.; Pairon, J.C.; Jaurand, M.C.; et al. *FGFR3* and *TP53* gene mutations define two distinct pathways in urothelial cell carcinoma of the bladder. *Cancer Res.* **2003**, *63*, 8108–8112. [PubMed]
12. Hernandez, S.; Lopez-Knowles, E.; Lloreta, J.; Kogevinas, M.; Jaramillo, R.; Amorós, A.; Tardón, A.; García-Closas, R.; Serra, C.; Carrato, A.; et al. *FGFR3* and *Tp53* mutations in T1G3 transitional bladder carcinomas: Independent distribution and lack of association with prognosis. *Clin. Cancer Res.* **2005**, *11*, 5444–5450. [CrossRef] [PubMed]
13. Rosser, C.J.; Dai, Y.; Miyake, M.; Zhang, G.; Goodison, S. Simultaneous multi-analyte urinary protein assay for bladder cancer detection. *BMC Biotechnol.* **2014**, *14*, 24. [CrossRef] [PubMed]
14. Ecke, T.H. Focus on urinary bladder cancer markers: A review. *Minerva Urol. Nefrol.* **2008**, *60*, 237–246. [PubMed]
15. Shariat, S.F.; Karam, J.A.; Lotan, Y.; Karakiewizc, P.I. Critical evaluation of urinary markers for bladder cancer detection and monitoring. *Rev. Urol.* **2008**, *10*, 120–135. [PubMed]
16. Lopez-Beltran, A.; Montironi, R. Non-invasive urothelial neoplasms: According to the most recent WHO classification. *Eur. Urol.* **2004**, *46*, 170–176. [CrossRef] [PubMed]
17. Montironi, R.; Lopez-Beltran, A. The 2004 WHO classification of bladder tumors: A summary and commentary. *Int. J. Surg. Pathol.* **2005**, *13*, 143–153. [CrossRef] [PubMed]
18. Lokeshwar, V.B.; Habuchi, T.; Grossman, H.B.; Murphy, W.M.; Hautmann, S.H.; Hemstreet, G.P., 3rd; Bono, A.V.; Getzenberg, R.H.; Goebell, P.; Schmitz-Dräger, B.J.; et al. Bladder tumor markers beyond cytology: International Consensus Panel on bladder tumor markers. *Urology* **2005**, *66*, 35–63. [CrossRef] [PubMed]

19. Agarwal, P.K.; Black, P.C.; Kamat, A.M. Considerations on the use of diagnostic markers in management of patients with bladder cancer. *World J. Urol.* **2008**, *26*, 39–44. [CrossRef] [PubMed]
20. Botteman, M.F.; Pashos, C.L.; Redaelli, A.; Laskin, B.; Hauser, R. The health economics of bladder cancer: A comprehensive review of the published literature. *Pharmacoeconomics* **2003**, *21*, 1315–1330. [CrossRef] [PubMed]
21. Mitra, N.; Indurkhya, A. A propensity score approach to estimating the cost-effectiveness of medical therapies from observational data. *Health Econ.* **2005**, *14*, 805–815. [CrossRef] [PubMed]

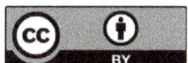

© 2017 by the authors. Licensee MDPI, Basel, Switzerland. This article is an open access article distributed under the terms and conditions of the Creative Commons Attribution (CC BY) license (http://creativecommons.org/licenses/by/4.0/).

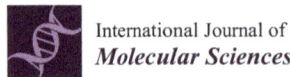

Article

UBC® *Rapid* Test—A Urinary Point-of-Care (POC) Assay for Diagnosis of Bladder Cancer with a focus on Non-Muscle Invasive High-Grade Tumors: Results of a Multicenter-Study

Thorsten H. Ecke [1,*], Sarah Weiß [2], Carsten Stephan [2,3], Steffen Hallmann [1], Christian Arndt [4], Dimitri Barski [4], Thomas Otto [4] and Holger Gerullis [5]

1. HELIOS Hospital, Department of Urology, Bad Saarow D-15526, Germany; steffen.hallmann@helios-gesundheit.de
2. Department of Urology, Charité University Hospital, Berlin D-10117, Germany; sarah.weiss2@helios-gesundheit.de (S.W.); carsten.stephan@charite.de (C.S.)
3. Berlin Institute for Urological Research, Berlin D-10115, Germany
4. Department of Urology, Lukas Hospital Neuss, Neuss D-41464, Germany; arndt_christian@web.de (C.A.); barskidimitri@gmail.com (D.B.); thomas_otto@lukasneuss.de (T.O.)
5. University Hospital for Urology, Klinikum Oldenburg, School of Medicine and Health Sciences Carl von Ossietzky University Oldenburg, Oldenburg D-26133, Germany; holger.gerullis@gmx.net
* Correspondence: thorsten.ecke@helios-kliniken.de; Tel.: +49-336-317-2267; Fax: +49-336-317-3136

Received: 11 September 2018; Accepted: 29 November 2018; Published: 2 December 2018

Abstract: Objectives: UBC® *Rapid* Test measures soluble fragments of cytokeratins 8 and 18 in urine. We present results of a multicenter study using an updated version of UBC® *Rapid* Test in bladder cancer patients, patients with urinary bladder cancer positive history, and healthy controls. Material and Methods: In total 530 urine samples have been included in this study. Clinical urine samples were used from 242 patients with tumors of the urinary bladder (134 non-muscle-invasive low-grade tumors (NMI-LG), 48 non-muscle-invasive high-grade tumors (NMI-HG), and 60 muscle-invasive high-grade tumors (MI-HG)), 62 patients with non-evidence of disease (NED), and 226 healthy controls. Urine samples were analyzed by the UBC® Rapid point-of-care (POC) assay and evaluated by Concile Omega 100 POC Reader. All statistical analyses have been performed using R version 3.2.3. Results: Elevated levels of UBC® Rapid Test in urine are higher in patients with bladder cancer in comparison to the control group ($p < 0.001$). The sensitivity for the whole bladder cancer cohort was 53.3% (positive predictive value (PPV) 90.2%, negative predictive value (NPV) 65.2%) and was 38.8% (PPV 78.8%, NPV 72.1%) for non-muscle-invasive low-grade bladder cancer; 75.0% (PPV 72.0%, NPV 94.7%) for non-muscle-invasive high-grade bladder cancer and 68.3% (PPV 74.6%, NPV 91.8%) for muscle-invasive high-grade bladder cancer. The specificity for the statistical calculations was 93.8%. The cut-off value (10 µg/L) was evaluated for the whole patient cohort. The area under the curve of the quantitative UBC® Rapid Test using the optimal threshold obtained by receiver operating characteristics (ROC) analysis was 0.774. Elevated values of UBC® *Rapid* Test in urine are higher in patients with high-grade bladder cancer in comparison to low-grade tumors and the healthy control group. Conclusions: UBC® *Rapid* Test has potential to be a clinically valuable urinary protein biomarker for detection of high-grade bladder cancer patients and could be added in the management of NMI-HG tumors. UBC® *Rapid* results generated in both study centers in the present multicenter study are very similar and reproducible. Furthermore UBC® *Rapid* Test is standardized and calibrated and thus independent of used batch of test as well as study site.

Keywords: bladder cancer; tumor markers; urinary based diagnostics

1. Introduction

In Europe bladder cancer (BCa) is the fifth most frequent cancer. Its incidence rate was 151,200 and its annual mortality rate was 51,400 cases in 2012 [1]. Around 30% of bladder cancer patients suffered from muscle-invasive bladder cancer (MIBC) at the time of first diagnosis [2]. Radical cystectomy (RC) is the gold standard to treat patients with MIBC.

Non-muscle invasive high-grade bladder cancer has a particularly high rate of recurrence and will progress to muscle-invasive disease. The ideal urine-soluble marker should be used for primary diagnosis, follow-up, and screening of high-risk populations; replacing cystoscopy during follow-up or decreasing the number of control cystoscopies during follow-up would be a worthwhile goal. Due to its contact with urine, malignant cells are shed into the urine, and this urine contains the carcinogens producing the malignancy. Some of these urinary based tests have a higher specificity and sensitivity than classical urine cytology and could be important for screening and case findings [3].

Intermediate filaments of the cytoskeleton of epithelial cells containing cytokeratins are often overexpressed in urothelial tumors. In humans twenty different cytokeratins have been identified, and cytokeratins 8, 18, and 19 are known to be important in urothelial cells [4]. The expressions of cytokeratins such as 8, 18, and 19 are higher in urothelial cells and may be elevated because of a higher cell turnover rate [5,6]. Immunohistochemical features of urothelial dysplasia include aberrant cytokeratin 20 expression at different levels of the urothelium, however, there is also usually overexpression of p53 and high Ki-67 index [7].

UBC® Rapid Test is based upon an immunochromatographic method and measures fragments of cytokeratin 8 and 18 qualitatively. The measured levels are lower in low-grade tumors and benign urological diseases [8,9]. Cytokeratins 8 and 18 are soluble in urine and can be detected quantitatively with monoclonal antibodies using sandwich ELISA as well as UBC® Rapid assay with a photometric reader. It is important to highlight that this version of UBC® Rapid Test is a modified and updated version of fast cytokeratin determination in urine in comparison to the assay introduced 15 years ago. Furthermore this new version of UBC® Rapid Test is used in combination with a reader to quantitate the signal quite comparably with an ELISA assay, but it is a point-of-care (POC) assay. Previous UBC Rapid assays were only assays for visual evaluation of results.

In the last publication of our group we had a focus on carcinoma in situ (CIS), and we could show excellent results for UBC® Rapid Test for detecting CIS [10]. Regarding these facts, it is mandatory to include new tests into bladder cancer diagnostics, specifically a test that could detect flat, high-risk tumors difficult to detect in cystoscopy would be a step to ameliorate the finding of these tumors. The aim of this multicenter study is to report the final results with the highest number of measured samples for UBC® Rapid Test and to evaluate the usefulness of UBC® Rapid Test in patients with urinary bladder cancer with a focus on non-muscle invasive high-grade (NMI-HG) tumors and compare with healthy individuals.

2. Results

A total of 530 patients were included in the study; 242 with confirmed bladder cancer, 62 with non-evidence of disease (NED), and 226 healthy controls with no history of bladder cancer. The median age of the study population was 73 (range 26–98) years. Of these patients, 391 (73.8%) were men and 139 (26.3%) were women. Among the 242 patients with confirmed bladder cancer, 134 had non-muscle-invasive low-grade (NMI-LG), 48 had NMI-HG, and 60 had muscle-invasive high-grade (MI-HG) BCa; 182 (75.2%) had non-muscle-invasive bladder cancer (pTa and pT1 tumors), 60 (24.8%) had stage pT2–4. Carcinoma in situ (CIS) was detected in 23 cases (9.5%). A detailed analysis of the CIS patients in this study had already been published [10].

The number of patients and healthy controls are listed in Table 1 for study center I (HELIOS Hospital Bad Saarow) and study center II (Lukaskrankenhaus Neuss). Both groups enrolled a similar number of patients in the study. Table 2 shows all relevant data for center 1 and center 2 separately.

We could show that elevated concentrations of UBC® Rapid Test are detectable in urine of bladder cancer patients (Tables 1 and 2). Elevated levels of UBC® Rapid Test in urine are higher in patients with bladder cancer in comparison to the control group. In 134 NMI-LG tumors the mean value of UBC® Rapid Test was 30.9 µg/L, for NMI-HG tumors 95.5 µg/L, for MI-HG tumors 66.9 µg/L, for NED patients 10.0 µg/L, and for the healthy individuals 7.7 µg/L. Elevated levels of UBC® Rapid Test in urine are statistically significantly higher in patients with bladder cancer in comparison to the control group ($p < 0.0001$). The high-risk group showed a markedly higher UBC® Rapid signal than the low-risk group. The area under the curve (AUC) of the quantitative UBC® Rapid Test using the optimal threshold obtained by receiver operating characteristics curve (ROC) analysis (cut-off 10.0 µg/L) was 0.774 as shown in Figure 1. ROC analyses of patients from center 1, center 2, and all patients together is shown in Figure 2, and demonstrated very similar outcomes. Figure 3 shows the distribution of UBC® Rapid values in boxplots in the different patient groups (overall $p < 0.001$). It shows also that most of the elevated values are definitely higher than the cut-point, especially for NMI-HG tumors.

Table 1. Patient characteristics and results of UBC® Rapid. Abbreviations: non-muscle-invasive low grade (NMI-LG), non-muscle-invasive high grade (NMI-HG), muscle-invasive high grade (MI-HG), non-evidence of disease (NED), positive predictive value (PPV), negative predictive value (NPV).

	NMI-LG	NMI-HG	MI-HG	NED	Control	p-Value
n	134	48	60	62	226	
Age						
Mean	71.0	73.8	73.6	70.8	68.9	
(SD)	(11.9)	(10.6)	(10.0)	(11.4)	(12.2)	0.036
Median	73.5	75	74.5	72	71	
Range	26–92	51–94	52–98	46–88	31–93	
Sex						
Female (%)	34 (25.4)	6 (12.5)	19 (31.7)	10 (16.1)	70 (31.0)	0.021
Male (%)	100 (74.6)	42 (87.5)	41 (68.3)	52 (83.9)	156 (69.0)	
Diabetes	25 (18.7%)	8 (16.7%)	12 (20%)	10(16.1%)	34 (15%)	0.849
Erythrocyte (urine dipstick)	83 (61.9%)	44 (91.7%)	58 (96.7%)	38 (61.3%)	73 (32.3%)	<0.001
Leucocytes (urine dipstick)						
Mean	84.6	109.9	229.7	127.8	64.3	
(SD)	(172.6)	(167.6)	(228.1)	(206.6)	(150.3)	<0.001
Median	0	25	100	20	0	
Range	0–500	0–500	0–500	0–500	0–500	
Nitrite pos.	5 (3.7%)	5 (10.4%)	8 (13.3%)	3 (4.8%)	12 (5.3%)	0.085
Cystoscopy	100 (74.6%)	33 (68.8%)	42 (70%)	49 (79%)	36 (15.9%)	<0.001
UBC (µg/L)						
Mean	30.9	95.5	66.9	10	7.7	
(SD)	(63.4)	(104.6)	(90.1)	(9.79)	(13.92)	<0.001
Median	6.4	46	24.85	5	5	
Range	5–300	5–300	5–300	5–56.5	5–166	
Sensitivity	38.8%	75.0%	68.3%	22.6%		
Specificity	93.8%	93.8%	93.8%	93.8%		
PPV	78.8%	72.0%	74.6%	50%		
NPV	72.1%	94.6%	94.6%	81.5%		

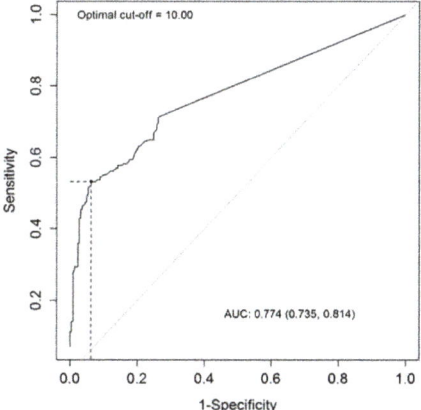

Figure 1. Analysis of the predictive ability—receiver operating (ROC) curve analysis for UBC® Rapid at cut-off value 10.0 µg/L with AUC 0.774 for the whole population.

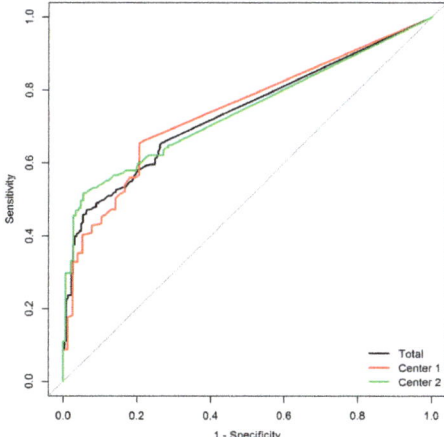

Figure 2. Analysis of the predictive ability—ROC curve analysis for UBC® Rapid at cut-off value 10.0 µg/L for the center 1 (red), center 2 (green), and whole population (black). p-value for comparison between centers = 0.874.

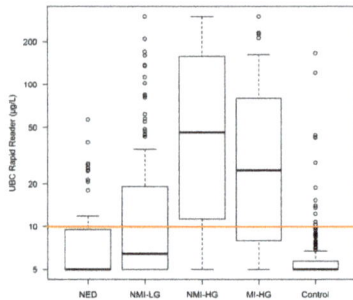

Figure 3. Box plot for non-evidence of disease (NED), non-muscle-invasive low grade (NMI-LG), non-muscle-invasive high grade (NMI-HG), muscle-invasive high grade (MI-HG), control. Orange line for cut-off at 10 µg/L.

Sensitivity was calculated as 38.8% for NMI-LG, 75.0% for NMI-HG, and 68.3% for MI-HG bladder cancer, and the UBC® *Rapid* specificity was 93.8% for all calculations.

Data of sensitivity, specificity, positive, and negative predictive values using a cut-off 10.0 µg/L for UBC® *Rapid* Test including the 95% confidence interval are also listed in Tables 1 and 2.

The data, which were generated in the two centers separately and reported in Figure 2, show impressively that ROC analysis is very similar and the sensitivity and specificity in both centres demonstrate no significant differences (Table 2). In the clinical data base it is obvious that center 1 has a higher rate of patients with diabetes and the rate of cystoscopies is higher in center 2. Though the rate of nitrite positive urine samples in center 2 is higher, the mean value of leucocytes is similar in both centers. Nevertheless, the results for UBC© *Rapid* Test are very similar in both centers demonstrating the robustness and stability of UBC® *Rapid* Test POC assay.

Table 2. Patient characteristics and results of UBC® Rapid separated for center 1 and center 2.

	NMI-LG		NMI-HG		MI-HG		NED		Control		p-Value	
	Center 1	Center 2	Center 1	Center 2	Center 1	Center 2	Center 1	Center 2	Center 1	Center 2	Center 1	Center 2
n	78	56	26	22	25	35	30	32	78	148		
Age												
Mean	71.1	70.8	74.9	72.5	74.2	73.2	73.0	68.8	67.6	69.6	0.042	0.554
(SD)	(11.6)	(12.4)	(11.6)	(9.4)	(11.0)	(9.3)	(8.8)	(13.1)	(12.64)	(11.94)		
Median	74	72	78.5	75	75	74	73.5	70.5	69.5	71.5		
Range	33–90	26–92	52–94	51–92	52–98	53–88	46–88	46–88	31–86	33–93		
Gender												
Female (%)	20 (25.6)	14 (25.0)	4 (15.4)	2 (9.1)	6 (24.0)	13 (37.1)	3 (10.0)	7 (21.9)	23 (29.5)	47 (31.8)	0.220	0.127
Male (%)	58 (74.4)	42 (75.0)	22 (84.6)	20 (90.9)	19 (76.0)	22 (62.9)	27 (90.0)	25 (78)	55 (70.5)	101 (68.2)		
Diabetes	22 (28.2%)	3 (5.4%)	6 (23.1)	2 (9.1%)	6 (24%)	6 (17.1%)	5 (16.7%)	5 (15.6%)	13 (16.7%)	21 (14.2%)	0.469	0.337
Erythrocyte pos.	45 (57.7%)	38 (67.9%)	24 (92.3%)	20 (91.0%)	24 (96.0%)	34 (97.1%)	17 (56.7%)	21 (65.6%)	34 (43.6%)	39 (26.4%)	<0.001	<0.001
Leucocytes												
Mean	79.17	92.39	142.3	71.6	249.0	215.4	142.50	113.55	76.6	57.7	<0.001	<0.001
(SD)	(165.2)	(183.8)	(182.04)	(143.4)	(229.41)	(229.5)	(220.1)	(195.2)	(165.60)	(141.68)		
Median	0	0	100	25	100	100	25	0	0	0		
Range	0–500	0–500	0–500	0–500	0–500	0–500	0–500	0–500	0–500	0–500		
Nitrite pos.	3 (3.8%)	2 (3.6%)	4 (15.1%)	1 (1.8%)	2 (8%)	6 (17.1%)	1 (3.3%)	2 (6.3%)	3 (3.8%)	9 (6.1%)	0.199	0.185
Cystoscopy	47 (60.3%)	53 (94.6%)	11 (42.3%)	22 (100%)	11 (44%)	31 (88.6%)	20 (66.7%)	29 (90.6%)	16 (20.5%)	20 (13.5%)	<0.001	<0.001
UBC [μg/L]												
Mean	21.1	44.6	83.9	109.3	61.4	70.9	7.48	12.37	7.8	7.6	<0.001	<0.001
(SD)	(43.7)	(81.9)	(94.8)	(115.8)	(80.9)	(97.1)	(7.06)	(11.4)	(13.9)	(14.0)		
Median	6.5	6.2	41.4	59.4	28.9	20.7	5	6.5	5	5		
Range	5–300	5–300	5–300	5–300	5–300	5–300	5–39.1	5–56.5	5–121	5–166		
Sensitivity	38.5%	39.3%	73.1%	77.3%	68.0%	68.6%	6.7%	37.5%				
Specificity	92.3%	94.6%	92.3%	94.6%	92.3%	94.6%	92.3%	94.6%				
PPV	83.3%	73.3%	76.0%	68.0%	73.9%	75.0%	25%	60%				
NPV	60.0%	80.5%	91.1%	96.6%	90.0%	92.7%	72%	87.5%				

3. Discussion

The main purpose of this multi-center study was to evaluate the clinical usefulness of UBC® Rapid Test for diagnosis of bladder cancer with a specific focus on patients with NMI-HG tumors of the urinary bladder compared with healthy individuals. The results of the present study show that cytokeratin concentrations determined by UBC® Rapid Test measured by POC reader are statistically significant for patients with bladder cancer and healthy controls. Values of UBC® Rapid Test in high-grade tumors are significantly higher than in low-grade tumors, NED patients, and healthy individuals. The AUC as a parameter of diagnostic quality was calculated with 0.774. UBC® Rapid Test determined quantitatively could be applied to determine the risk for bladder cancer, but also the risk of having a high-grade tumor with increased risk for recurrence. The need for quantitative urinary markers like UBC® Rapid Test had also been published before [11]. The results of this study are showing again high values for UBC® Rapid Test especially for patients with high-grade bladder cancer [9,12–14]. Following from a previously published study with a high number of samples, the results of this study show that this test could be useful for combination in a diagnostic panel for patients of the high-risk group for bladder cancer. In previous reports of UBC® Rapid, a sensitivity of 65% and a specificity of 92% was calculated [15,16]. In the study of Mian et al. [16] only the older version UBC® Rapid with only visual evaluation was available. In our study, the new version of UBC® Rapid Test as cytokeratin assay was used; an improved lateral flow method resulted in a clearer test and control bands to evaluate. In this study UBC® Rapid Test was used with the Omega 100 reader to quantify the results.

Data presented in newer UBC® Rapid studies reported a cut-off of 12.3 µg/L, a sensitivity, specificity, PPV, and NPV of 60.7%, 70.1%, 46.8%, and 79.3%, respectively, and with an AUC of 0.68 [9]. According to other previous reported UBC® Rapid studies in the literature, the sensitivity of the qualitative UBC® Rapid Test ranged from 46.2% to 78.4%, and its specificity from 82.4% to 97.4% [9,12,16–20]. These data concur with our own results, whereas the sensitivity was low with 38.8% for detecting non-muscle invasive low-grade tumors. It increased to 75% for non-muscle invasive high-grade tumors and 68.3% for muscle-invasive tumors at a specificity of 93.8%. Therefore, it achieved the highest sensitivity of a single urinary marker test for detecting high-grade bladder cancer. The diagnostic accuracy of the quantitative UBC® Rapid Test POC system has been assessed in just five studies, which reported a sensitivity of 46.6% to 64.5% and a specificity ranging from 70.1% to 86.3%, respectively [9,12,17,19,20]. In this multicenter study, we could measure a high number of samples and the results for UBC© Rapid Test are very similar in both study centers. There is no significant difference in the ROC analyses, showing that the test is very stable and reproducible.

Currently, many different urinary POC test systems are available on the market, permitting non-invasive and rapid determination of urinary markers. Their diagnostic accuracy, however, is mostly controversially discussed in a small number of studies [21,22]. The sensitivities are usually higher than those reported for urinary cytology alone, but at a lower specificity [5,22]. Nevertheless, additional costs of urinary markers in surveillance protocols are ultimately not justified [23].

According to EAU guidelines, the examination of voided urine to detect cancer cells by cytology has a high sensitivity in high-grade tumors and CIS [2]. The major limitations for cytology are that specimens could be hampered by low cellular yield, urinary tract infections, stones, or intravesical instillations. Regardless, experienced readers can exceed specificity of up to 90% [5,24]. However, negative cytology does not exclude a tumor. As method cytology is subjective, on the other side UBC® Rapid Test is an objective method that is standardized and reproducible [22].

The use of those urinary markers for routine follow-up is not recommended in clinical practice by current guidelines and remains a debated issue [22,25]. The use of urine markers is only recommended as an adjunct to cystoscopy in current guidelines [26–28]. Other tests like Fluorescence in situ hybridization (FISH) and immunocytology have shown improved sensitivity compared with cytology [29–31]. These tests are complex and difficult to perform and they require specialized laboratory facilities.

It is common that new urine tests are compared with the results of cytology. Across a large number of studies, the results varied a lot. Sensitivity for G1-tumors is lower than 30%, for G2-tumors around 60%, and for G3-tumors 90%. Specificity is around 90–95% [32]. In the study of Ritter et al., UBC® *Rapid* Test was also compared with cytology, showing better results for UBC® *Rapid* Test [9]. One limitation of our study is that we had no comparison to cytology, mainly due to the focus on high-grade bladder cancer. But it is also known that urinary cytology is of limited diagnostic value for detecting low-grade bladder tumors compared to high-grade tumors (up to 84% [33]). In the reported study by Pichler et al., the sensitivity of bladder wash cytology was only 21.4%; the sensitivity of high-grade tumors can reach sensitivities of up to 84% [33]. Urinary cytology had been evaluated in many studies previously, and sensitivities and specificities are limited by the experience of the pathologists. This well-known fact has also been reported in recent references. Furthermore, it could also be interesting to include a combination of different tumor markers into BCa diagnostics. How to combine UBC® *Rapid* with other markers has been shown by Gleichenhagen et al. [13]. In this study a combination of UBC® *Rapid* and survivin increased the sensitivity to 66% with a specificity of 95%. For high-grade tumors, the combination showed a sensitivity of 82% and a specificity of 95%. A combination of both assays confirmed the benefit of using marker panels.

In contrast to dichotomized urinary tests, the quantitative character of the UBC® *Rapid* Test enables risk stratification for bladder cancer based on the absolute UBC® *Rapid* Test value. UBC® *Rapid* Test might not only contribute to improved detection of bladder cancer, but also to improved prediction of high-risk tumors. This has also been shown for other quantitative protein-based urinary tests [34]. An approach to objectify risk stratification should include a number of different parameters including quantitative UBC® *Rapid* Test, grade of haematuria, smoking status, age, and gender for developing a nomogram [35].

Of course, there are many other markers on the market, and genetic testing looks especially promising. Regardless, at the moment these markers are a rapid diagnostic tool too complicated to be included into basic and fast diagnostics. Currently, we still must stick to the proteins when we discuss quick testing. However, the "ideal urine-based marker" for detecting bladder cancer recurrence during surveillance would be rapid, non-invasive, and easy to perform and interpret. Furthermore, the assay should possess not only a high specificity to reduce superfluous cystoscopies on oncological follow-up, but also a high sensitivity so that no patient with low-grade and high-grade bladder cancer will be missed [34].

4. Materials and Methods

4.1. Patients

For this prospective study, 530 urine samples from bladder cancer patients and healthy controls have been collected between January 2014 and October 2015 at the Department of Urology, HELIOS, Hospital Bad Saarow (study center 1), and Lukas Hospital Neuss (study center 2), Germany. The study was approved by the local Institutional Review Board of national Medical Association Brandenburg (AS 147(bB)/2013). All patients with confirmed bladder cancer underwent cystoscopy, bladder ultrasound, and transurethral resection of bladder tumor in case of abnormal findings. Exclusion criteria were any kind of mechanical manipulation (cystoscopy, transrectal ultrasound, and catheterization) within 10 days before urine sampling. Other exclusion criteria were benign prostate enlargement, urolithiasis, other tumor diseases, severe infections, and pregnancy. All these criteria could influence the test to produce false positive results. Less than 10% of the possible study cohort had to be excluded based on exclusion criteria.

4.2. Procedure

Voided urine samples were collected in a sterile plastic container and subsequently processed. Urine samples were analyzed by the UBC® *Rapid* Test (Concile GmbH, Freiburg/Breisgau, Germany).

All tests were carried out as recommended by the manufacturer's instructions. The presence of a test band after 10 minutes of incubation was checked. After visual evaluation, the test cartridges were analyzed by the photometric point-of-care (POC) system Concile Omega 100 reader (Concile GmbH, Freiburg/Breisgau, Germany) for quantitative analysis. The cut-off value used for calculation of statistical parameters was based upon the evaluation of the receiver operating characteristics curve (ROC) and defined as 10.0 µg/L. The Omega 100 reader illuminates the test field with a complementary colored light to reduce interference in the analysis. The built-in charge-coupled device–matrix sensor takes a photograph of the light reflected, which is analyzed by the device.

4.3. Statistical Analysis

All statistical analyses have been performed using R version 3.2.3 (R Core Team (2015). R: A language and environment for statistical computing. R Foundation for Statistical Computing, Vienna, Austria. URL https://www.R-project.org/). Data are presented descriptively using means and standard deviations for numerical variables and absolute and relative frequencies for categorical variables. Comparison between groups at baseline has been performed using analysis of variance (ANOVA) for numerical variables and chi-square tests for categorical variables.

The predictive ability of UBC® *Rapid* Test measurements to detect bladder cancer was evaluated using Receiver Operating Characteristics (ROC) analysis, where the optimal cut-point was determined using the Youden index [36]. Sensitivity, specificity, positive, and negative predictive value was then calculated for the optimal cut-off and presented with exact 95% confidence intervals.

4.4. Ethics

The study was performed according to the Declaration of Helsinki. The study was approved by the local Institutional Review Board of National Medical Association Brandenburg (No. AS 147(bB)/2013 dated by 17 November 2013). Written and informed consent was obtained from each participant.

5. Conclusions

Elevated values of UBC® *Rapid* Test in urine are higher in patients with non-muscle invasive high-grade bladder cancer in comparison to low-grade tumors and the healthy control group. Sensitivity for non-muscle invasive high-grade tumors is very high with 75% at a specificity of 93.8%. Thus, UBC® *Rapid* Test has the potential to be a more sensitive and specific urinary protein biomarker to identify patients with high-grade tumors that are difficult to detect in cystoscopy. Results for UBC® *Rapid* Test in both study centers of the present multicenter study are very similar and reproducible. UBC® *Rapid* Test is standardized and calibrated, and thus independent of use, batch of test, as well as study site. UBC® *Rapid* Test should be added in the diagnostics and follow-up for NMI-HG tumors of urinary bladder cancer, though cystoscopy is still an important part of monitoring of bladder cancer.

Author Contributions: T.H.E. and H.G. conceived and designed the experiments; T.H.E., C.A. and D.B. performed the experiments; T.H.E. and C.S. analyzed the data; S.W., S.H. and T.O. contributed analysis tools; T.H.E. wrote the paper.

funding: The author(s) disclosed receipt of the following financial support for the research: The test systems were sponsored by the local distributor Concile GmbH, Freiburg/ Breisgau, Germany; the main company is IDL Biotech AB, Bromma, Sweden.

Acknowledgments: We thank the staff of the Urological Departments at HELIOS Hospital Bad, Saarow and Lukas Hospital Neuss, Germany, for their excellent help while collecting the samples. Statistical calculations have been performed by Marcus Thuresson from Statisticon, Uppsala, Sweden. The test systems were sponsored by Concile GmbH, Freiburg/Breisgau, Germany, and IDL Biotech AB, Bromma, Sweden.

Conflicts of Interest: The authors declare no conflict of interest.

References

1. Ferlay, J.; Steliarova-Foucher, E.; Lortet-Tieulent, J.; Rosso, S.; Coebergh, J.W.; Comber, H.; Forman, D.; Bray, F. Cancer incidence and mortality patterns in Europe: Estimates for 40 countries in 2012. *Eur. J. Cancer* **2013**, *49*, 1374–1403. [CrossRef] [PubMed]
2. Witjes, J.A.; Comperat, E.; Cowan, N.C.; de Santis, M.; Gakis, G.; Lebret, T.; Ribal, M.J.; Van der Heijden, A.G.; Sherif, A. EAU guidelines on muscle-invasive and metastatic bladder cancer: Summary of the 2013 guidelines. *Eur. Urol.* **2014**, *65*, 778–792. [CrossRef] [PubMed]
3. Lotan, Y.; Roehrborn, C.G. Sensitivity and specificity of commonly available bladder tumor markers versus cytology: Results of a comprehensive literature review and meta-analyses. *Urology* **2003**, *61*, 109–118. [CrossRef]
4. Southgate, J.; Harnden, P.; Trejdosiewicz, L.K. Cytokeratin expression patterns in normal and malignant urothelium: A review of the biological and diagnostic implications. *Histol. Histopathol.* **1999**, *14*, 657–664. [PubMed]
5. Lokeshwar, V.B.; Habuchi, T.; Grossman, H.B.; Murphy, W.M.; Hautmann, S.H.; Hemstreet, G.P., III; Bono, A.V.; Getzenberg, R.H.; Goebell, P.; Schmitz-Drager, B.J.; et al. Bladder tumor markers beyond cytology: International Consensus Panel on bladder tumor markers. *Urology* **2005**, *66*, 35–63. [CrossRef] [PubMed]
6. Siracusano, S.; Niccolini, B.; Knez, R.; Tiberio, A.; Benedetti, E.; Bonin, S.; Ciciliato, S.; Pappagallo, G.L.; Belgrano, E.; Stanta, G. The simultaneous use of telomerase, cytokeratin 20 and CD4 for bladder cancer detection in urine. *Eur. Urol.* **2005**, *47*, 327–333. [CrossRef] [PubMed]
7. Hodges, K.B.; Lopez-Beltran, A.; Davidson, D.D.; Montironi, R.; Cheng, L. Urothelial dysplasia and other flat lesions of the urinary bladder: Clinicopathologic and molecular features. *Hum. Pathol.* **2010**, *41*, 155–162. [CrossRef] [PubMed]
8. Schroeder, G.L.; Lorenzo-Gomez, M.F.; Hautmann, S.H.; Friedrich, M.G.; Ekici, S.; Huland, H.; Lokeshwar, V. A side by side comparison of cytology and biomarkers for bladder cancer detection. *J. Urol.* **2004**, *172*, 1123–1126. [CrossRef] [PubMed]
9. Ritter, R.; Hennenlotter, J.; Kuhs, U.; Hofmann, U.; Aufderklamm, S.; Blutbacher, P.; Deja, A.; Hohneder, A.; Gerber, V.; Gakis, G.; et al. Evaluation of a new quantitative point-of-care test platform for urine-based detection of bladder cancer. *Urol. Oncol.* **2014**, *32*, 337–344. [CrossRef] [PubMed]
10. Ecke, T.H.; Weiss, S.; Stephan, C.; Hallmann, S.; Barski, D.; Otto, T.; Gerullis, H. UBC® Rapid Test for detection of carcinoma in situ for bladder cancer. *Tumour Biol.* **2017**, *39*, 1010428317701624. [CrossRef] [PubMed]
11. Shariat, S.F.; Casella, R.; Wians, F.H., Jr.; Ashfaq, R.; Balko, J.; Sulser, T.; Gasser, T.C.; Sagalowsky, A.I. Risk stratification for bladder tumor recurrence, stage and grade by urinary nuclear matrix protein 22 and cytology. *Eur. Urol.* **2004**, *45*, 304–313, author reply 313. [CrossRef] [PubMed]
12. Ecke, T.H.; Arndt, C.; Stephan, C.; Hallmann, S.; Lux, O.; Otto, T.; Ruttloff, J.; Gerullis, H. Preliminary Results of a Multicentre Study of the UBC Rapid Test for Detection of Urinary Bladder Cancer. *Anticancer Res.* **2015**, *35*, 2651–2655. [PubMed]
13. Gleichenhagen, J.; Arndt, C.; Casjens, S.; Meinig, C.; Gerullis, H.; Raiko, I.; Bruning, T.; Ecke, T.; Johnen, G. Evaluation of a New Survivin ELISA and UBC® Rapid for the Detection of Bladder Cancer in Urine. *Int. J. Mol. Sci.* **2018**, *19*, 226. [CrossRef] [PubMed]
14. Styrke, J.; Henriksson, H.; Ljungberg, B.; Hasan, M.; Silfverberg, I.; Einarsson, R.; Malmstrom, P.U.; Sherif, A. Evaluation of the diagnostic accuracy of UBC® Rapid in bladder cancer: A Swedish multicentre study. *Scand. J. Urol.* **2017**, *51*, 293–300. [CrossRef] [PubMed]
15. Sanchez-Carbayo, M.; Herrero, E.; Megias, J.; Mira, A.; Soria, F. Initial evaluation of the new urinary bladder cancer rapid test in the detection of transitional cell carcinoma of the bladder. *Urology* **1999**, *54*, 656–661. [CrossRef]
16. Mian, C.; Lodde, M.; Haitel, A.; Vigl, E.E.; Marberger, M.; Pycha, A. Comparison of the monoclonal UBC-ELISA test and the NMP22 ELISA test for the detection of urothelial cell carcinoma of the bladder. *Urology* **2000**, *55*, 223–226. [CrossRef]

17. Hakenberg, O.W.; Fuessel, S.; Richter, K.; Froehner, M.; Oehlschlaeger, S.; Rathert, P.; Meye, A.; Wirth, M.P. Qualitative and quantitative assessment of urinary cytokeratin 8 and 18 fragments compared with voided urine cytology in diagnosis of bladder carcinoma. *Urology* **2004**, *64*, 1121–1126. [CrossRef] [PubMed]
18. Sanchez-Carbayo, M.; Herrero, E.; Megias, J.; Mira, A.; Espasa, A.; Chinchilla, V.; Soria, F. Initial evaluation of the diagnostic performance of the new urinary bladder cancer antigen test as a tumor marker for transitional cell carcinoma of the bladder. *J. Urol.* **1999**, *161*, 1110–1115. [CrossRef]
19. Babjuk, M.; Kostirova, M.; Mudra, K.; Pecher, S.; Smolova, H.; Pecen, L.; Ibrahim, Z.; Dvoracek, J.; Jarolim, L.; Novak, J.; et al. Qualitative and quantitative detection of urinary human complement factor H-related protein (BTA stat and BTA TRAK) and fragments of cytokeratins 8, 18 (UBC rapid and UBC IRMA) as markers for transitional cell carcinoma of the bladder. *Eur. Urol.* **2002**, *41*, 34–39. [CrossRef]
20. Pichler, R.; Tulchiner, G.; Fritz, J.; Schaefer, G.; Horninger, W.; Heidegger, I. Urinary UBC Rapid and NMP22 Test for Bladder Cancer Surveillance in Comparison to Urinary Cytology: Results from a Prospective Single-Center Study. *Int. J. Med. Sci.* **2017**, *14*, 811. [CrossRef]
21. Chou, R.; Gore, J.L.; Buckley, D.; Fu, R.; Gustafson, K.; Griffin, J.C.; Grusing, S.; Selph, S. Urinary Biomarkers for Diagnosis of Bladder Cancer: A Systematic Review and Meta-analysis. *Ann. Intern. Med.* **2015**, *163*, 922–931. [CrossRef] [PubMed]
22. Van Rhijn, B.W.; van der Poel, H.G.; van der Kwast, T.H. Urine markers for bladder cancer surveillance: A systematic review. *Eur. Urol.* **2005**, *47*, 736–748. [CrossRef] [PubMed]
23. Kamat, A.M.; Karam, J.A.; Grossman, H.B.; Kader, A.K.; Munsell, M.; Dinney, C.P. Prospective trial to identify optimal bladder cancer surveillance protocol: Reducing costs while maximizing sensitivity. *BJU Int.* **2011**, *108*, 1119–1123. [CrossRef] [PubMed]
24. Raitanen, M.P.; Aine, R.; Rintala, E.; Kallio, J.; Rajala, P.; Juusela, H.; Tammela, T.L. Differences between local and review urinary cytology in diagnosis of bladder cancer. An interobserver multicenter analysis. *Eur. Urol.* **2002**, *41*, 284–289. [CrossRef]
25. Babjuk, M.; Bohle, A.; Burger, M.; Capoun, O.; Cohen, D.; Comperat, E.M.; Hernandez, V.; Kaasinen, E.; Palou, J.; Roupret, M.; et al. EAU Guidelines on Non-Muscle-invasive Urothelial Carcinoma of the Bladder: Update 2016. *Eur. Urol.* **2017**, *71*, 447–461. [CrossRef]
26. Babjuk, M.; Oosterlinck, W.; Sylvester, R.; Kaasinen, E.; Bohle, A.; Palou-Redorta, J.; Roupret, M. EAU guidelines on non-muscle-invasive urothelial carcinoma of the bladder, the 2011 update. *Eur. Urol.* **2011**, *59*, 997–1008. [CrossRef]
27. Sturgeon, C.M.; Duffy, M.J.; Hofmann, B.R.; Lamerz, R.; Fritsche, H.A.; Gaarenstroom, K.; Bonfrer, J.; Ecke, T.H.; Grossman, H.B.; Hayes, P.; et al. National Academy of Clinical Biochemistry Laboratory Medicine Practice Guidelines for use of tumor markers in liver, bladder, cervical, and gastric cancers. *Clin. Chem.* **2010**, *56*, e1–e48. [CrossRef]
28. Hall, M.C.; Chang, S.S.; Dalbagni, G.; Pruthi, R.S.; Seigne, J.D.; Skinner, E.C.; Wolf, J.S., Jr.; Schellhammer, P.F. Guideline for the management of nonmuscle invasive bladder cancer (stages Ta, T1, and Tis): 2007 update. *J. Urol.* **2007**, *178*, 2314–2330. [CrossRef]
29. Banek, S.; Schwentner, C.; Tager, D.; Pesch, B.; Nasterlack, M.; Leng, G.; Gawrych, K.; Bonberg, N.; Johnen, G.; Kluckert, M.; et al. Prospective evaluation of fluorescence-in situ-hybridization to detect bladder cancer: Results from the UroScreen-Study. *Urol. Oncol.* **2013**, *31*, 1656–1662. [CrossRef]
30. Friedrich, M.G.; Hellstern, A.; Hautmann, S.H.; Graefen, M.; Conrad, S.; Huland, E.; Huland, H. Clinical use of urinary markers for the detection and prognosis of bladder carcinoma: A comparison of immunocytology with monoclonal antibodies against Lewis X and 486p3/12 with the BTA STAT and NMP22 tests. *J. Urol.* **2002**, *168*, 470–474. [CrossRef]
31. Van Rhijn, B.W.; Catto, J.W.; Goebell, P.J.; Knuchel, R.; Shariat, S.F.; van der Poel, H.G.; Sanchez-Carbayo, M.; Thalmann, G.N.; Schmitz-Drager, B.J.; Kiemeney, L.A. Molecular markers for urothelial bladder cancer prognosis: Toward implementation in clinical practice. *Urol. Oncol.* **2014**, *32*, 1078–1087. [CrossRef] [PubMed]
32. Ecke, T.H. Focus on urinary bladder cancer markers: A review. *Ital. J. Urol. Nephrol.* **2008**, *60*, 237–246.
33. Yafi, F.A.; Brimo, F.; Steinberg, J.; Aprikian, A.G.; Tanguay, S.; Kassouf, W. Prospective analysis of sensitivity and specificity of urinary cytology and other urinary biomarkers for bladder cancer. *Urol. Oncol.* **2015**, *33*, 66.e25–66.e31. [CrossRef] [PubMed]

34. Shariat, S.F.; Karam, J.A.; Lotan, Y.; Karakiewizc, P.I. Critical evaluation of urinary markers for bladder cancer detection and monitoring. *Rev. Urol.* **2008**, *10*, 120–135. [PubMed]
35. Lotan, Y.; Capitanio, U.; Shariat, S.F.; Hutterer, G.C.; Karakiewicz, P.I. Impact of clinical factors, including a point-of-care nuclear matrix protein-22 assay and cytology, on bladder cancer detection. *BJU Int.* **2009**, *103*, 1368–1374. [CrossRef] [PubMed]
36. Youden, W.J. Index for rating diagnostic tests. *Cancer* **1950**, *3*, 32–35. [CrossRef]

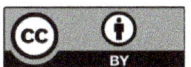

© 2018 by the authors. Licensee MDPI, Basel, Switzerland. This article is an open access article distributed under the terms and conditions of the Creative Commons Attribution (CC BY) license (http://creativecommons.org/licenses/by/4.0/).

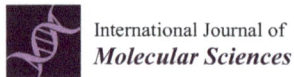

Article

mRNA-Expression of *KRT5* and *KRT20* Defines Distinct Prognostic Subgroups of Muscle-Invasive Urothelial Bladder Cancer Correlating with Histological Variants

Markus Eckstein [1,*,†], Ralph Markus Wirtz [2,3,†], Matthias Gross-Weege [4,†], Johannes Breyer [5,†], Wolfgang Otto [5,†], Robert Stoehr [1,†], Danijel Sikic [6,†], Bastian Keck [6,†], Sebastian Eidt [3,†], Maximilian Burger [5,†], Christian Bolenz [7,†], Katja Nitschke [4,†], Stefan Porubsky [8,†], Arndt Hartmann [1,†] and Philipp Erben [4,†]

[1] Institute of Pathology, University of Erlangen-Nuremberg, 91054 Erlangen, Germany; robert.stoehr@uk-erlangen.de (R.S.); arndt.hartmann@uk-erlangen.de (A.H.)
[2] STRATIFYER Molecular Pathology GmbH, 50935 Cologne, Germany; ralph.wirtz@stratifyer.de
[3] Institute of Pathology at the St Elisabeth Hospital Köln-Hohenlind, 50935 Cologne, Germany; Sebastian.eidt@stratifyer.de
[4] Department of Urology, University Medical Centre Mannheim, Medical Faculty Mannheim, University of Heidelberg, 68167 Mannheim, Germany; matthias.gross-weege@umm.de (M.G.-W.); katja.nitschke@medma.uni-heidelberg.de (K.N.); Philipp.Erben@medma.uni-heidelberg.de (P.E.)
[5] Department of Urology, University of Regensburg, 93053 Regensburg, Germany; Johannes.breyer@ukr.de (J.B.); wolfgang.otto@ukr.de (W.O.); maximilian.burger@ukr.de (M.B.)
[6] Department of Urology and Pediatric Urology, University Hospital Erlangen, 91058 Erlangen, Germany; danijel.sikic@uk-erlangen.de (D.S.); Bastian.keck@web.de (B.K.)
[7] Department of Urology, University of Ulm, 89081 Ulm, Germany; Christian.Bolenz@uniklinik-ulm.de
[8] Department of Pathology, University Medical Centre Mannheim, Medical Faculty Mannheim, University of Heidelberg, 68167 Mannheim, Germany; Stefan.porubsky@medma.uni-heidelberg.de
* Correspondence: markus.eckstein@uk-erlangen.de; Tel.: +49-9131-8522525
† On behalf of the BRIDGE Consortium.

Received: 22 September 2018; Accepted: 22 October 2018; Published: 30 October 2018

Abstract: Recently, muscle-invasive bladder cancer (MIBC) has been subclassified by gene expression profiling, with a substantial impact on therapy response and patient outcome. We tested whether these complex molecular subtypes of MIBC can be determined by mRNA detection of keratin 5 (*KRT5*) and keratin 20 (*KRT20*). Reverse transcriptase quantitative polymerase chain reaction (RT-qPCR) was applied to quantify gene expression of *KRT5* and *KRT20* using TaqMan®-based assays in 122 curatively treated MIBC patients (median age 68.0 years). Furthermore, in silico analysis of the MD Anderson Cancer Center (MDACC) cohort (GSE48277 + GSE47993) was performed. High expression of *KRT5* and low expression of *KRT20* were associated with significantly improved recurrence-free survival (RFS) and disease-specific survival disease specific survival (DSS: 5-year DSS for *KRT5* high: 58%; 5-year DSS for *KRT20* high: 29%). *KRT5* and *KRT20* were associated with rates of lymphovascular invasion and lymphonodal metastasis. The combination of *KRT5* and *KRT20* allowed identification of patients with a very poor prognosis ($KRT20^+/KRT5^-$, 5-year DSS 0%, $p < 0.0001$). In silico analysis of the independent MDACC cohorts revealed congruent results (5-year DSS for *KRT20* low vs. high: 84% vs. 40%, $p = 0.042$). High *KRT20*-expressing tumors as well as $KRT20^+/KRT^-$ tumors were significantly enriched with aggressive urothelial carcinoma variants (micropapillary, plasmacytoid, nested).

Keywords: Bladder cancer; muscle-invasive bladder cancer; molecular diagnostics; molecular subtyping; *KRT5*; *KRT20*

1. Introduction

Urothelial bladder cancer (UBC) is one of the 10 most common malignancies worldwide, with nearly 386,000 new cases and nearly 150,200 deaths per year [1]. Non-muscle-invasive bladder cancer (NMIBC) variants (70%) are not immediately life-threatening but often progress, while muscle-invasive bladder cancer (MIBC) tumors account only for nearly 30%, but are responsible for most deaths [2]. Due to the high cost of treatment modalities and the often necessary lifelong surveillance, UBC is one of the most expensive tumor entities [3].

The current standard of care in MIBC is radical cystectomy with perioperative platinum-based chemotherapy in selected cases. At present, clinical management of MIBC suffers from two major problems: First, the therapy selection is heavily influenced by a limited clinicopathological staging system, resulting in high rates of inadequate treatment [4]. Second, due to limited insight into molecular variants, it is not yet possible to identify potential (chemo)therapy responders [2,5]. Therefore, several groups have started to characterize UBC by gene expression profiling, as was previously done for breast cancer [6,7], which identified highly prognostic molecular signatures [5,8–19]. The MD Anderson Cancer Center (MDACC) subtypes resembled those identified for breast cancer and showed typical mRNA expression profiles of basal and luminal markers, with keratin 5 (*KRT5*) expression being highly upregulated in basal and keratin 20 (*KRT20*) being upregulated in luminal tumors. The third subtype (p53-like) is characterized by either a luminal or basal expression profile and an activated p53 wild-type pathway, which might be caused by prominent immune cell infiltration [14,20]. Recently, we demonstrated the high prognostic relevance of assessing *KRT5* and *KRT20* expression in high-risk NMIBC [21]. High *KRT5* mRNA expression identified a subgroup of nonluminal NMIBC that showed superior recurrence-free survival (RFS) and progression-free survival (PFS) despite being World Health Organization (WHO) grade 3 and stage pT1. In contrast, NMIBC with high *KRT20* mRNA expression was accompanied by significantly increased rates of tumor progression.

Here, we tested whether molecular subtyping by *KRT20* and *KRT5* mRNA expression is also applicable in MIBC. The main aim of this study was to prove the possibility and feasibility of introducing those two markers into the clinicopathological routine.

2. Material and Methods

2.1. Patient Population, Specimen Collection, and Histopathological Evaluation

Formalin-fixed paraffin-embedded (FFPE) tumor tissue samples were obtained from 169 patients with histologically confirmed MIBC (pT2-4) who were treated with radical cystectomy in conjunction with bilateral lymphadenectomy at a single center between 1999 and 2007 by 2 oncological surgeons with substantial cystectomy experience. Thirty-two patients received adjuvant platinum-containing chemotherapy (in the final study cohort, 22 patients received adjuvant platinum-containing chemotherapy). None of the patients underwent neoadjuvant radiation or chemotherapy. Hematoxylin and Eosin stained HE sections were reevaluated according to the 2017 Union internationale contre le cancer (UICC) staging manual and graded according to the common grading systems (World Health Organization1973 and 2016) by 3 experienced uropathologists (A.H., S.P., M.E.) [22]. Primary squamous cell carcinomas, pure neuroendocrine carcinomas, tumors originating from other organs (metastases or arising from neighboring organs), samples with low calmodulin 2 (CALM2) housekeeping gene expression (Ct values $\geq$ 28.0) and cases with missing follow-up data were excluded (n = 47). The final cohort consisted of 122 patients. The median follow-up period was 26.5 months (range 0.7–180.8 months). Follow-up data were achieved from local tumor registries and clinical case files, and by telephone calls to last known treating private practices.

In total, 59 patients had a recurrence: 44 patients with distant metastases, 5 patients with isolated local recurrences with delayed distant metastases, and 10 patients with co-occurrence of local and distant recurrence. The date of recurrence was defined as first confirmation of local and/or distant metastasis. Most recurrences were confirmed by computed tomography, but due to the retrospective nature of this study, in several cases we did not know the modality of recurrence detection. None of the patients received local resection of local recurrences or distant metastases.

All patients gave informed consent, and the study was approved by the institutional review board under numbers 2013-517N-MA (approval date: 21.02.2013) and 2016-814R-MA (approval date: 05.04.2016). To validate RT-qPCR-data, array gene expression data (Illumina HumanHT-12 WG-DASL V4.0 R2 expression beadchip) of 44 MIBC patients from the MDACC cohort (GSE48276) were analyzed (median age 67.6, range 41–89.6 years) [14].

2.2. RNA Isolation from FFPE Tissue

RNA was extracted from FFPE tissue using 10 µm sections, which were processed in a fully automated manner by a commercially available bead-based extraction method (XTRACT kit; STRATIFYER Molecular Pathology GmbH, Cologne, Germany). RNA was eluted with 100 µL elution buffer and RNA eluates were analyzed. The section was taken from a paraffin block containing a tumor area of at least 5 × 5 mm with a total tumor content of at least 30% tumor cells.

2.3. mRNA Quantification by RT-qPCR

RT-qPCR was applied for relative quantification of *KRT5* and *KRT20* mRNA as well as *CALM2* (calmodulin 2; housekeeping gene) expression by using gene-specific TaqMan®-based assays as described previously [21,23]. *CALM2* is a stably expressed gene among breast cancer tumor tissue samples and has been applied successfully to bladder cancer specimens [21,24,25]. Each patient sample or control was analyzed in triplicate. Experiments were run on a Siemens Versant (Siemens, Germany) according to the following protocol: 5 min at 50 °C, 20 s at 95 °C, followed by 40 cycles of 15 s at 95 °C and 60 s at 60 °C. Forty amplification cycles were applied and the cycle quantification threshold (Ct) values of 3 markers and 1 reference gene for each sample were estimated as the mean of the 3 measurements. Ct values were normalized by subtracting the Ct value of the housekeeping gene CALM2 from the Ct value of the target gene (ΔCt).

2.4. Statistical Analysis

All *p*-values were calculated 2-sided, and values of <0.05 were considered to be significant. Survival analyses were performed by univariate Kaplan–Meier regressions and tested for significance with the log-rank. Results were considered to be significant if the test revealed significance levels <0.05. Multivariate analyses were performed by Cox proportional hazard regression model, including all relevant clinicopathological characteristics (pT-Stage, pN-Stage, lymphovascular invasion (L), blood vessel invasion (V), age, gender, receipt of adjuvant platinum-containing chemotherapy, status of resection margins, and tumor grading (WHO 2016 and WHO 1973)). Statistical analyses of numeric continuous variables were performed by nonparametric tests (Wilcoxon rank-sum test, Kruskal–Wallis test). Contingency analysis of nominal variables was performed by Pearson's chi-squared test. Correlation analysis of numeric continuous variables was performed using Spearman rank correlations. All statistical analyses were performed with GraphPad Prism 7.2 (GraphPad Software Inc., La Jolla, CA, USA) and JMP SAS 13.2 (SAS, Cary, NC, USA).

3. Results

3.1. Clinicopathological Data and Expression of KRT5 and KRT20 mRNA in MIBC

The distribution of clinicopathological data of the entire cohort and respective *KRT*-expression subgroups (*KRT5* high vs. low; *KRT20* high vs. low; Epi-Typer Class 1, Epi-Typer Class 2) including age, gender, pT-Stage, pN-Stage, and grading (WHO 1973, WHO 2004/2016) is depicted in Table 1.

Table 1. Clinicopathological characteristics of the Mannheim cohort (overall and respective subgroups). KRT, keratin; L, lymphovascular invasion; V, blood vessel invasion; R, resection margin; WHO, World Health Organization; n.s., not significant; G, Grade; T, Tumor. * p-Value a: $KRT5_{high}$ vs. $KRT5_{low}$; p-value b: $KRT20_{high}$ vs. $KRT20_{low}$.

Characteristic	Total	KRT5 High	KRT5 Low	KRT20 High	KRT20 Low	p-Value
Cohort size (n)	122	89	33	48	74	
Mean age (years)	67.9	67.9	68.4	67.5	67.9	a: n.s. b: n.s.
Gender (n)						
Male	89 (73%)	66 (74%)	23 (70%)	34 (71%)	55 (74%)	a: n.s.
Female	33 (27%)	23 (26%)	10 (30%)	14 (29%)	19 (26%)	b: n.s.
Adjuvant chemotherapy	22 (18%)	14 (16%)	8 (24%)	9 (19%)	13 (17%)	n.s.
Pathological characteristics						
pTis (concomitant)	43 (35%)	34 (38%)	9 (27%)	19 (40%)	24 (32%)	a: n.s. b: n.s.
pT2	33 (27%)	28 (31%)	5 (15%)	14 (29%)	19 (26%)	a: 0.027
pT3	62 (51%)	44 (50%)	18 (55%)	25 (52%)	37 (50%)	b: n.s.
pT4	27 (22%)	17 (19%)	10 (30%)	9 (19%)	18 (24%)	
pN0	74 (60%)	60 (67%)	14 (42%)	20 (42%)	54 (73%)	a: 0.0005
pN1-2	48 (37%)	29 (33%)	19 (57%)	28 (58%)	20 (27%)	b: 0.002
L0	62 (51%)	52 (58%)	10 (30%)	17 (35%)	45 (61%)	a: 0.005
L1	60 (49%)	37 (52%)	23 (70%)	31 (65%)	29 (39%)	b: 0.006
V0	104 (85%)	81 (91%)	23 (70%)	42 (87%)	61 (84%)	a: 0.005
V1	18 (15%)	8 (9%)	10 (30%)	6 (13%)	12 (16%)	b: n.s.
R0	105 (86%)	77 (86%)	28 (85%)	42 (88%)	63 (85%)	a: n.s.
R1	17 (14%)	12 (14%)	5 (15%)	6 (12%)	11 (15%)	b: n.s.
Grading						
WHO 1973						
G1	0 (0%)	0 (0%)	0 (0%)	0 (0%)	0 (0%)	
G2	27 (22%)	21 (24%)	6 (18%)	11 (23%)	16 (22%)	a: n.s.
G3	95 (78%)	68 (76%)	27 (82%)	37 (77%)	58 (78%)	b: n.s.
WHO 2004						
Low grade	0 (0%)	0 (0%)	0 (0%)	0 (0%)	0 (0%)	a: n.s.
High grade	122 (100%)	89 (100%)	33 (100%)	48 (100%)	74 (100%)	b: n.s.

Characteristic	Epi-Typer Class 1	Epi-Typer Class 2	p-Value
Cohort size (n)	103	19	
Mean age (years)	67.9	71	n.s.
Gender (n)			
Male	75 (73%)	14 (74%)	n.s.
Female	28 (27%)	5 (26%)	
Adjuvant chemotherapy	17 (17%)	5 (26%)	n.s.
Pathological T stage			

Table 1. Cont.

Characteristic	Total	KRT5 High	KRT5 Low	KRT20 High	KRT20 Low	p-Value
pTis (concomitant)		37 (36%)		6 (31%)		n.s.
pT2						
pT3						
pT4						
Pathological characteristics						
pN0		69 (67%)		5 (26%)		0.0009
pN1-2		34 (33%)		14 (74%)		
L0		58 (56%)		4 (21%)		0.004
L1		45 (44%)		15 (79%)		
V0		90 (87%)		14 (74%)		n.s.
V1		13 (13%)		5 (26%)		
R0		89 (86%)		16 (84%)		n.s.
R1		14 (14%)		3 (16%)		
Grading WHO 1973						
G1		0 (0%)		0 (0%)		n.s.
G2		22 (21%)		5 (26%)		n.s.
G3		81 (79%)		14 (74%)		n.s.
Grading WHO 2004						
Low grade		0 (0%)		0 (0%)		n.s.
High grade		103 (100%)		19 (100%)		n.s.

Distribution of clinic-pathological determinants across the entire cohort and respective subgroups. p-value a: $KRT5_{high}$ vs. $KRT5_{low}$; p-value b: $KRT20_{high}$ vs. $KRT20_{low}$.

Data distribution of normalized *KRT5* and *KRT20* expression levels had a broad dynamic range (Figure 1A). Expression of *KRT5* and *KRT20* correlated inversely ($r = -0.42$, $p < 0.0001$; Figure 1A). Consistent with previous studies, there was a significant association between high *KRT5* expression and squamous and sarcomatoid differentiation (Figure 1C) [14]. Tumors with variant histology (micropapillary, nested, plasmacytoid) showed an interesting keratin expression pattern: they showed high expression of *KRT20*, while the expression of *KRT5* was very low in these cases (Figure 1C,D). High expression of *KRT5* was associated with a lower rate of lymphovascular invasion (LVI) ($p = 0.0004$) and lymphonodal metastasis ($p = 0.002$; Figure 1B), while high *KRT20* expression correlated positively with LVI/nodal status (Figure 1B). Furthermore, luminal bladder cancer variants (micropapillary, plasmacytoid, nested) exhibited significantly lower levels of *KRT5* and significantly higher levels of *KRT20* expression than conventional UBC or basal variants (sarcomatoid, squamous; Figure 1E).

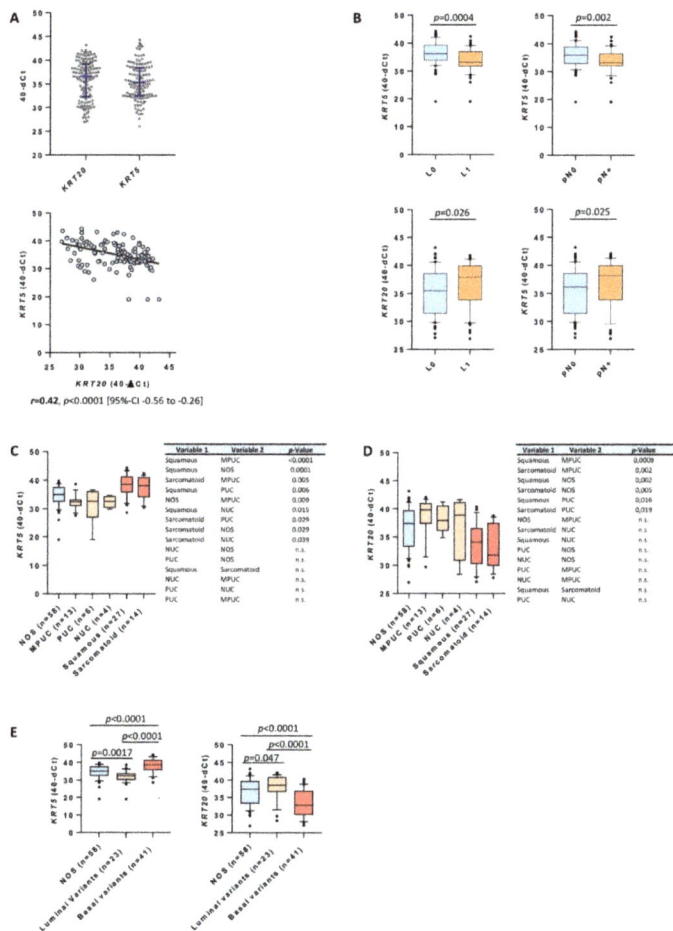

Figure 1. (**A**) Data distribution of *KRT5* and *KRT20* mRNA levels in patients with muscle-invasive bladder cancer (MIBC) treated with radical cystectomy and correlation of *KRT5* and *KRT20* mRNA levels. Blue bars within the boxplot indicate median value and 25%/75% quartiles. The black line in the correlation plot indicates the strength of correlation. (**B**) Correlation of *KRT5* mRNA expression levels with N-stage and lymphovascular invasion (L; L1 = lymphovascular invasion present; L0 = lymphovascular invasion absent; pN0 = no lymphnode metastasis present; pN+ = lymphnode metastasis present). High expression of *KRT5* mRNA is associated with significantly lower rates of LVI and nodal metastasis. (**C,D**) Distribution of *KRT5* and *KRT20* in conventional (not otherwise specified; NOS), micropapillary (MPUC), plasmacytoid (PUC), nested (NUC), squamous, and sarcomatoid differentiated urothelial carcinomas. (**E**) Distribution of *KRT20* and *KRT5* stratified by conventional urothelial carcinomas, luminal variants (including nested, plasmacytoid, and micropapillary carcinomas), and basal variants (including squamous and sarcomatoid carcinomas).

3.2. KRT5 and KRT20 mRNA Expression Defines Highly Prognostic Relevant Subgroups of MIBC

As shown in Figure 2A,B the differential expression of *KRT5* and *KRT20* clearly defines two distinct subgroups. High *KRT20* mRNA expression was significantly associated with worse RFS (multivariate hazard ratio (HR) = 2.33) and DSS (multivariate = HR 2.24; Figure 2A, Supplementary Table S1). Low *KRT5* expression level was associated with unfavorable RFS (multivariate HR = 1.47) and DSS (multivariate HR = 1.59; Figure 2B, Supplementary Table S1). Next, an algorithm (Epi-Typer) based on the above calculated cutoffs for *KRT5* and *KRT20* mRNA expression was used to further subclassify the tumors, as depicted in Figure 2C. *KRT5* and *KRT20* cutoffs were calculated by a predictive monoforest algorithm stratified by disease-specific survival status (disease-specific death vs. no disease-specific death). There was no statistically significant difference between the $KRT5^+/KRT20^-$ and $KRT5^+/KRT20^+$ subtypes with regard to RFS and DSS when these two groups were summarized to the $KRT5^+/KRT20^{+/-}$ phenotype (data not shown). The $KRT20^+/KRT5^-$ (class 2) subgroup showed a very poor prognosis with 5-year RFS (multivariate HR = 2.10; Figure 2C) and DSS of 0% (multivariate HR = 3.20; Figure 2C), whereas the $KRT5^+/KRT20^{+/-}$ (class 1) subgroup showed a favorable prognosis with 5-year RFS of 52% and 5-year DSS of 58% (Figure 2C).

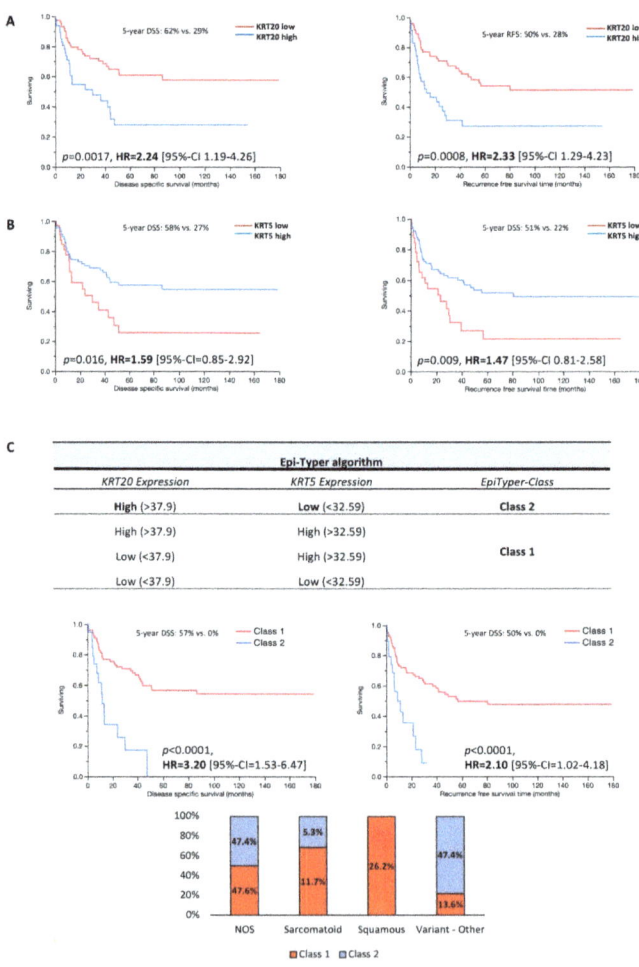

Figure 2. Kaplan–Meier analysis for recurrence-free survival (RFS) and disease-specific survival (DSS) based on (**A**) *KRT20* and (**B**) *KRT5* mRNA expression levels. (**C**) Epi-Typer algorithm and Kaplan–Meier analysis in the MIBC cohort for RFS and DSS based on marker combination (Epi-Typer) of *KRT5* and *KRT20* mRNA expression levels (red color: tumors within Epi-Typer Class 1; blue color: tumors within Epi-Typer Class 2).

3.3. Multivariate Data Analysis

Multivariate Cox–proportional hazard models were calculated including fixed clinicopathological variables: pT-Stage, pN-Stage, Grading WHO 1973, Grading WHO 2016 (no impact; all included tumors were high grade), lymphovascular invasion, blood vessel invasion, age at cystectomy, gender, resection margin status, receipt of adjuvant platinum-containing chemotherapy, and presence of urothelial carcinoma in situ. Models were calculated for each respective cutoff group (*KRT5* high vs. low, *KRT20* high vs. low, Epi-Typer classes). Detailed multivariate analyses are depicted in Supplementary Table S1, including multivariate hazard ratios, significance levels, and 95% confidence intervals.

3.4. KRT5 and KRT20 mRNA Expression in the MDACC Cohort

Data validation was performed using in silico MDACC data (GSE48276; GSE = gene set enrichment) [14]. The basal subtype was significantly enriched with *KRT5* ($p = 0.0002$), whereas the luminal subtype showed significant enrichment with *KRT20* ($p = 0.0005$) (Figure 3). High expression of *KRT20* mRNA was associated with significantly worse DSS, while *KRT5* mRNA expression had no prognostic impact ($p = 0.042$ for *KRT20* and $p = 0.075$ for *KRT5*; Figure 3). In addition, the Epi-Typer algorithm added no prognostic impact to the *KRT20*/*KRT5* cutoff (data not shown).

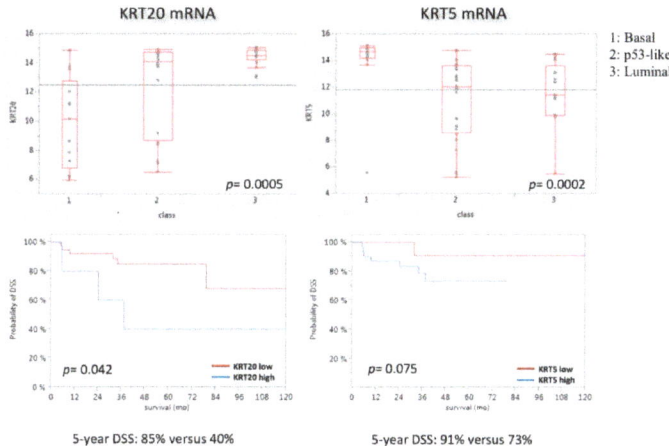

Figure 3. Association of *KRT5* and *KRT20* mRNA expression levels with MDACC molecular subtypes (MDACC cohort). Class 1 = basal, Class 2 = p53-like, Class 3 = luminal. As expected, luminal tumors were enriched with *KRT20* and basal tumors were enriched with *KRT5*. p53-like subtype shows a broad expression range of both genes. Basal tumors show a slightly higher proliferation rate. Kaplan–Meier regression analysis is unfavorable for highly *KRT20*-expressing tumors.

4. Discussion

Treatment options for UBC have evolved minimally over the last decades. Recent genome-wide mRNA expression analyses have revealed molecular subtypes with huge prognostic and predictive impact. Here, we show the possibility of stratifying MIBC into relevant subgroups by using two of the most prominent markers of the genome-wide approaches, the inversely related cytokeratins *KRT5* and *KRT20*, as surrogate markers for nonluminal and luminal differentiation. *KRT5* is a marker of stem or progenitor cells and can be found in basal-like carcinoma subtypes, often with squamous/sarcomatoid histological features, whereas *KRT20*, a marker of superficial umbrella cells, is enriched in luminal subtypes [8,9,12–15,17,20,26–28].

Most interestingly, the *KRT20* positive luminal subtype displayed worse RFS and DSS in MIBC, similar to previously published results in NMIBC [17,21]. This association between improved survival and keratin mRNA expression was also evident in the MDACC cohort (Figure 3) [14]. Furthermore, high expression of *KRT5* and low expression of *KRT20* were associated with a lower prevalence of lymphovascular invasion and lymphonodal metastasis, which is consistent with the favorable prognosis of *KRT5*-enriched MIBC in our cohort. At first glance, these results seem paradoxical, since the luminal subtype including *KRT20* was previously shown to be associated with a favorable prognosis [14], but are explainable due to characteristics of our cohort: (1) the *KRT20* high phenotype contains 23 cases with variant histology, of which are 13 micropapillary, 6 plasmacytoid, and 4 nested UBCs, which have been shown to be highly aggressive luminal variants with poor prognosis [29–33]; (2) many luminal tumors with and without variant histology are enriched with epithelial to mesenchymal transition (EMT) like gene expression pathways [18,29]. In a recent TCGA (=the cancer genome atlas) publication, Robertson et al. demonstrated that the luminal tumor family can be further subdivided into a luminal papillary cluster (no EMT-like pattern, favorable prognosis) and two luminal phenotypes with highly aggressive behavior (luminal, luminal infiltrated), which showed worse prognosis than basal differentiated tumors [18]. Luminal tumors with variant histology clustered into the aggressive luminal tumor families. Interestingly, Hedegaard et al. demonstrated that luminal NMIBC with poor PFS exhibited a strongly activated cancer-stem-cell-like and EMT signature and showed a huge parallel to the genomically unstable and infiltrated subtypes defined by the Lund group [13,17]. Additionally, in the past, several studies demonstrated the association between high *KRT20* expression and high tumor stage and grade [34]. High *KRT20* expression in lymph nodes after radical cystectomy is associated with a higher tumor stage, a higher rate of micrometastasis, and a worse outcome [35]. Moreover, high expression of *KRT20* in the bone marrow prior to radical cystectomy is associated with a worse outcome [36]. However, luminal tumors with favorable prognosis and *KRT20*/*KRT5* expression above the cutoff threshold are included in the favorable Epi-Typer class 1. This could mean that highly aggressive luminal tumors exhibit a strong *KRT20* polarized luminal-only phenotype with very low *KRT5* expression, while less aggressive luminal tumors show a mixed expression phenotype, reflecting differentiation that is still more closely related to the normal urothelial expression phenotype. Interestingly, we could prove that luminal variants exhibit significantly higher levels of *KRT20* and significantly lower levels of *KRT5* than conventional or basal variants (squamous/sarcomatoid). On the other hand, highly *KRT5*-expressing tumors are suggested to be of basal subtype and to respond better to neoadjuvant chemotherapy [5], which did not show worse survival than conventional luminal UBC in our cohort. However, the Epi-Typer algorithm is able to stratify class 1 basal and luminal tumors to identify patients who could benefit from neoadjuvant chemotherapy. Due to the lack of patients with neoadjuvant treatment in our cohort, the predictive potential of our RT-qPCR assay has to be investigated in an upcoming study.

As demonstrated previously in NMIBC, the assessment of cytokeratin (CK) 5 and CK20 protein expression by immunohistochemistry correlates well with *KRT5* and *KRT20* mRNA expression but lacks prognostic value [21], which is in line with previous breast cancer studies investigating *MKI67 (marker of proliferation Ki-67)*, *ER (estrogen receptor)*, *ERBB2 (Erb-B2 Receptor Tyrosine Kinase 2)*, and *PR (progesterone receptor)* mRNA and protein expression [37]. Therefore, RT-qPCR has been considered as a possible alternative for immunohistochemistry, as it is objective and not affected by interobserver variability [37–40]. Furthermore, simple gene expression assays in a ready-to-use format are quite simple to establish and to perform on small devices (e.g., Cepheid approaches) compared to immunohistochemistry on expansive autostainers. Tests on such platforms are very cheap and highly standardized, and need little hands-on time. Furthermore, no big laboratory inventory is needed to perform these ready-to-use assays, and therefore they are also suitable for small centers, private practices, or labs that do not have the opportunity to establish the extremely expensive infrastructure for next-generation sequencing or immunohistochemistry. On the other hand, there are several disadvantages with such tests: Due to the increased treatment individualization, they tend to oversimplify biological backgrounds. Furthermore, important predictive genetic alterations—e.g., microsatellite instability for response to checkpoint inhibition [41], recombinant DNA mismatch repair deficiency status for neoadjuvant chemotherapy [42], and others—are not assessable with such simple tests. Taken together, simple tests may play a big role in initial risk stratification to stratify which patients could benefit from further large-scale analysis after initial curative treatment.

Taken together, our data suggest that RT-qPCR-based molecular subtyping of UBC by *KRT5* and *KRT20* mRNA expression is a suitable method to predict RFS and DSS of MIBC patients (Epi-Typer) and could be used in small centers without access to huge immunohistochemistry facilities. Since our study is limited by its retrospective nature, small study cohort, and data from a single center, our results have to be further investigated in upcoming prospective trials with regard to specific treatment modalities.

Supplementary Materials: Supplementary materials can be found at http://www.mdpi.com/1422-0067/19/11/3396/s1.

Author Contributions: Study conduction: B.K., C.B., M.B., A.H., P.E.; Study supervision: B.K., C.B., M.B., A.H., P.E.; Data acquisition—Follow-up data: M.G.W., K.N., P.E., C.B.; Pathological reevaluation: M.E., S.P., A.H.; qPCR assessments: R.M.W., R.S., D.S., S.E., K.N.; Data analysis: M.E., J.B., W.O., D.S., P.E.; Manuscript writing: M.E., P.E.; Critical revision of the manuscript: All contributing authors.

funding: This study was funded by the German Cancer Aid (DKG), grant number 110541.

Conflicts of Interest: The authors declare no conflict of interest.

Abbreviations

UBC	urothelial bladder cancer
MIBC	muscle-invasive bladder cancer
CK	cytokeratin
KRT	keratin
MKI67	marker of proliferation Ki67
CALM2	calmodulin 2
FFPE	formalin-fixed paraffin-embedded
MDACC	MD Anderson Cancer Center
PFS	progression-free survival
RFS	recurrence-free survival
DSS	disease-specific survival
NMIBC	non-muscle-invasive bladder cancer
RT-qPCR	reverse-transcription quantitative polymerase chain reaction

References

1. Jemal, A.; Bray, F.; Center, M.M.; Ferlay, J.; Ward, E.; Forman, D. Global cancer statistics. *CA Cancer J. Clin.* **2011**, *61*, 69–90. [CrossRef] [PubMed]
2. Shah, J.B.; McConkey, D.J.; Dinney, C.P. New strategies in muscle-invasive bladder cancer: On the road to personalized medicine. *Clin. Cancer Res.* **2011**, *17*, 2608–2612. [CrossRef] [PubMed]
3. Svatek, R.S.; Hollenbeck, B.K.; Holmang, S.; Lee, R.; Kim, S.P.; Stenzl, A.; Lotan, Y. The economics of bladder cancer: Costs and considerations of caring for this disease. *Eur. Urol.* **2014**, *66*, 253–262. [CrossRef] [PubMed]
4. Svatek, R.S.; Shariat, S.F.; Novara, G.; Skinner, E.C.; Fradet, Y.; Bastian, P.J.; Kamat, A.M.; Kassouf, W.; Karakiewicz, P.I.; Fritsche, H.M.; et al. Discrepancy between clinical and pathological stage: External validation of the impact on prognosis in an international radical cystectomy cohort. *BJU Int.* **2011**, *107*, 898–904. [CrossRef] [PubMed]
5. Seiler, R.; Ashab, H.A.; Erho, N.; van Rhijn, B.W.; Winters, B.; Douglas, J.; Van Kessel, K.E.; Fransen van de Putte, E.E.; Sommerlad, M.; Wang, N.Q.; et al. Impact of Molecular Subtypes in Muscle-invasive Bladder Cancer on Predicting Response and Survival after Neoadjuvant Chemotherapy. *Eur. Urol.* **2017**, *72*, 544–554. [CrossRef] [PubMed]
6. Perou, C.M.; Sorlie, T.; Eisen, M.B.; van de Rijn, M.; Jeffrey, S.S.; Rees, C.A.; Pollack, J.R.; Ross, D.T.; Johnsen, H.; Akslen, L.A.; et al. Molecular portraits of human breast tumours. *Nature* **2000**, *406*, 747–752. [CrossRef] [PubMed]

7. Cancer Genome Atlas Network. Comprehensive molecular portraits of human breast tumours. *Nature* **2012**, *490*, 61–70. [CrossRef] [PubMed]
8. Blaveri, E.; Simko, J.P.; Korkola, J.E.; Brewer, J.L.; Baehner, F.; Mehta, K.; Devries, S.; Koppie, T.; Pejavar, S.; Carroll, P.; et al. Bladder cancer outcome and subtype classification by gene expression. *Clin. Cancer Res.* **2005**, *11*, 4044–4055. [CrossRef] [PubMed]
9. Dyrskjot, L.; Thykjaer, T.; Kruhoffer, M.; Jensen, J.L.; Marcussen, N.; Hamilton-Dutoit, S.; Wolf, H.; Orntoft, T.F. Identifying distinct classes of bladder carcinoma using microarrays. *Nat. Genet.* **2003**, *33*, 90–96. [CrossRef] [PubMed]
10. Kim, W.J.; Kim, E.J.; Kim, S.K.; Kim, Y.J.; Ha, Y.S.; Jeong, P.; Kim, M.J.; Yun, S.J.; Lee, K.M.; Moon, S.K.; et al. Predictive value of progression-related gene classifier in primary non-muscle invasive bladder cancer. *Mol. Cancer* **2010**, *9*, 3. [CrossRef] [PubMed]
11. Lee, J.S.; Leem, S.H.; Lee, S.Y.; Kim, S.C.; Park, E.S.; Kim, S.B.; Kim, S.K.; Kim, Y.J.; Kim, W.J.; Chu, I.S. Expression signature of E2F1 and its associated genes predict superficial to invasive progression of bladder tumors. *J. Clin. Oncol.* **2010**, *28*, 2660–2667. [CrossRef] [PubMed]
12. Sanchez-Carbayo, M.; Socci, N.D.; Lozano, J.; Saint, F.; Cordon-Cardo, C. Defining molecular profiles of poor outcome in patients with invasive bladder cancer using oligonucleotide microarrays. *J. Clin. Oncol.* **2006**, *24*, 778–789. [CrossRef] [PubMed]
13. Sjodahl, G.; Lauss, M.; Lovgren, K.; Chebil, G.; Gudjonsson, S.; Veerla, S.; Patschan, O.; Aine, M.; Ferno, M.; Ringner, M.; et al. A molecular taxonomy for urothelial carcinoma. *Clin. Cancer Res.* **2012**, *18*, 3377–3386. [CrossRef] [PubMed]
14. Choi, W.; Porten, S.; Kim, S.; Willis, D.; Plimack, E.R.; Hoffman-Censits, J.; Roth, B.; Cheng, T.; Tran, M.; Lee, I.L.; et al. Identification of distinct basal and luminal subtypes of muscle-invasive bladder cancer with different sensitivities to frontline chemotherapy. *Cancer Cell* **2014**, *25*, 152–165. [CrossRef] [PubMed]
15. Cancer Genome Atlas Research Network. Comprehensive molecular characterization of urothelial bladder carcinoma. *Nature* **2014**, *507*, 315–322. [CrossRef] [PubMed]
16. Breyer, J.; Otto, W.; Wirtz, R.M.; Wullich, B.; Keck, B.; Erben, P.; Kriegmair, M.C.; Stoehr, R.; Eckstein, M.; Laible, M.; et al. ERBB2 Expression as Potential Risk-Stratification for Early Cystectomy in Patients with pT1 Bladder Cancer and Concomitant Carcinoma in situ. *Urol. Int.* **2016**, *98*, 282–289. [CrossRef] [PubMed]
17. Hedegaard, J.; Lamy, P.; Nordentoft, I.; Algaba, F.; Hoyer, S.; Ulhoi, B.P.; Vang, S.; Reinert, T.; Hermann, G.G.; Mogensen, K.; et al. Comprehensive Transcriptional Analysis of Early-Stage Urothelial Carcinoma. *Cancer Cell* **2016**, *30*, 27–42. [CrossRef] [PubMed]
18. Robertson, A.G.; Kim, J.; Al-Ahmadie, H.; Bellmunt, J.; Guo, G.; Cherniack, A.D.; Hinoue, T.; Laird, P.W.; Hoadley, K.A.; Akbani, R.; et al. Comprehensive Molecular Characterization of Muscle-Invasive Bladder Cancer. *Cell* **2017**, *171*, 540–556. [CrossRef] [PubMed]
19. Rinaldetti, S.; Rempel, E.; Worst, T.S.; Eckstein, M.; Steidler, A.; Weiss, C.A.; Bolenz, C.; Hartmann, A.; Erben, P. Subclassification, survival prediction and drug target analyses of chemotherapy-naive muscle-invasive bladder cancer with a molecular screening. *Oncotarget* **2018**, *9*, 25935–25945. [CrossRef] [PubMed]
20. Dadhania, V.; Zhang, M.; Zhang, L.; Bondaruk, J.; Majewski, T.; Siefker-Radtke, A.; Guo, C.C.; Dinney, C.; Cogdell, D.E.; Zhang, S.; et al. Meta-Analysis of the Luminal and Basal Subtypes of Bladder Cancer and the Identification of Signature Immunohistochemical Markers for Clinical Use. *EBioMedicine* **2016**, *12*, 105–117. [CrossRef] [PubMed]
21. Breyer, J.; Wirtz, R.M.; Otto, W.; Erben, P.; Kriegmair, M.C.; Stoehr, R.; Eckstein, M.; Eidt, S.; Denzinger, S.; Burger, M.; et al. In stage pT1 non-muscle-invasive bladder cancer (NMIBC), high KRT20 and low KRT5 mRNA expression identify the luminal subtype and predict recurrence and survival. *Virchows Arch.* **2017**, *470*, 267–274. [CrossRef] [PubMed]
22. Moch, H.; Humphrey, P.A.; Ulbright, T.M.; Reuter, V.E. WHO Classification of Tumours of the Urinary System and Male Genital Organs. 2016. Available online: https://www.ncbi.nlm.nih.gov/pubmed/26935559 (accessed on 28 February 2018).
23. Eckstein, M.; Wirtz, R.M.; Pfannstil, C.; Wach, S.; Stoehr, R.; Breyer, J.; Erlmeier, F.; Gunes, C.; Nitschke, K.; Weichert, W.; et al. A multicenter round robin test of PD-L1 expression assessment in urothelial bladder cancer by immunohistochemistry and RT-qPCR with emphasis on prognosis prediction after radical cystectomy. *Oncotarget* **2018**, *9*, 15001–15014. [CrossRef] [PubMed]

24. Tramm, T.; Sorensen, B.S.; Overgaard, J.; Alsner, J. Optimal reference genes for normalization of qRT-PCR data from archival formalin-fixed, paraffin-embedded breast tumors controlling for tumor cell content and decay of mRNA. *Diagn. Mol. Pathol.* **2013**, *22*, 181–187. [CrossRef] [PubMed]
25. Kriegmair, M.C.; Balk, M.; Wirtz, R.; Steidler, A.; Weis, C.A.; Breyer, J.; Hartmann, A.; Bolenz, C.; Erben, P. Expression of the p53 Inhibitors MDM2 and MDM4 as Outcome Predictor in Muscle-invasive Bladder Cancer. *Anticancer Res.* **2016**, *36*, 5205–5213. [CrossRef] [PubMed]
26. Chan, K.S.; Espinosa, I.; Chao, M.; Wong, D.; Ailles, L.; Diehn, M.; Gill, H.; Presti, J., Jr.; Chang, H.Y.; van de Rijn, M.; et al. Identification, molecular characterization, clinical prognosis, and therapeutic targeting of human bladder tumor-initiating cells. *Proc. Natl. Acad. Sci. USA* **2009**, *106*, 14016–14021. [CrossRef] [PubMed]
27. Ho, P.L.; Kurtova, A.; Chan, K.S. Normal and neoplastic urothelial stem cells: Getting to the root of the problem. *Nat. Rev. Urol.* **2012**, *9*, 583–594. [CrossRef] [PubMed]
28. Reis-Filho, J.S.; Simpson, P.T.; Martins, A.; Preto, A.; Gartner, F.; Schmitt, F.C. Distribution of p63, cytokeratins 5/6 and cytokeratin 14 in 51 normal and 400 neoplastic human tissue samples using TARP-4 multi-tumor tissue microarray. *Virchows Arch.* **2003**, *443*, 122–132. [PubMed]
29. Guo, C.C.; Dadhania, V.; Zhang, L.; Majewski, T.; Bondaruk, J.; Sykulski, M.; Wronowska, W.; Gambin, A.; Wang, Y.; Zhang, S.; et al. Gene Expression Profile of the Clinically Aggressive Micropapillary Variant of Bladder Cancer. *Eur. Urol.* **2016**, *70*, 611–620. [CrossRef] [PubMed]
30. Comperat, E.; Roupret, M.; Yaxley, J.; Reynolds, J.; Varinot, J.; Ouzaid, I.; Cussenot, O.; Samaratunga, H. Micropapillary urothelial carcinoma of the urinary bladder: A clinicopathological analysis of 72 cases. *Pathology* **2010**, *42*, 650–654. [CrossRef] [PubMed]
31. Ghoneim, I.A.; Miocinovic, R.; Stephenson, A.J.; Garcia, J.A.; Gong, M.C.; Campbell, S.C.; Hansel, D.E.; Fergany, A.F. Neoadjuvant systemic therapy or early cystectomy? Single-center analysis of outcomes after therapy for patients with clinically localized micropapillary urothelial carcinoma of the bladder. *Urology* **2011**, *77*, 867–870. [CrossRef] [PubMed]
32. Kamat, A.M.; Gee, J.R.; Dinney, C.P.; Grossman, H.B.; Swanson, D.A.; Millikan, R.E.; Detry, M.A.; Robinson, T.L.; Pisters, L.L. The case for early cystectomy in the treatment of nonmuscle invasive micropapillary bladder carcinoma. *J. Urol.* **2006**, *175*, 881–885. [CrossRef]
33. Bertz, S.; Wach, S.; Taubert, H.; Merten, R.; Krause, F.S.; Schick, S.; Ott, O.J.; Weigert, E.; Dworak, O.; Rodel, C.; et al. Micropapillary morphology is an indicator of poor prognosis in patients with urothelial carcinoma treated with transurethral resection and radiochemotherapy. *Virchows Arch.* **2016**, *469*, 339–344. [CrossRef] [PubMed]
34. Christoph, F.; Muller, M.; Schostak, M.; Soong, R.; Tabiti, K.; Miller, K. Quantitative detection of cytokeratin 20 mRNA expression in bladder carcinoma by real-time reverse transcriptase-polymerase chain reaction. *Urology* **2004**, *64*, 157–161. [CrossRef] [PubMed]
35. Gazquez, C.; Ribal, M.J.; Marin-Aguilera, M.; Kayed, H.; Fernandez, P.L.; Mengual, L.; Alcaraz, A. Biomarkers vs conventional histological analysis to detect lymph node micrometastases in bladder cancer: A real improvement? *BJU Int.* **2012**, *110*, 1310–1316. [CrossRef] [PubMed]
36. Retz, M.; Rotering, J.; Nawroth, R.; Buchner, A.; Stockle, M.; Gschwend, J.E.; Lehmann, J. Long-term follow-up of bladder cancer patients with disseminated tumour cells in bone marrow. *Eur. Urol.* **2011**, *60*, 231–238. [CrossRef] [PubMed]
37. Wirtz, R.M.; Sihto, H.; Isola, J.; Heikkila, P.; Kellokumpu-Lehtinen, P.L.; Auvinen, P.; Turpeenniemi-Hujanen, T.; Jyrkkio, S.; Lakis, S.; Schlombs, K.; et al. Biological subtyping of early breast cancer: A study comparing RT-qPCR with immunohistochemistry. *Breast Cancer Res. Treat.* **2016**, *157*, 437–446. [CrossRef] [PubMed]
38. Atmaca, A.; Al-Batran, S.E.; Wirtz, R.M.; Werner, D.; Zirlik, S.; Wiest, G.; Eschbach, C.; Claas, S.; Hartmann, A.; Ficker, J.H.; et al. The validation of estrogen receptor 1 mRNA expression as a predictor of outcome in patients with metastatic non-small cell lung cancer. *Int. J. Cancer* **2014**, *134*, 2314–2321. [CrossRef] [PubMed]
39. Sikic, D.; Breyer, J.; Hartmann, A.; Burger, M.; Erben, P.; Denzinger, S.; Eckstein, M.; Stöhr, R.; Wach, S.; Wullich, B.; et al. High androgen receptor mRNA expression is independently associated with prolonged cancer-specific and recurrence-free survival in stage T1 bladder cancer. *Transl. Oncol.* **2017**, *10*, 340–345. [CrossRef] [PubMed]

40. Wilson, T.R.; Xiao, Y.; Spoerke, J.M.; Fridlyand, J.; Koeppen, H.; Fuentes, E.; Huw, L.Y.; Abbas, I.; Gower, A.; Schleifman, E.B.; et al. Development of a robust RNA-based classifier to accurately determine ER, PR, and HER2 status in breast cancer clinical samples. *Breast Cancer Res. Treat.* **2014**, *148*, 315–325. [CrossRef] [PubMed]
41. Le, D.T.; Durham, J.N.; Smith, K.N.; Wang, H.; Bartlett, B.R.; Aulakh, L.K.; Lu, S.; Kemberling, H.; Wilt, C.; Luber, B.S.; et al. Mismatch repair deficiency predicts response of solid tumors to PD-1 blockade. *Science* **2017**, *357*, 409–413. [CrossRef] [PubMed]
42. Iyer, G.; Balar, A.V.; Milowsky, M.I.; Bochner, B.H.; Dalbagni, G.; Donat, S.M.; Herr, H.W.; Huang, W.C.; Taneja, S.S.; Woods, M.; et al. Multicenter Prospective Phase II Trial of Neoadjuvant Dose-Dense Gemcitabine Plus Cisplatin in Patients With Muscle-Invasive Bladder Cancer. *J. Clin. Oncol.* **2018**, *36*, 1949–1956. [CrossRef] [PubMed]

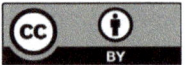

© 2018 by the authors. Licensee MDPI, Basel, Switzerland. This article is an open access article distributed under the terms and conditions of the Creative Commons Attribution (CC BY) license (http://creativecommons.org/licenses/by/4.0/).

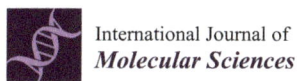 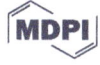

Article

Diagnostic and Prognostic Implications of FGFR3^{high}/Ki67^{high} Papillary Bladder Cancers

Mirja Geelvink [1], Armin Babmorad [1], Angela Maurer [1], Robert Stöhr [2], Tobias Grimm [3], Christian Bach [4], Ruth Knuechel [1], Michael Rose [1,†] and Nadine T. Gaisa [1,*,†]

1. Institute of Pathology, RWTH Aachen University, Pauwelsstrasse 30, 52074 Aachen, Germany; mirja.geelvink@rwth-aachen.de (M.G.); armin.babmorad@rwth-aachen.de (A.B.); amaurer@ukaachen.de (A.M.); rknuechel-clarke@ukaachen.de (R.K.); mrose@ukaachen.de (M.R.)
2. Institute of Pathology, University Hospital Erlangen, Friedrich-Alexander University Erlangen-Nürnberg (FAU), 91054 Erlangen, Germany; Robert.Stoehr@uk-erlangen.de
3. Department of Urology, Ludwig Maximilian University Munich, 81377 Munich, Germany; Tobias_Grimm@med.uni-muenchen.de
4. Department of Urology, RWTH Aachen University, 52074 Aachen, Germany; chbach@ukaachen.de
* Correspondence: ngaisa@ukaachen.de; Tel.: +49-241-8036118; Fax: +49-241-8082439
† These authors are contributed equally.

Received: 30 July 2018; Accepted: 24 August 2018; Published: 28 August 2018

Abstract: Prognostic/therapeutic stratification of papillary urothelial cancers is solely based upon histology, despite activated FGFR3-signaling was found to be associated with low grade tumors and favorable outcome. However, there are FGFR3-overexpressing tumors showing high proliferation—a paradox of coexisting favorable and adverse features. Therefore, our study aimed to decipher the relevance of FGFR3-overexpression/proliferation for histopathological grading and risk stratification. N = 142 (n = 82 pTa, n = 42 pT1, n = 18 pT2-4) morphologically G1–G3 tumors were analyzed for immunohistochemical expression of FGFR3 and Ki67. Mutation analysis of *FGFR3* and *TP53* and FISH for *FGFR3* amplification and rearrangement was performed. SPSS 23.0 was used for statistical analysis. Overall FGFR3^{high}/Ki67^{high} status (n = 58) resulted in a reduced Δmean progression-free survival (PFS) (p < 0.01) of 63.92 months, and shorter progression-free survival (p < 0.01; mean PFS: 55.89 months) in pTa tumors (n = 50). *FGFR3*^{mut}/*TP53*^{mut} double mutations led to a reduced Δmean PFS (p < 0.01) of 80.30 months in all tumors, and *FGFR3*^{mut}/*TP53*^{mut} pTa tumors presented a dramatically reduced PFS (p < 0.001; mean PFS: 5.00 months). Our results identified FGFR3^{high}/Ki67^{high} papillary pTa tumors as a subgroup with poor prognosis and encourage histological grading as high grade tumors. Tumor grading should possibly be augmented by immunohistochemical stainings and suitable clinical surveillance by endoscopy should be performed.

Keywords: FGFR3; Ki67; TP53; bladder cancer; prognosis

1. Introduction

Bladder cancer is the second most common genitourinary malignancy [1]. At primary diagnosis, most of the tumors are papillary non-invasive cancers (pTa) which are mostly well differentiated but show a high rate of recurrence. Those tumors are characterized by certain molecular alterations as for example FGFR3 activation [2–5]. Up to 30% of all patients have invasive disease at diagnosis. These tumors frequently derive from flat carcinoma in situ (CIS) of the urothelium (a high grade lesion, often *TP53*-mutated) and quickly develop muscle-invasion and metastasis [6,7]. Current prognostic and therapeutic stratification in urothelial cancers is therefore based on tumor staging and grading at histological examination. Staging criteria is the depth of invasion defined by the tumor node metastasis (TNM)-classification of the Union Internationale Contre le Cancer (UICC) [8]. The tumor grading is based upon architectural order and nuclear shape features, which have been thoroughly defined as diagnostic criteria in the 2004 WHO classification of bladder cancer in order to achieve reproducible and comparable diagnoses worldwide. Low grade (LG) tumors show uniform, slightly enlarged nuclei in an orderly, polarized architecture, sometimes with a prominent palisading of the basal layer. Mitotic figures are infrequent [9,10]. High grade (HG) tumors show more pleomorphic nuclei with multiple mitotic features and various extent of architectural disarray [10]. Based on previous genetic analyses and clinical observations, it has been proposed that the histological appearance (grading) of tumors correlates with the underlying genetic alterations, and low grade tumors were regarded genetically stable, whereas high grade tumors, harboring a high number of genetic alterations, were considered genetically "unstable" [7]. Proposed prognostic markers in papillary non-invasive tumors have been the Ki67 labeling index (marker for cell proliferation) and keratin 20 expression (marker for cell differentiation). Tumors with Ki67 $\geq$ 15% were regarded as highly proliferative [11–13] and aberrant expression of keratin 20 was linked to disease recurrence in pTa tumors [14]. Lately, Hurst et al. conducted a comprehensive molecular study on n = 141 papillary non-invasive bladder cancers (low grade, G1 and G2 according to WHO 1973) and found lower overall mutation rates, but more mutations in chromatin modifying genes than in muscle-invasive bladder cancer, and two distinct genomic subgroups of tumors (genomic subtype 1 and 2). The majority of tumors with genomic subtype 1 showed no or only few copy-number alterations. Genomic subtype 2 was characterized by loss of 9q (including the mTORC1 regulator TSC1), increased Ki67 labeling index, upregulated mTORC1 signaling (comprising the overrepresentation of genes in processes that are involved in the unfolded protein response, glycolysis, and cholesterol homeostasis) as well as enrichment for DNA repair and cell-cycle genes [15]. *FGFR3* mutations were not found to be significantly different in both subgroups (72% vs. 89%) and *TP53* mutations were absent [15]. The authors did not show a correlation of molecular profiles with specific histological features.

However, in routine histological diagnostics, pathologists often see papillary non-invasive tumors with quite uniform, relatively small nuclei, which give a "crowded" impression, but seem to be of "low nuclear grade". Interestingly, Ki67 labeling in these tumors is often enhanced and from this point of view a reconsideration of a possible "high grade"-biology is implicated. Opposite to the negative predictive impact of a high Ki67 index, these tumors often show a strong expression of FGFR3, which indicates an activation of the signaling pathway resulting in cellular proliferation, but is generally associated with a benign course of disease with higher recurrence rates but less progression [7]. Being aware of this diagnostic-biological "dilemma", we delineated in this study the immunohistochemical and genetic basis of such FGFR3^{high}/Ki67^{high} papillary bladder cancers in order to reveal their prognostic impact.

2. Results

2.1. Immunohistochemical Combination of Ki67-Index and FGFR3 Levels Defines Worse Patients' Outcome

Overall, FGFR3 and Ki67 protein expression was analyzed by immunohistochemistry (Figure 1A–I) in n = 142 primary bladder tumors comprising n = 82 papillary non-invasive tumors (for cohort characteristics, see Table S1). In this cohort, 87/142 patients (61.3%) showed a high Ki67-index ($\geq$15% positivity) and 100/142 bladder cancer patients (70.4%) were characterized by strong FGFR3 expression (Tomlinson Score 3) (Figure S1A,C). In papillary non-invasive pTa tumors, 82.9% showed strong FGFR3 and 54.9% increased Ki67 expression (Figure S1B,D).

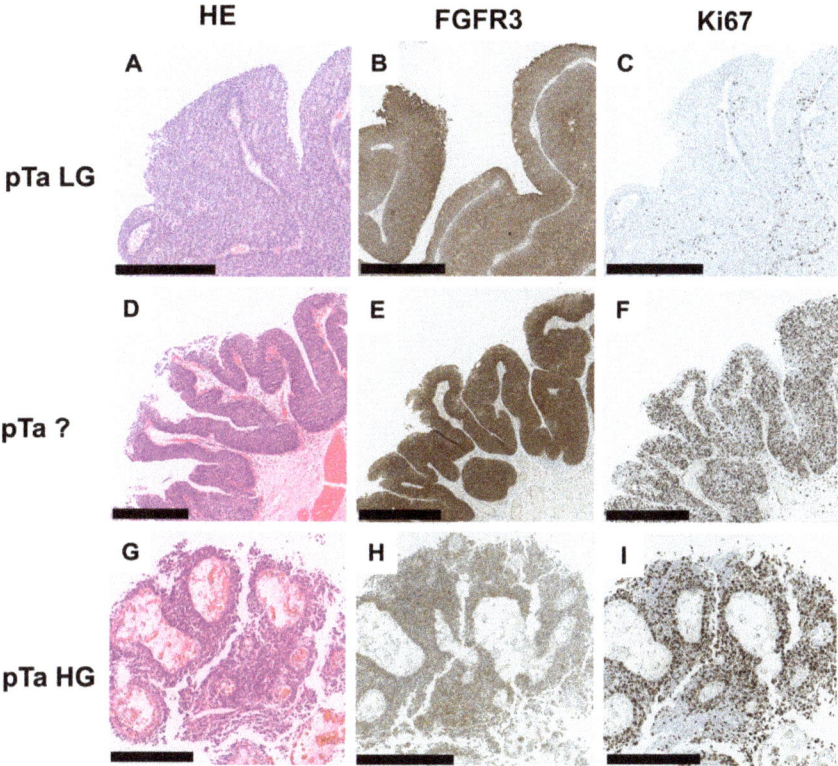

Figure 1. FGFR3 and Ki67 protein expression in papillary non-invasive (pTa) bladder tumors. Immunohistochemical staining for FGFR3 and Ki67 protein of representative tumors are shown. (**A–C**) pTa low grade (LG) tumor: (**A**) Hematoxylin and Eosin (HE) staining; (**B**) strong FGFR3 immunoreactivity; and (**C**) only a few cell nuclei are positive for Ki67 expression. (**D–F**) pTa tumor with "crowded low nuclear grade" (pTa?) morphology: (**D**) HE staining; (**E**) strong FGFR3 immunoreactivity; and (**F**) high nuclear Ki67 protein staining. (**G–I**) pTa high grade (HG) tumor: (**G**) HE staining; (**H**) moderate FGFR3 protein expression; and (**I**) high nuclear Ki67 staining. Scale bar: 500 µm; original digital magnifications vary from 5× to 7×.

Next, associations between clinico-pathological characteristics and both FGFR3 and Ki67 protein expression were tested. FGFR3 expression and Ki67 index correlated with tumor grading (FGFR3: $p < 0.001$, Ki67: $p < 0.001$), but only FGFR3 expression was significantly associated with tumor stage (FGFR3: $p < 0.001$) (Tables 1 and 2). No association was found between FGFR3/Ki67 and age at diagnosis or gender.

Table 1. Clinico-pathological parameters in correlation to FGFR3 protein expression.

		FGFR3 Expression [a]			
	n	0–2	3	p-Value [b]	Spearman ρ
Parameter:					
Age at diagnosis					
<70 years	67	20	47	0.946	0.006
≥70 years	75	22	53		
Gender					
female	31	10	21	0.372	0.031
male	111	32	79		
Histological tumor grade					
low grade	49	3	46	**<0.001**	−0.373
high grade	93	39	54		
Tumor stage					
pTa	82	14	68	**<0.001**	−0.320
pT1–pT4	60	28	32		

[a] Tomlinson score according to [16]; [b] Fisher's exact test; Significant p-values are marked in bold face.

Table 2. Clinico-pathological parameters in correlation to Ki67 protein expression.

		Ki67 Expression [a]			
	n	<15%	≥15%	p-Value [b]	Spearman ρ
Parameter:					
Age at diagnosis					
<70 years	67	31	36	0.083	0.146
≥70 years	75	24	51		
Gender					
female	31	14	17	0.408	0.070
male	111	41	70		
Histological tumor grade					
low grade	49	34	15	**<0.001**	0.457
high grade	93	21	72		
Tumor stage					
pTa	82	37	45	0.069	0.175
pT1–pT4	60	18	42		

[a] According to [11]; [b] Fisher's exact test; Significant p-values are marked in bold face.

To assess the clinical impact, Kaplan–Meier analyses were performed. FGFR3 expression had no significant impact on progression-free survival (PFS) (Figure 2A). In contrast, enhanced Ki67 expression (≥15%) significantly predicted shorter progression-free survival (Δmean PFS: 2.71 months, $p = 0.043$). Finally, we aimed to decipher the potential prognostic impact of combined FGFR3 expression and Ki67 index: FGFR3^{high}/Ki67^{high} status was found in $n = 58$ cases. A combined analysis of FGFR3/Ki67 positivity (Figure 2C and Figure S2A) resulted in a reduced Δmean PFS ($p < 0.01$) of 63.92 months when comparing FGFR3^{high}/Ki67^{high} tumors (mean PFS: 54.87 months ± 6.73; 95% CI: 41.78 to 68.05) with all other combinations (mean PFS: 118.78 months ± 6.95; 95% CI: 105.17 to 132.40). If, for example, both markers were expressed at low levels, bladder cancer patients showed no progressive disease at all (Figure S2A). Therefore, our results identify FGFR3^{high}/Ki67^{high} tumors as an aggressive subgroup.

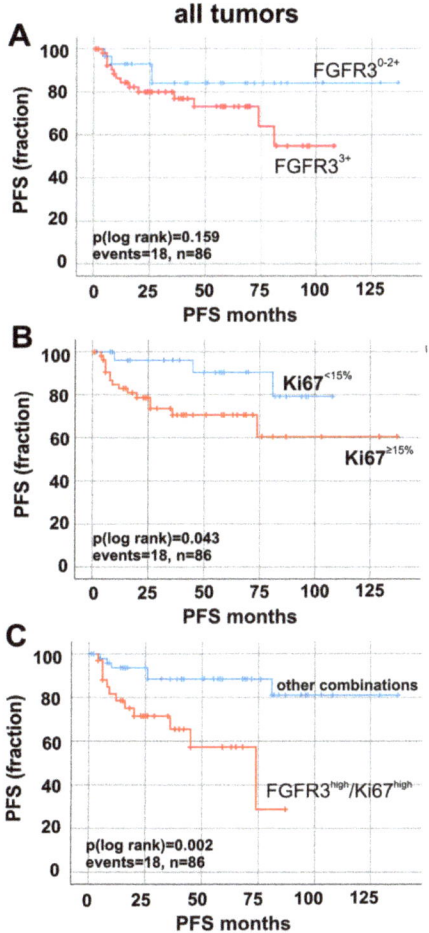

Figure 2. Prognostic impact of FGFR3 and Ki67 protein expression in all tumors (pTa, pT1 and pT2–4). Kaplan–Meier survival curves display progression-free survival (PFS). (**A**) Survival curves of patients with high FGFR3 expression (red curve, $n = 56$) compared to low FGFR3 expression (blue curve, $n = 30$). (**B**) Kaplan–Meier analysis of patients with high Ki67 expression (red curve, $n = 56$) compared to low Ki67 expression (blue curve, $n = 30$). (**C**) Survival curve analysis of FGFR3^{high}/Ki67^{high} expression (red curve, $n = 34$) compared to all other combinations of FGFR3 and Ki67 expression (blue curve, $n = 32$). n: overall number of cases; events: overall events of tumor progression.

The calculated Cox regression model (including the potentially prognostic parameters stage, grade, age, keratin 20 and keratin 5/6) confirmed independency of the clinical impact of a FGFR3^{high}/Ki67^{high} status on progression-free survival. Patients displaying a combined overexpression of FGFR3 and Ki67 showed an approximately four-fold higher risk for tumor progression (multivariate hazard ratio (HR): 3.943, 95% CI: 1.247 to 12.466, $p = 0.019$) (Table 3).

Table 3. Multivariate Cox regression analysis of immunohistochemical markers including all factors potentially influencing PFS.

Variable	HR	p-Value	95%CI	
			Lower	Upper
FGFR3 ^{high}/Ki67^{high}	3.943	**0.019**	1.247	12.466
pT status	0.957	0.941	0.295	3.105
Tumor grade	0.846	0.823	0.196	3.653
Keratin 5/6	0.482	0.280	0.128	1.812
Keratin 20	0.424	0.115	0.146	1.232
Age	1.773	0.347	0.537	5.847

2.2. Prognostic Impact of Ki67-Index and FGFR3 Overexpression in Papillary Non-Invasive (pTa) Tumors

Stratifying our cohort by invasiveness, i.e., into papillary non-invasive (pTa) and invasive tumors (pT1–pT4), FGFR3 overexpression (Tomlinson Score 3) was not associated with tumor progression in pTa bladder cancer ($p > 0.05$ for PFS) (Figure 3A).

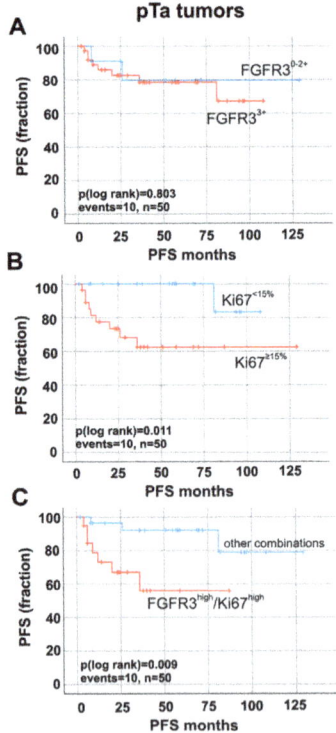

Figure 3. Prognostic impact of FGFR3 and Ki67 protein expression in papillary non-invasive (pTa) tumors. Kaplan–Meier survival curves demonstrate progression-free survival (PFS). (**A**) Survival curves of patients with high FGFR3 expression (red curve, $n = 39$) compared to low FGFR3 expression (blue curve, $n = 11$). (**B**) Kaplan–Meier analysis of patients with high Ki67 expression (red curve, $n = 28$) compared to low Ki67 expression (blue curve, $n = 22$). (**C**) Impact of combined markers on risk stratification of tumor progression is shown. Survival curve analysis of FGFR3^{high}/Ki67^{high} expression (red curve, $n = 20$) compared to all other combinations of FGFR3 and Ki67 expression (blue curve, $n = 30$) in pTa tumors. n, overall number of cases; events, overall events of tumor progression.

Single marker analysis of high Ki67-index correlated with progression-free survival (Δmean PFS: 17.06 months, $p = 0.011$) (Figure 3B). Now, combining the two immunohistochemical markers, univariate Kaplan–Meier curve revealed a significant impact of FGFR3^{high}/Ki67^{high} expression on patients' outcome only in pTa tumors. In fact, patients with high FGFR3^{high}/Ki67^{high} showed a significantly ($p < 0.01$) shorter progression-free survival (mean PFS: 55.89 months ± 9.23; 95% CI: 37.82 to 73.98) compared to those patients with all other combinations of FGFR3/Ki67 expression (mean PFS: 113.85 months ± 8.12; 95% CI: 97.94 to 129.77, $p = 0.009$) (Figure 3C).

2.3. Altered Molecular FGFR3/TP53 Status Predicts Worse Patients' Survival

Since we hypothesized that FGFR3-overexpression and high cell proliferation might indicate a higher risk for progression in papillary non-invasive tumors, we further investigated the molecular status of our cohort by studying both mutations for *FGFR3* as papillary and *TP53* as invasive markers (for detailed mutation data, see Table S2). In total, 48 out of 99 (48.5%) analyzed patients harbored mutations within the *FGFR3* gene (Figure 4A).

The most frequent mutation was p.S249C (pTa: 13/21, pT1: 10/22, pT2–4: 2/5). *FGFR3* mutations showed no significant association with clinico-pathological parameters like tumor stage or grade (Table S3). *TP53* mutations were present in $n = 23/98$ (23.5%) patients (Figure 4A). There were $n = 18/23$ (78.3%) tumors which solely showed missense mutations (pTa: 6/6, pT1: 7/11, pT2–4: 5/6) and $n = 5/23$ (21.7%) tumors with mutations leading to a premature transcription stop either due to the appearance of a stop codon or a frameshift (pTa: 0/6, pT1: 4/11, pT2–4: 1/6). *TP53* mutations correlated with tumor grade ($p < 0.05$) but not with stage (Table S4). Mutations in both genes (referred to as double mutations) were found in $n = 6/99$ (6.1%) patients.

Survival analysis revealed no significant association between single mutations, i.e., *FGFR3* or *TP53*, with patient's outcome for PFS (Figure 4B,C). However, mutations in both genes (*FGFR3*^{mut}/*TP53*^{mut}) predicted unfavorable prognosis for PFS. Double mutations led to a reduced Δmean PFS ($p < 0.01$) of 80.30 months: *FGFR3*^{mut}/*TP53*^{mut} tumors (mean PFS: 27.08 months ± 8.41; 95% CI: 10.59 to 43.57) showed shorter PFS in contrast with all other combinations (mean PFS: 107.83 months ± 8.62; 95% CI: 90.49.17 to 124.28) (Figure 4D and Figure S2B).

Multivariate analysis confirmed the prognostic impact of *FGFR3*^{mut}/*TP53*^{mut} tumors. Double mutated tumors exhibited a 6.6 times higher risk for tumor progression (multivariate hazard ratio (HR): 6.563, 95% CI: 1.694 to 25.425, $p = 0.006$) (Table 4).

2.4. Prognostic Impact of FGFR3 and TP53 Mutations in Papillary Non-Invasive (pTa) Tumors

Next, we focused on pTa tumors, in particular those with FGFR3-overexpression and high cell proliferation. In pTa tumors, the following distribution was found: $n = 17/42$ (40.5%) *FGFR3*^{wt}/*TP53*^{wt}, $n = 19/42$ (45.2%) *FGFR3*^{mut}/*TP53*^{wt}, $n = 4/42$ (9.5%) *FGFR3*^{wt}/*TP53*^{mut} and $n = 2/42$ (4.8%) *FGFR3*^{mut}/*TP53*^{mut}. On the contrary, pT1 tumors showed $n = 9/39$ (23.1%) *FGFR3*^{wt}/*TP53*^{wt}, $n = 19/39$ (48.7%) *FGFR3*^{mut}/*TP53*^{wt}, $n = 8/39$ (20.5%) *FGFR3*^{wt}/*TP53*^{mut} and $n = 3/39$ (7.7%) *FGFR3*^{mut}/*TP53*^{mut}. pT2–4 tumors represented with the following mutational pattern: $n = 8/18$ (44.4%) *FGFR3*^{wt}/*TP53*^{wt}, $n = 4/18$ (22.2%) *FGFR3*^{mut}/*TP53*^{wt}, $n = 5/18$ (27.8%) *FGFR3*^{wt}/*TP53*^{mut} and $n = 1/18$ (5.6%) *FGFR3*^{mut}/*TP53*^{mut}.

Survival analyses revealed a correlation between *FGFR3* mutations and shorter PFS ($p = 0.041$) in pTa tumors (Figure 5A). *TP53* mutations did not show any effects ($p > 0.05$) on PFS (Figure 5B). Interestingly, tumors exhibiting double mutation status *FGFR3*^{mut}/*TP53*^{mut} ($n = 6$) presented a dramatically reduced Δmean PFS ($p < 0.001$) of 102.52 months (mean PFS: 5.00 months ± 1.00; 95% CI: 3.04 to 6.96) in pTa tumors (Figure 5C) compared with all other combinations (mean PFS: 107.52 months ± 9.72; 95% CI: 88.46 to 126.57).

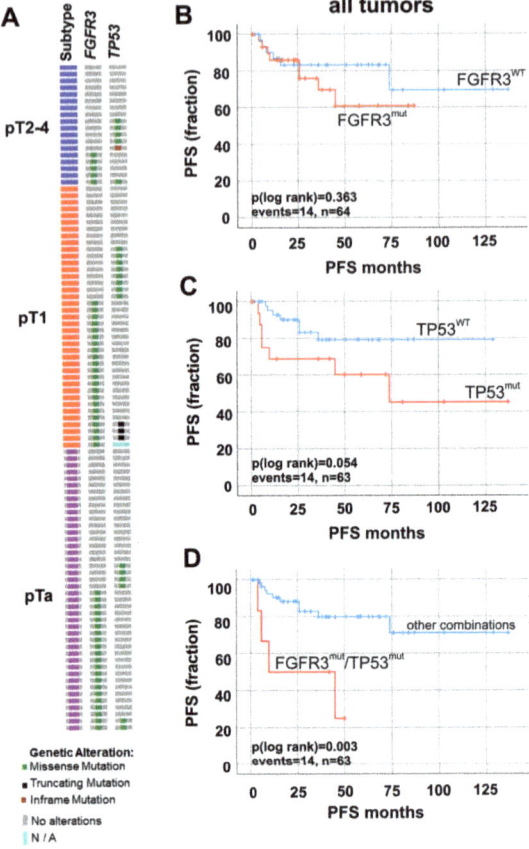

Figure 4. *FGFR3* and *TP53* mutation frequency and prognostic impact on tumor progression. (**A**) Oncoprint graph for *FGFR3* and *TP53* mutation analysis. (**B–D**) Kaplan–Meier survival curves display progression-free survival (PFS). (**B**) Survival curves of tumors with detected *FGFR3* mutations (red curve, $n = 30$) compared to non-mutated *FGFR3* gene status (blue curve, $n = 34$). (**C**) Kaplan–Meier analysis of tumors with mutated *TP53* (red curve, $n = 17$) compared to wildtype *TP53* (blue curve, $n = 46$). (**D**) Impact of double mutations on risk stratification of tumor progression is demonstrated. Univariate analysis of double mutations (red curve, $n = 6$) compared to all other combinations of mutated and non-mutated *FGFR3* and *TP53* genes (blue curve, $n = 57$). n, overall number of cases; events, overall events of tumor progression.

Table 4. Multivariate Cox regression analysis of molecular markers including all factors potentially influencing PFS.

Variable	HR	p-Value	95%CI	
			Lower	Upper
FGFR3^{mut}/*TP53*^{mut}	6.563	**0.006**	1.694	25.425
pT status	1.179	0.821	0.284	4.896
Tumor grade	0.241	0.138	0.037	1.580
Keratin 5/6	0.714	0.621	0.188	2.712
Keratin 20	0.872	0.814	0.279	2.730
Age	1.41	0.584	0.412	2.809

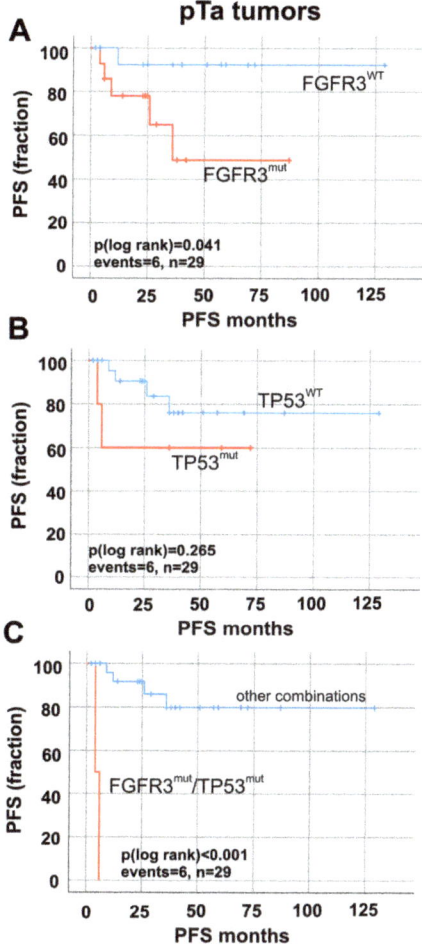

Figure 5. Prognostic impact of *FGFR3* and *TP53* mutations on tumor progression in papillary non-invasive (pTa) tumors. Progression-free survival (PFS) is shown. (**A**) Univariate survival analysis illustrates that detected *FGFR3* mutations (red curve, $n = 14$) predict shorter PFS compared to non-mutated *FGFR3* gene status (blue curve, $n = 15$). (**B**) Kaplan–Meier analysis of tumors with mutated *TP53* (red curve, $n = 5$) compared to wildtype *TP53* (blue curve, $n = 24$). (**C**) Impact of double mutations on risk stratification of tumor progression is shown. Survival analysis of double mutations (red curve, $n = 2$) compared to all other combinations of mutated and non-mutated *FGFR3* and *TP53* genes (blue curve, $n = 27$) in pTa tumors. n: overall number of cases; events: overall events of tumor progression.

Finally, we assessed the clinical impact of immunohistochemical and mutational status as a combined approach. Survival analysis displayed that *FGFR3*^{mut}/*TP53*^{mut} double mutated tumors were significantly associated with worse patients' outcome only in FGFR3 and Ki67 overexpressing tumors: reduced PFS in FGFR3^{high}/Ki67^{high} double mutated tumors compared with all other combinations of molecular status of *TP53* and *FGFR3* (FGFR3^{wt}/TP53^{wt} $p = 0.001$; FGFR3^{mut}/TP53^{wt} $p < 0.001$; FGFR3^{wt}/TP53^{mut} $p = 0.116$) (data not shown). However, it has to be noted that the number of double mutations is very low, and, hence, statistical validity should be enhanced in future studies.

2.5. FGFR3^{high}/Ki67^{high} Tumors Define a Subset of pTa Tumors Including Lesions with Molecular FGFR3 Pathway Activation

Prognostic stratification of bladder cancer patients in routine histopathological diagnostics claims simple and cost-effective means, therefore, we evaluated the concordance of immunohistochemical staining results and molecular status.

The majority of FGFR3^{high}/Ki67^{high} tumors was characterized by conjunct *FGFR3* mutations with a significant correlation only in papillary non-invasive tumors (pTa n = 19/27 (70.4%), $p < 0.001$) but not in pT1 and pT2–4 tumors (Table S5). There was no significant correlation between FGFR3^{high}/Ki67^{high} tumors and *TP53* mutations independently of the given tumor stage (data not shown).

To evaluate the diagnostic potential of immunohistochemical markers covering the molecular FGFR3 pathway, we performed ROC (Receiver operating characteristics) curve statistics to calculate sensitivity and specificity. Accordingly, both immunohistochemical markers detect *FGFR3* mutations with 90.5% sensitivity and 61.9% specificity (area under curve (AUC): 0.776, p = 0.004, positive predictive value (PPV): 70.4%, negative predictive value (NPV): 85.7%). These data show that FGFR3^{high}/Ki67^{high} tumors include papillary lesions with mutation-based altered FGFR3 signaling, but also tumors without molecular alterations (pTa n = 8/27 (29.6%)). Hence, our data give evidence that FGFR3^{high}/Ki67^{high} tumors define a subset of pTa tumors associated with poor prognosis potentially decoupled from the described protective effect of FGFR3 activation [7].

3. Discussion

In our study, we systematically analyzed papillary non-invasive and invasive tumors for distinct prognostic immunohistochemical and molecular markers. We focused on a subgroup of immunohistochemically FGFR3^{high}/Ki67^{high} tumors in order to reveal their prognostic impact on patient survival and re-evaluate their histological classification/grading.

Although, according to nuclear and architectural criteria, these papillary tumors appear to be orderly and more "nuclear low grade", we found them associated with worse PFS compared with FGFR3^{high}/Ki67^{low} tumors. This was especially evident in pTa tumors, where mean progression-free survival was reduced to 55 instead of 113 months. Therefore, we asked whether these tumors harbor a special molecular phenotype turning them into aggressive ones. In literature *FGFR3* and *TP53* mutations were initially thought to be mutually exclusive as *FGFR3* mutations were associated with pTa and LG tumors ("papillary pathway"), whereas the *TP53* mutations were often found in invasive and HG carcinomas ("CIS/invasive pathway") [17,18]. Notwithstanding, Hernandez et al. reported *FGFR3* and *TP53* mutations to be independently distributed in a large series of pT1G3 tumors, that were consequently interpreted as a particular group of bladder tumors that could not be classified into either one pathway or the other [4]. In our study, we saw a similar trend with well-known inverse relationships between *FGFR3* and *TP53* mutations for both stage and grade, while mutations in *FGFR3* and *TP53* revealed an independent but not mutually exclusive assignment (six tumors with double mutations). Biologically activated FGFR3 signaling promotes cell proliferation and tumor growth, however interestingly, highest numbers of FGFR3-alterations are found in benign papillary or low grade papillary tumors with usually low proliferation (Ki67) index [19–21]. TP53 inactivation results in reduced cellular apoptosis and thus maintains tumor growth via reduced cell death [22–25]. We hypothesized that a FGFR3^{high}/Ki67^{high} phenotype might be resulting from inactivated p53, however we found no sufficient molecular evidence for this theory in our cohort. Recent comprehensive sequencing data of papillary non-invasive bladder tumors revealed a genomic subtype 2, which is characterized by loss of 9q (including TSC1), increased Ki67 labeling index, upregulated mTORC1 signaling, glycolysis, features of the unfolded protein response, altered cholesterol homeostasis and DNA repair [15]. Therefore, high proliferation might be explained by mutations in DNA repair genes or the deletion/mutation of *TSC1*, which consequently leads towards an upregulation of mTORC1 and *PIK3CA* mutations. Further analyses to strengthen this theory have to be performed in the future.

Comprehensive molecular data of bladder cancer has been gained in the recent years [15,26,27], however, complex multigene analysis and RNA expression analysis are costly and laborious, and therefore cost-effective simple analyses for routine histological examination are needed. In our study, we analyzed whether fast and simple immunohistochemical analyses are suitable to detect a more aggressive molecular subtype. We found a highly significant correlation between strong FGFR3/Ki67 immunohistochemical staining and *FGFR3* mutation status, which indicates that FGFR3 protein expression is more frequent than mutational activation [16]. Moreover, our FGFR3^{high}/Ki67^{high} subgroup also comprises those neoplasms without any molecular (*FGFR3* and/or *TP53*) alterations defining in this combination a subset of pTa tumors with poor prognosis, i.e., FGFR3 overexpression was associated with unfavorable outcome as previously shown, for instance, for invasive bladder tumors treated with adjuvant chemotherapy [28]. Thus, our data support the proposed clinical significance of these two immunohistochemical markers for diagnostic and prognostic stratification of more aggressive papillary non-invasive bladder tumors.

Taken together, we found immunohistochemically FGFR3^{high}/Ki67^{high} pTa tumors associated with worse prognosis/survival, despite appearing histologically of "lower nuclear grade"/G2. Even if these tumors appear to be "low grade" (according to the 2004 WHO classification), we recommend classifying them as "high grade" pTa tumors. In light of our findings, we suggest immunohistochemical staining for FGFR3 and Ki67 in order to gain evidence for this more aggressive molecular subgroup with worse prognosis. These patients probably could profit from close endoscopic follow-up, as especially urine cytology might also be challenging/less sensitive due to their minimal nuclear changes.

4. Materials and Methods

4.1. Patient Samples, Tissue Microarrays and DNA

We retrospectively selected urothelial bladder cancer cases (mutational analysis: n = 42 pTa, n = 39 pT1, n = 18 pT2–4; immunohistochemical analysis: n = 82 pTa, n = 42 pT1, n = 18 pT2–4) from our pathology archive and from the archive of the Institute of Pathology in Erlangen. Formalin-fixed paraffin-embedded (FFPE) surgical specimens were used to construct tissue microarrays (all samples) and extract DNA (n = 99 samples) using Qiagen kits (Qiagen, Hilden, Germany) as previously described [29–31]. Patient information was obtained by the Department of Urology and the local ethics committee approved a retrospective, pseudonymized study of archival tissues (RWTH EK 009/12). Histological tumor grade and stage was classified according to WHO 2004 classification [8].

4.2. Immunohistochemistry

For immunohistochemical stainings, TMA sections were pretreated with DAKO PT-Link heat induced antigen retrieval with Low pH (pH 6) or High pH (pH 9) Target Retrieval Solution (DAKO, Hamburg, Germany) and incubated for 30 min at room temperature with respective antibodies in a DAKO Autostainer (DAKO). For stainings anti-FGFR3 (clone B9, PTlink pH6, dilution 1:25, Flex+M; Santa Cruz Biotechnology, Heidelberg, Germany), anti-Ki67 (clone MIB-1, PTlink pH 6, dilution 1:400, Flex+M; DAKO), anti-CK 20 (clone Ks20.8, PTlink pH 6, dilution 1:200, Flex+M; DAKO), and anti-CK5/6 (clone D5/16 B4, PTlink pH 9, dilution 1:100, Flex+M; DAKO) were used. Appropriate linker molecules EnVision^{TM}FLEX+ (mouse/rabbit), EnVision FLEX/HRP detection system and counterstaining with EnVision FLEX Hematoxylin were applied. Stainings were evaluated by an experienced uropathologist (NTG) who was blinded for patient identity, diagnosis and clinical follow-up results. FGFR3 positivity was reported according to a semiquantitative scoring system developed by Tomlinson et al. [16]. All other stainings were evaluated for staining intensities (0 = no staining, 1 = weak staining, 2 = moderate staining, 3 = strong staining) and percentages of positive stained tumor cells. Results were judged as follows: Keratin 20 positive $\geq$10% stained cells [14,32], Keratin 5/6 positive $\geq$10% [32], Ki67 positive $\geq$15% [11,13] stained cells.

4.3. Fluorescence In Situ Hybridization

ZytoLight Dual Color Probe SPEC FGFR3/*CEN* 4 and *ZytoLight* Dual Color Break Apart Probe SPEC FGFR3 (Zytovision, Bremerhaven, Germany) were hybridized onto 3 µm TMA sections according to the manufacturer's protocols. Slides were evaluated with a Zeiss Axiovert 135 fluorescence microscope (Carl Zeiss, Oberkochen, Germany), and Diskus Software (MIL 7.5, 4.80) (Büro Hilgers, Königswinter, Germany) using appropriate channels/filters (AHF ZyGreen F36-720, AHF ZyOrange F36-740, AHF DAPI, AHF F56-700). Signals of 60 nuclei of tumor cells were counted at high magnification ($\times 1000$) and judged as described previously [33].

4.4. Sanger Sequencing

PCR-amplification of exons 7, 10 and 15 of the *FGFR3* gene and exons 5, 6, 7, 8 and 9 of *TP53* were carried out using routine protocols. Primers and annealing temperatures are given in Table S6. PCR products were purified by either ExoSAP-IT (Affymetrix, Lahr/Schwarzwald, Germany) or a PCR purification kit (PerkinElmer Chemagen, Baesweiler, Germany) according to the manufacturer's instructions. Sanger sequencing of both strands was run on an ABI PRISM 3500 Genetic Analyzer (Applied Biosystems, Weiterstadt, Germany) using the Big dye Terminator kit (Applied Biosystems), the same primer sets and the seq purification kit (PerkinElmer Chemagen).

4.5. Statistical Analysis

Statistical analysis was performed using SPSS (Statistical Package for the Social Sciences) software version 23.0 (SPSS Inc., Chicago, IL, USA). *p*-values < 0.05 were considered significant. Statistical associations between clinico-pathological and molecular factors were determined by Fisher's exact test. Correlation analysis was performed by calculating a Spearman's rank correlation coefficient. Survival (progression-free survival (PFS)) was calculated using the Kaplan–Meier method with log-rank statistics. Survival was measured from surgery until relapse, death or progression and was censored for patients alive without evidence of event at the last follow-up date. Multivariate Cox-regression analysis was performed to test for an independently prognostic value of FGFR3-Ki67 protein expression and *FGFR3-TP53* mutations. Receiver operating characteristics (ROC) curves were calculated to assess biomarker performance of immunohistochemical markers regarding molecular alterations.

Supplementary Materials: Supplementary materials can be found at http://www.mdpi.com/1422-0067/19/9/2548/s1.

Author Contributions: Conceptualization, R.K. and N.T.G; Methodology, M.G., A.B., A.M. and M.R.; Software, M.R.; Validation, R.S.; Resources, T.G. and C.B.; Writing—Original Draft Preparation, N.T.G., M.G. and M.R.; Writing—Review and Editing, A.M., A.B., R.S., T.G., and C.B.; Visualization, M.R.; and Supervision, R.K. and N.T.G.

funding: This research received no external funding.

Acknowledgments: The authors appreciate the excellent technical support of Ursula Schneider, Inge Losen, Patrick Kühl and Oliver Dohmen.

Conflicts of Interest: The authors declare that they have no conflict of interest.

References

1. Siegel, R.L.; Miller, K.D.; Jemal, A. Cancer statistics. *CA Cancer J. Clin.* **2018**, *68*, 7–30. [CrossRef]
2. Van Rhijn, B.W.; Lurkin, I.; Radvanyi, F.; Kirkels, W.J.; Van der Kwast, T.H.; Zwarthoff, E.C. The fibroblast growth factor receptor 3 (FGFR3) mutation is a strong indicator of superficial bladder cancer with low recurrence rate. *Cancer Res.* **2001**, *61*, 1265–1268. [PubMed]
3. Billerey, C.; Chopin, D.; Aubriot-Lorton, M.H.; Ricol, D.; Gil Diez de Medina, S.; van Rhijn, B.; Bralet, M.P.; Lefrere-Belda, M.A.; Lahaye, J.B.; Abbou, C.C.; et al. Frequent FGFR3 mutations in papillary non-invasive bladder (pTa) tumors. *Am. J. Pathol.* **2001**, *158*, 1955–1959. [CrossRef]

4. Hernandez, S.; Lopez-Knowles, E.; Lloreta, J.; Kogevinas, M.; Jaramillo, R.; Amoros, A.; Tardón, A.; García-Closas, R.; Serra, C.; Carrato, A.; et al. FGFR3 and Tp53 mutations in T1G3 transitional bladder carcinomas: Independent distribution and lack of association with prognosis. *Clin. Cancer. Res.* **2005**, *11*, 5444–5450. [CrossRef] [PubMed]
5. Neuzillet, Y.; van Rhijn, B.W.; Prigoda, N.L.; Bapat, B.; Liu, L.; Bostrom, P.J.; Fleshner, N.E.; Gallie, B.L.; Zlotta, A.R.; Jewett, M.A.; et al. FGFR3 mutations, but not FGFR3 expression and FGFR3 copy-number variations, are associated with favourable non-muscle invasive bladder cancer. *Virchows. Arch.* **2014**, *465*, 207–213. [CrossRef] [PubMed]
6. Wu, X.R. Urothelial tumorigenesis: A tale of divergent pathways. *Nat. Rev. Cancer.* **2005**, *5*, 713–725. [CrossRef] [PubMed]
7. Knowles, M.A.; Hurst, C.D. Molecular biology of bladder cancer: New insights into pathogenesis and clinical diversity. *Nat. Rev. Cancer* **2015**, *15*, 25–41. [CrossRef] [PubMed]
8. Brierley, J.; Gospodarowicz, M.K.; Wittekind, C. *TNM Classification of Malignant Tumours*, 8th ed.; John Wiley & Sons Inc.: Chichester, UK; Hoboken, NJ, USA, 2017; ISBN 9781119263579.
9. Montironi, R.; Lopez-Beltran, A.; Scarpelli, M.; Mazzucchelli, R.; Cheng, L. Morphological classification and definition of benign, preneoplastic and non-invasive neoplastic lesions of the urinary bladder. *Histopathology* **2008**, *53*, 621–633. [CrossRef] [PubMed]
10. Moch, H.; Humphrey, P.A.; Ulbright, T.M.; Reuter, V.E. *International Agency for Research on Cancer. WHO Classification of Tumours of the Urinary System and Male Genital Organs*, 4th ed.; International Agency for Research on Cancer: Lyon, France, 2016; ISBN 9789283224372.
11. Cina, S.J.; Lancaster-Weiss, K.J.; Lecksell, K.; Epstein, J.I. Correlation of Ki-67 and p53 with the new World Health Organization/International Society of Urological Pathology Classification System for Urothelial Neoplasia. *Arch. Pathol. Lab. Med.* **2001**, *125*, 646–651. [CrossRef] [PubMed]
12. Hentic, O.; Couvelard, A.; Rebours, V.; Zappa, M.; Dokmak, S.; Hammel, P.; Maire, F.; O'Toole, D.; Lévy, P.; Sauvanet, A.; et al. Ki-67 index, tumor differentiation, and extent of liver involvement are independent prognostic factors in patients with liver metastases of digestive endocrine carcinomas. *Endocr. Relat. Cancer* **2011**, *18*, 51–59. [CrossRef] [PubMed]
13. Bertz, S.; Otto, W.; Denzinger, S.; Wieland, W.F.; Burger, M.; Stohr, R.; Link, S.; Hofstädter, F.; Hartmann, A. Combination of CK20 and Ki-67 immunostaining analysis predicts recurrence, progression, and cancer-specific survival in pT1 urothelial bladder cancer. *Eur. Urol.* **2014**, *65*, 218–226. [CrossRef] [PubMed]
14. Harnden, P.; Mahmood, N.; Southgate, J. Expression of cytokeratin 20 redefines urothelial papillomas of the bladder. *Lancet* **1999**, *353*, 974–977. [CrossRef]
15. Hurst, C.D.; Alder, O.; Platt, F.M.; Droop, A.; Stead, L.F.; Burns, J.E.; Burghel, G.J.; Jain, S.; Klimczak, L.J.; Lindsay, H.; et al. Genomic Subtypes of Non-invasive Bladder Cancer with Distinct Metabolic Profile and Female Gender Bias in KDM6A Mutation Frequency. *Cancer Cell* **2017**, *32*, 701–715. [CrossRef] [PubMed]
16. Tomlinson, D.C.; Baldo, O.; Harnden, P.; Knowles, M.A. FGFR3 protein expression and its relationship to mutation status and prognostic variables in bladder cancer. *J. Pathol.* **2007**, *213*, 91–98. [CrossRef] [PubMed]
17. Van Rhijn, B.W.; van der Kwast, T.H.; Vis, A.N.; Kirkels, W.J.; Boeve, E.R.; Jobsis, A.C.; Zwarthoff, E.C. FGFR3 and P53 characterize alternative genetic pathways in the pathogenesis of urothelial cell carcinoma. *Cancer. Res.* **2004**, *64*, 1911–1914. [CrossRef] [PubMed]
18. Bakkar, A.A.; Wallerand, H.; Radvanyi, F.; Lahaye, J.B.; Pissard, S.; Lecerf, L.; Kouyoumdjian, J.C.; Abbou, C.C.; Pairon, J.C.; Jaurand, M.C.; et al. FGFR3 and TP53 gene mutations define two distinct pathways in urothelial cell carcinoma of the bladder. *Cancer. Res.* **2003**, *63*, 8108–8112. [PubMed]
19. Hernandez, S.; Lopez-Knowles, E.; Lloreta, J.; Kogevinas, M.; Amoros, A.; Tardon, A.; Carrato, A.; Serra, C.; Malats, N.; Real, F.X. Prospective study of FGFR3 mutations as a prognostic factor in nonmuscle invasive urothelial bladder carcinomas. *J. Clin. Oncol.* **2006**, *24*, 3664–3671. [CrossRef] [PubMed]
20. Junker, K.; van Oers, J.M.; Zwarthoff, E.C.; Kania, I.; Schubert, J.; Hartmann, A. Fibroblast growth factor receptor 3 mutations in bladder tumors correlate with low frequency of chromosome alterations. *Neoplasia* **2008**, *10*, 1–7. [CrossRef] [PubMed]

21. Van Rhijn, B.W.; Zuiverloon, T.C.; Vis, A.N.; Radvanyi, F.; van Leenders, G.J.; Ooms, B.C.; Kirkels, W.J.; Lockwood, G.A.; Boevé, E.R.; Jöbsis, A.C.; et al. Molecular grade (FGFR3/MIB-1) and EORTC risk scores are predictive in primary non-muscle-invasive bladder cancer. *Eur. Urol.* **2010**, *58*, 433–441. [CrossRef] [PubMed]
22. Sigal, A.; Rotter, V. Oncogenic mutations of the p53 tumor suppressor: The demons of the guardian of the genome. *Cancer. Res.* **2000**, *60*, 6788–6793. [PubMed]
23. Zuckerman, V.; Wolyniec, K.; Sionov, R.V.; Haupt, S.; Haupt, Y. Tumour suppression by p53: The importance of apoptosis and cellular senescence. *J. Pathol.* **2009**, *219*, 3–15. [CrossRef] [PubMed]
24. Oren, M.; Rotter, V. Mutant p53 gain-of-function in cancer. *Cold Spring Harb. Perspect Biol.* **2010**, *2*, a001107. [CrossRef] [PubMed]
25. Rivlin, N.; Brosh, R.; Oren, M.; Rotter, V. Mutations in the p53 Tumor Suppressor Gene: Important Milestones at the Various Steps of Tumorigenesis. *Genes Cancer* **2011**, *2*, 466–474. [CrossRef] [PubMed]
26. Weinstein, J.N.; Akbani, R.; Broom, B.M.; Wang, W.; Verhaak, R.G.; McConkey, D.; Lerner, S.; Morgan, M.; Creighton, C.J.; Smith, C.; et al. Comprehensive molecular characterization of urothelial bladder carcinoma. *Nature* **2014**, *507*, 315–322. [CrossRef]
27. Hedegaard, J.; Lamy, P.; Nordentoft, I.; Algaba, F.; Hoyer, S.; Ulhoi, B.P.; Vang, S.; Reinert, T.; Hermann, G.G.; Mogensen, K.; et al. Comprehensive Transcriptional Analysis of Early-Stage Urothelial Carcinoma. *Cancer Cell* **2016**, *30*, 27–42. [CrossRef] [PubMed]
28. Sung, J.Y.; Sun, J.M.; Chang, J.B.; Seo, S.I.; Soo, J.S.; Moo, L.H.; Yong, C.H.; Young, K.S.; Choi, Y.L.; Young, K.G. FGFR3 overexpression is prognostic of adverse outcome for muscle-invasive bladder carcinoma treated with adjuvant chemotherapy. *Urol. Oncol.* **2014**, *32*, e23–e31. [CrossRef]
29. Gaisa, N.T.; Graham, T.A.; McDonald, S.A.; Canadillas-Lopez, S.; Poulsom, R.; Heidenreich, A.; Jakse, G.; Tadrous, P.J.; Knuechel, R.; Wright, N.A. The human urothelium consists of multiple clonal units, each maintained by a stem cell. *J Pathol.* **2011**, *225*, 163–171. [CrossRef] [PubMed]
30. Fischbach, A.; Rogler, A.; Erber, R.; Stoehr, R.; Poulsom, R.; Heidenreich, A.; Schneevoigt, B.S.; Hauke, S.; Hartmann, A.; Knuechel, R.; et al. Fibroblast growth factor receptor (FGFR) gene amplifications are rare events in bladder cancer. *Histopathology* **2015**, *66*, 639–649. [CrossRef] [PubMed]
31. Molitor, M.; Junker, K.; Eltze, E.; Toma, M.; Denzinger, S.; Siegert, S.; Knuechel, R.; Gaisa, N.T. Comparison of structural genetics of non-schistosoma-associated squamous cell carcinoma of the urinary bladder. *Int. J. Clin. Exp. Pathol.* **2015**, *8*, 8143–8158. [PubMed]
32. Gaisa, N.T.; Braunschweig, T.; Reimer, N.; Bornemann, J.; Eltze, E.; Siegert, S.; Toma, M.; Villa, L.; Hartmann, A.; Knuechel, R. Different immunohistochemical and ultrastructural phenotypes of squamous differentiation in bladder cancer. *Virchows. Arch.* **2011**, *458*, 301–312. [CrossRef] [PubMed]
33. Baldia, P.H.; Maurer, A.; Heide, T.; Rose, M.; Stoehr, R.; Hartmann, A.; Williams, S.V.; Knowles, M.A.; Knuechel, R.; Gaisa, N.T. Fibroblast growth factor receptor (FGFR) alterations in squamous differentiated bladder cancer: A putative therapeutic target for a small subgroup. *Oncotarget* **2016**, *7*, 71429–71439. [CrossRef] [PubMed]

© 2018 by the authors. Licensee MDPI, Basel, Switzerland. This article is an open access article distributed under the terms and conditions of the Creative Commons Attribution (CC BY) license (http://creativecommons.org/licenses/by/4.0/).

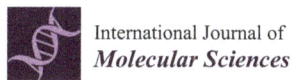

Article

Diagnostic and Prognostic Potential of MicroRNA Maturation Regulators Drosha, AGO1 and AGO2 in Urothelial Carcinomas of the Bladder

Anja Rabien [1,2,*], Nadine Ratert [1,2], Anica Högner [3], Andreas Erbersdobler [4], Klaus Jung [1,2], Thorsten H. Ecke [5,†] and Ergin Kilic [3,6,†]

1. Department of Urology, Charité—Universitätsmedizin Berlin, Corporate Member of Freie Universität Berlin, Humboldt-Universität zu Berlin, and Berlin Institute of Health, 10117 Berlin, Germany; n.ratert@gmx.de (N.R.); klaus.jung@charite.de (K.J.)
2. Berlin Institute for Urologic Research, 10117 Berlin, Germany
3. Institute of Pathology, Charité—Universitätsmedizin Berlin, Corporate Member of Freie Universität Berlin, Humboldt-Universität zu Berlin, and Berlin Institute of Health, 10117 Berlin, Germany; anica.hoegner@charite.de (A.H.); e.kilic@pathologie-leverkusen.de (E.K.)
4. Institute of Pathology, University Medicine Rostock, 18055 Rostock, Germany; andreas.erbersdobler@med.uni-rostock.de
5. Department of Urology, HELIOS Hospital Bad Saarow, 15526 Bad Saarow, Germany; thorsten.ecke@helios-kliniken.de
6. Institute of Pathology, Hospital Leverkusen, 51375 Leverkusen, Germany
* Correspondence: anja.rabien@charite.de; Tel.: +49-30-450515035; Fax: +49-30-450515904
† These authors contributed equally to this work.

Received: 16 May 2018; Accepted: 30 May 2018; Published: 31 May 2018

Abstract: Bladder cancer still requires improvements in diagnosis and prognosis, because many of the cases will recur and/or metastasize with bad outcomes. Despite ongoing research on bladder biomarkers, the clinicopathological impact and diagnostic function of miRNA maturation regulators Drosha and Argonaute proteins AGO1 and AGO2 in urothelial bladder carcinoma remain unclear. Therefore, we conducted immunohistochemical investigations of a tissue microarray composed of 112 urothelial bladder carcinomas from therapy-naïve patients who underwent radical cystectomy or transurethral resection and compared the staining signal with adjacent normal bladder tissue. The correlations of protein expression of Drosha, AGO1 and AGO2 with sex, age, tumor stage, histological grading and overall survival were evaluated in order to identify their diagnostic and prognostic potential in urothelial cancer. Our results show an upregulation of AGO1, AGO2 and Drosha in non-muscle-invasive bladder carcinomas, while there was increased protein expression of only AGO2 in muscle-invasive bladder carcinomas. Moreover, we were able to differentiate between non-muscle-invasive and muscle-invasive bladder carcinoma according to AGO1 and Drosha expression. Finally, despite Drosha being a discriminating factor that can predict the probability of overall survival in the Kaplan–Meier analysis, AGO1 turned out to be independent of all clinicopathological parameters according to Cox regression. In conclusion, we assumed that the miRNA processing factors have clinical relevance as potential diagnostic and prognostic tools for bladder cancer.

Keywords: bladder cancer; Drosha; AGO1; AGO2; biomarkers; immunohistochemistry

1. Introduction

In 2012, 430,000 new cases of bladder cancer were diagnosed worldwide. Thus, bladder cancer is the ninth most common cancer in the world with the highest incidence in Northern America,

Europe and some countries in Northern Africa and Western Asia [1]. Despite their heterogeneity, several characteristics have been found, which distinguish the subgroups of less aggressive, but often recurring non-muscle-invasive bladder cancer (NMIBC) and the more progressive muscle-invasive bladder cancer (MIBC). The latter holds an overall survival rate of 60% at most [2]. NMIBC develops from urothelial hyperplasia to low-grade carcinoma, with up to 15% proceeding to high-grade tumors. These cancers show characteristic alterations in the Ras-MAPK and PI3K-Akt pathways. The pathway leading to MIBC often includes dysplasia/carcinoma in situ and high-grade non-invasive carcinoma that accumulates common defects, e.g., in tumor suppressors, such as p53 or pRb, or in matrix metalloproteinases [2,3]. Although several potential biomarkers have been tested for their diagnostic and prognostic potential, targets for routine use are still needed.

A recent field of biomarker research has focused on microRNAs (miRNAs), which are involved in various biological processes, including tumorigenesis [4,5]. Several studies profiled the miRNA expression patterns in bladder cancer tissue and indicated some interesting findings regarding its diagnostic and/or prognostic potential [6,7]. The biogenesis of miRNAs is a multistep process involving a couple of protein complexes [8]. In the nucleus, miRNA genes are transcribed by RNA polymerase II/III into a long single or multiple primary miRNA, which is subsequently processed by the "Drosha microprocessor" into hairpin precursor miRNA (pre-miRNA). This "Drosha microprocessor" is a complex of the RNase III enzyme Drosha, its cofactor DiGeorge syndrome critical region gene 8 (DGCR8/Pasha) and other components. The pre miRNA is actively exported by exportin 5/Ras-related nuclear protein-guanosine triphosphate (Ran-GTP) to the cytoplasm. In this cellular compartment, RNase III enzyme Dicer converts pre miRNA to a mature double-stranded miRNA duplex that contains both the mature and its complementary strand and consists of about 20 nucleotides. The mature miRNA is subsequently loaded onto the miRNA Induced Silencing Complex (miRISC). The Argonaute (AGO) family proteins AGO1–AGO4 are the central components of the miRISC complex, which stabilize the mature miRNA strand. The other strand is degraded. AGO2 is the only protein with endonucleolytic activity that mediates the inhibition of target mRNA expression. The subsequent rate of miRNA complementarity and target mRNA affects the repression of translation or cleavage of mRNA. Additionally, there is some evidence indicating an alternative biogenesis pathway in which pre miRNAs are directly loaded onto the miRISC complex after Drosha processing, omitting Dicer processing [9].

As mentioned above, AGO1 and AGO2 are needed for the process of degrading mRNAs or impairing their translation, while Drosha plays a role in initial miRNA maturation. Consequently, it is postulated that they also play a key role in tumor behavior. Some studies have already reported a tumor specific expression of AGO1, AGO2, Dicer and Drosha in the urogenital tract. For example, the Argonautes have been implicated in clear cell renal cell carcinoma [10] and prostate cancer [11]. Meanwhile, the data for Argonautes and Drosha also exist for bladder carcinoma [12,13], but these are contradictory to our findings in major points and require discussion. The aim of our comprehensive immunohistochemical study was to investigate AGO1, AGO2 and Drosha expression in normal bladder urothelium and malignant bladder cancer tissue (NMIBC and MIBC) using a tissue microarray (TMA) as well as to correlate the expression of these proteins with clinicopathological parameters. We believe that our findings will support the potential of these three targets to become bladder carcinoma biomarkers but they will have to be carefully investigated further to avoid inaccurate conclusions indicated by the contradictory results in the literature.

2. Results

2.1. Immunostaining Pattern of AGO1, AGO2, and Drosha Expression in Bladder Tissue

All three targets appeared with a granular pattern in malignant and non-malignant tissue, while they were also often expressed in endothelial cells (Figures 1 and 2). AGO1 staining was found in the cytoplasm and partly in the nuclei of normal and tumor tissue (Figure 1A–C). AGO2 was mainly expressed in the cytoplasm and particularly in the pseudoluminal areas of tumors and adjacent normal tissue (Figure 1D–F). Furthermore, AGO2 was also found in lymphocytes (Figure 1F). Drosha staining was located in the cytoplasm and partly in the nucleus in normal and tumor tissue (Figure 2).

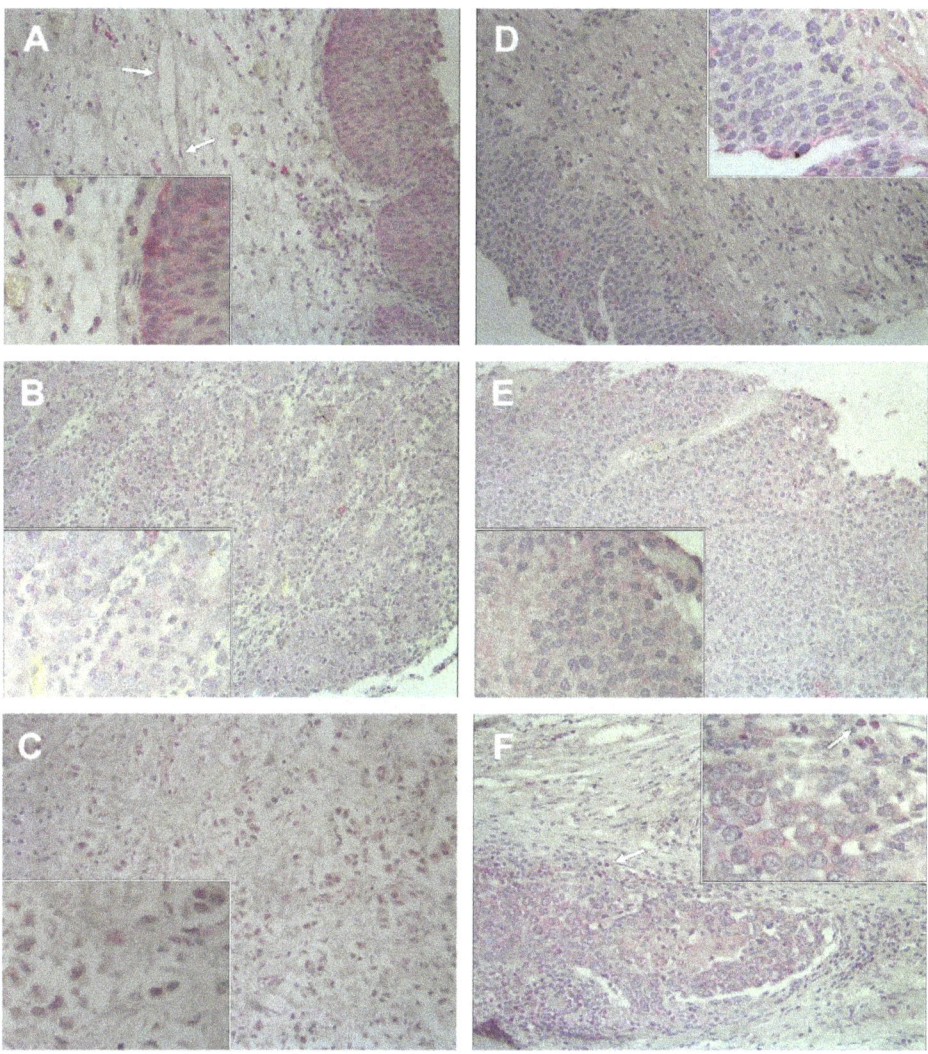

Figure 1. Immunohistochemical staining of AGO1 and AGO2 in bladder tissue. Representative images show the expression of AGO1 in non-malignant bladder tissue (**A**), in non-muscle-invasive pT1 tumor (**B**) and muscle-invasive pT3b tumor tissue (**C**); as well as the expression of AGO2 in normal bladder tissue (**D**), in non-muscle-invasive pTa tumor (**E**) and muscle-invasive pT3b tumor tissue (**F**). The arrows indicate the staining in endothelial cells (**A**) and AGO2 staining of lymphocytes (**F**). Pseudoluminal expression of AGO2 can be seen in (**D**). Magnification: 200×, inserts 400×.

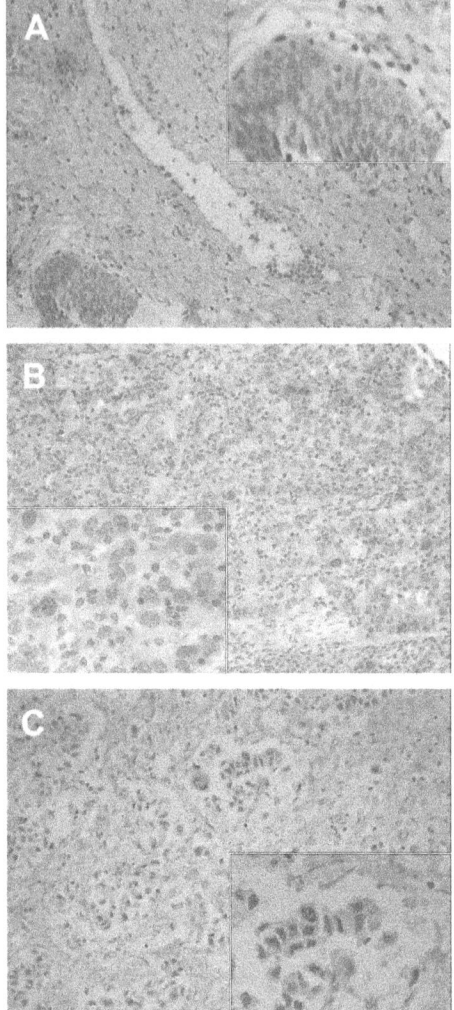

Figure 2. Immunohistochemical staining of Drosha in bladder tissue. Representative images show the expression of Drosha in non-malignant bladder tissue (**A**), in non-muscle-invasive pT1 tumor (**B**) and muscle-invasive pT3b tumor tissue (**C**). The staining of endothelial cells can be seen in (**A**). Magnification: 200×, inserts 400×.

2.2. AGO1, AGO2 and Drosha Expression in Bladder Carcinomas Compared to Non-Malignant Tissue and Association with Clinicopathological Parameters

The clinicopathological parameters of the bladder cancer cases are shown in Table 1. AGO1, AGO2 and Drosha were markedly upregulated in NMIBC compared to adjacent normal tissue. However, only AGO2 was significantly upregulated in MIBC (Table 2). Positive AGO2 staining identified 73/109 tumors (67%) without any difference between NMIBC and MIBC when calculating a Fisher's exact test (Table 3). However, AGO1 and Drosha expression was decreased in NMIBC compared to MIBC ($p < 0.001$, Table 3).

Table 1. Clinicopathological characteristics of the patients undergoing transurethral resection of the bladder or radical cystectomy.

Patient Characteristics (n = 112)	n (%)
Age, years [A]	
<69	52 (46.4)
≥69	60 (53.6)
Sex	
female	31 (27.7)
male	81 (72.3)
Tumor characteristics	
pT stage [B]	
pTa	42 (37.5)
pT1	20 (17.9)
pT2	26 (23.2)
pT3	18 (16.1)
pT4	6 (5.4)
WHO grade [B]	
low	37 (33.0)
high	75 (67.0)
Operative method	
TUR-B	85 (75.9)
RTX	27 (24.1)
Follow up, months [C]	
Mean	56
Median	53
Range	3–200
Status after follow-up time [C]	
alive	67 (60.9)
dead	43 (39.1)

[A] Age was dichotomized according to median; [B] WHO/ISUP criteria of 2016; [C] 110 cases available. WHO: World Health Organization; ISUP: International Society of Uropathology; TUR-B: transurethral resection of the bladder; RTX: radical cystectomy.

Table 2. Comparison of AGO1, AGO2, and Drosha expression in adjacent normal tissue to NMIBC as well as MIBC in valid cases.

Characteristics	Nonmalignant n (%)	NMIBC n (%)	MIBC n (%)
Argonaute 1	30 (100)	60 (100)	38 (100)
negative	22 (73.3)	23 (38.3)	30 (78.9)
positive	8 (26.7)	37 (61.7)	8 (21.1)
p value [A]		0.003	0.774
Argonaute 2	34 (100)	61 (100)	48 (100)
negative	27 (79.4)	21 (34.4)	15 (31.3)
positive	7 (20.6)	40 (65.6)	33 (68.8)
p value [A]		<0.001	<0.001
Drosha	35 (100)	61 (100)	45 (100)
negative	23 (65.7)	8 (13.1)	23 (51.1)
positive	12 (34.3)	53 (86.9)	22 (48.9)
p value [A]		<0.001	0.255

[A] Fisher's exact test. (N)MIBC: (non-)muscle-invasive bladder cancer.

None of the three targets was associated with the clinicopathological parameters of age and sex (Table 3). However, decreased expression of AGO1 (Chi-square test, $p = 0.001$) and Drosha (Chi-square test, $p < 0.001$) was associated with advanced pathological tumor stage and with MIBC compared to NMIBC (Fisher's exact test, $p < 0.001$) as mentioned above. Drosha levels were also associated with World Health Organization (WHO) grade (Fisher's exact test, $p = 0.045$). In order to assess the consistency between AGO1, AGO2 and Drosha expression, the McNemar test was utilized. We obtained significant differences between AGO1/AGO2 and AGO1/Drosha expression in bladder tumor tissue samples ($p < 0.001$; Table 3).

Table 3. Immunostaining of AGO1, AGO2 and Drosha associated with clinicopathological parameters of bladder cancer patients.

Para-meters n (%)	AGO1 n = 98			AGO2 n = 109			Drosha n = 106		
	neg 53 (54.1)	pos 45 (45.9)	p value	neg 36 (33.0)	pos 73 (67.0)	p value	neg 31 (29.2)	pos 75 (70.8)	p value
Age, years [A]									
<69	23 (23.5)	21 (21.4)	0.839 [B]	17 (15.6)	33 (30.3)	1.000 [B]	15 (14.2)	36 (34.0)	1.000 [B]
≥69	30 (30.6)	24 (24.5)		19 (17.4)	40 (36.7)		16 (15.1)	39 (36.8)	
Sex									
female	14 (14.3)	12 (12.2)	1.000 [B]	10 (9.2)	20 (18.3)	1.000 [B]	8 (7.5)	22 (20.8)	0.815 [B]
male	39 (39.8)	33 (33.7)		26 (23.9)	53 (48.6)		23 (21.7)	53 (50.0)	
pT stage									
pTa	18 (18.4)	23 (23.5)	0.001 [C]	17 (15.6)	24 (22.0)	0.437 [C]	3 (2.8)	38 (35.8)	<0.001 [C]
pT1	5 (5.1)	14 (14.3)		4 (3.7)	16 (14.7)		5 (4.7)	15 (14.2)	
pT2	15 (15.3)	5 (5.1)		9 (8.3)	16 (14.7)		10 (9.4)	13 (12.3)	
pT3	13 (13.3)	1 (1.0)		5 (4.6)	12 (11.0)		12 (11.3)	6 (5.7)	
pT4	2 (2.0)	2 (2.0)		1 (0.9)	5 (4.6)		1 (0.9)	3 (2.8)	
NMIBC	23 (23.5)	37 (37.8)	<0.001 [B]	21 (19.3)	40 (36.7)	0.838 [B]	8 (7.5)	53 (50.0)	<0.001 [B]
MIBC	30 (30.6)	8 (8.2)		15 (13.8)	33 (30.3)		23 (21.7)	22 (20.8)	
WHO grade [D]									
low	15 (15.3)	20 (20.4)	0.138 [B]	14 (12.8)	22 (20.2)	0.392 [B]	6 (5.7)	30 (28.3)	0.045 [B]
high	38 (38.8)	25 (25.5)		22 (20.2)	51 (46.8)		25 (23.6)	45 (42.5)	
AGO1 [E]									
neg	-	-	-	21 (21.9)	31 (32.3)	0.025 [B]	22 (23.7)	27 (29.0)	<0.001 [B]
pos	-	-	-	8 (8.3)	36 (37.5)		5 (5.4)	39 (41.9)	
AGO2 [E]									
neg	21 (21.9)	8 (8.3)	<0.001 [F]	-	-	-	11 (10.7)	23 (22.3)	0.649 [B]
pos	31 (32.3)	36 (37.5)		-	-	-	19 (18.4)	50 (48.5)	
Drosha [E]									
neg	22 (23.7)	5 (5.4)	<0.001 [F]	11 (10.7)	19 (18.4)	0.644 [F]	-	-	-
pos	27 (29.0)	39 (41.9)		23 (22.3)	50 (48.5)		-	-	-

[A] Age was dichotomized according to median; [B] Fisher's exact test ($p < 0.05$); [C] Chi-square test according to Pearson ($p < 0.05$); [D] WHO/ISUP criteria of 2016; [E] number of valid cases: Ago1/Ago2 $n = 96$, Ago1/Drosha $n = 93$, Ago2/Drosha $n = 103$; [F] McNemar test ($p < 0.05$). AGO: Argonaute; neg: negative, pos: positive staining; (N)MIBC: (non-)muscle-invasive bladder cancer; WHO: World Health Organization; ISUP: International Society of Uropathology.

2.3. Association of AGO1, AGO2 and Drosha Expression with Patient Survival

The overall survival times available for 110 cases were used in Kaplan–Meier survival analyses, and different subgroups were compared using Chi-square and the log-rank tests. As expected, higher pT stages and tumor grade were significantly associated with reduced patient survival time ($p < 0.001$). We also obtained significant associations by performing separate Kaplan–Meier analyses according to pTa and ≥pT1 tumors ($p < 0.001$) as well as for NMIBC and MIBC ($p = 0.001$). In order to assess the clinical relevance of AGO1, AGO2 and Drosha as prognostic markers in bladder cancer patients, the Kaplan–Meier analyses of dichotomized immunoreactivity data were conducted. AGO1 and AGO2 expression levels that were divided into negative and positive values did not show any significant differences for the available 96 cases and 107 cases, respectively (Figure 3A,B). However, Drosha had a significant correlation with the overall survival time, with a higher probability of survival associated with positive Drosha expression (73 cases, 20 events; 5-year survival of 73%) compared with negative expression (31 cases, 18 events; 5-year survival of 57%) (Figure 3C). Multivariate Cox regression analysis including the clinicopathological parameters of age, sex, pT stage and tumor grade combined with the three targets of AGO1, AGO2 and Drosha (alone or together) did not reveal any statistical significances, while AGO1 turned out to be independent of all patient parameters (Table S1).

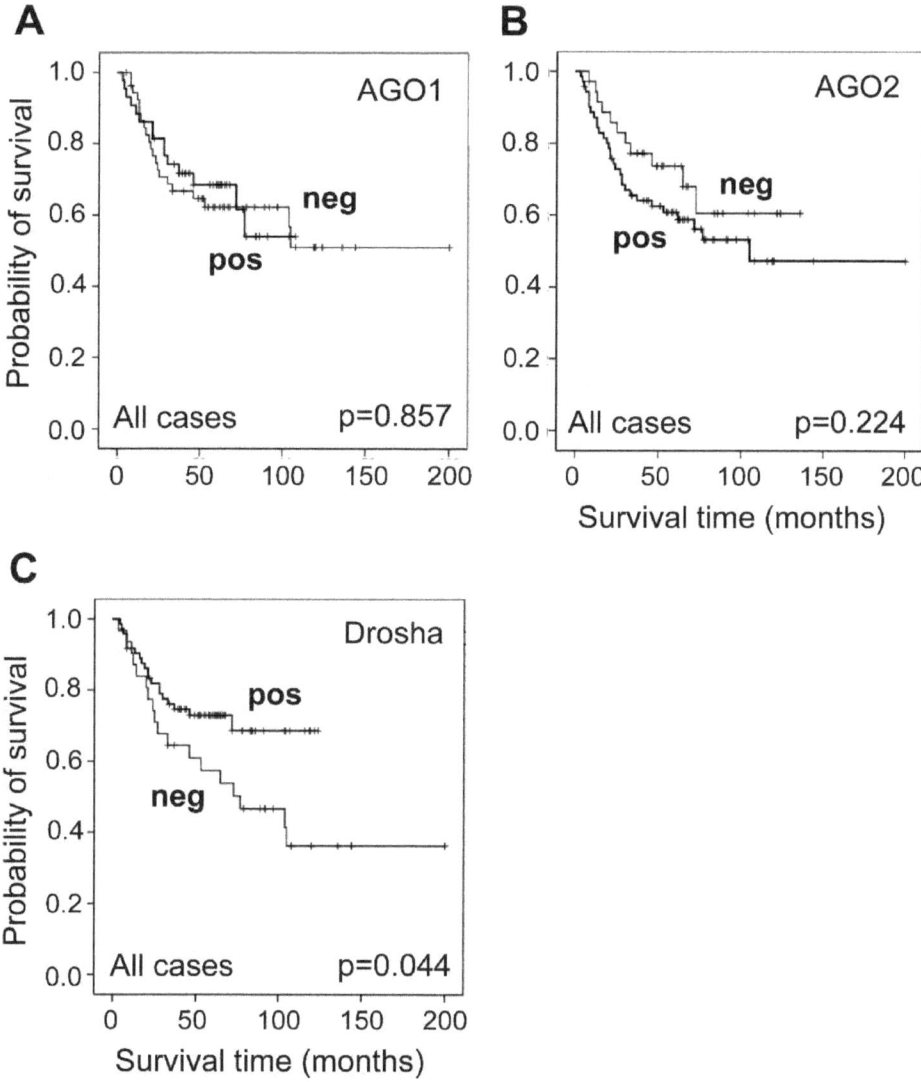

Figure 3. Kaplan–Meier analysis showing overall survival time of bladder cancer patients as a function of AGO1, AGO2 and Drosha levels. Dichotomized expression was not associated with overall survival for 96 cases of AGO1 (**A**) and 107 cases of AGO2 staining (**B**), but Drosha significantly indicated a higher probability of survival with positive expression regarding the 104 available cases (**C**). The overall survival time was defined as the months elapsed between transurethral resection or radical cystectomy and death or the last follow-up date. Censored cases were marked (+). Statistical significance was given as $p < 0.05$. Pos: positive, neg: negative.

3. Discussion

Nuclear cleavage of the primary miRNA by Drosha is an essential function in early miRNA maturation. The proteins of the Argonaute family, AGO1 and AGO2, define the next step in miRNA maturation in the cytoplasm and play a key role in post-transcriptional regulation, such as degrading mRNA or impairing its translation. There is an increasing number of studies examining the implication of miRNA maturation regulators in cancer pathobiology, whereas the contribution of Drosha and Argonautes to the diagnosis and clinicopathological behavior of bladder cancer still needs to be clarified. In this study, we investigated the immunohistochemical expression of Drosha, AGO1 and AGO2 proteins in bladder cancer and their association with clinicopathological parameters and overall survival in order to define the diagnostic and prognostic potentials of these miRNA processors for bladder carcinoma.

Higher expression levels of AGO1 and AGO2 associated with tumor progression have been found in different cancer entities, such as in epithelial skin cancer and ovarian cancer [14,15]. There was an upregulation of AGO2 expression in an estrogen receptor α-negative breast cancer cell line, in prostate cancer as well as in esophageal squamous cell carcinoma tissue, which indicates that AGO2 plays a key role in tumorigenesis [16,17]. Furthermore, in hematological cancers, such as multiple myeloma, high AGO2 levels have been reported as a marker of high-risk disease [18]. With regard to bladder carcinoma, previous studies have described the overexpression of Drosha, AGO1 and AGO2 compared to non-malignant bladder tissue [12,13], which we could attribute to NMIBC. In the case of AGO2, this overexpression was found both in NMIBC and MIBC. The differentiation of NMIBC and MIBC cases has not been considered in the earlier studies [12,13].

The association of AGO1 with AGO2 and Drosha according to our McNemar test hints at similar processes and changes of miRNA machinery in bladder cancer, although AGO2 and Drosha were different. With respect to clinicopathological parameters, we found decreased protein expression of AGO1 and Drosha to be significantly associated with higher tumor stage and with MIBC in comparison to NMIBC, although there were no differences for AGO2. In striking contrast, Yang et al. [12] detected a significant association of increased AGO2 levels with higher histological grade, lymph node metastasis and distant metastasis of bladder carcinoma. However, grade and statistical test were not further defined in this study. Zhang et al. [13] claimed that higher AGO2 and Drosha expression was associated with higher histological grade, pT stage ($\geq$T1) and recurrence of bladder carcinoma, although their table data indicated an association with lower grade. These results were inconsistent and the grade was not further defined but we could confirm an association of higher Drosha levels with the lower WHO grade according to criteria of 2016 if applicable to the study above. The decreased expression of AGO1 and Drosha in MIBC compared with NMIBC could suggest a shift from more active miRNA machinery to decreased activity. For bladder cancer, some increased oncogenic miRNAs and many decreased tumor-suppressive miRNAs have been described [19] and thus, a connection could be possible.

Higher Drosha [13] and AGO2 expressions [12,13] have been reported to correspond to shorter overall survival [12] or to shorter recurrence-free and cancer-specific survival [13] in Kaplan–Meier analysis although we only found Drosha to be significantly correlated with prolonged overall survival. Yang et al. [12] contains very few cases in the Kaplan–Meier curves so that the results, especially those indicating that AGO2 is an independent factor, are questionable. However, the other study [13] presents enough cases for sound results and stresses AGO2 as an independent prognostic factor in a reduced model with grade and pT stage only. We could not confirm the prognostic value of AGO2 in our analyses, which had a median observation time of 53 months in contrast to the 36 months [12] and 35 months [13] of the other studies. In contrast, our calculations just proved that AGO1 was independent of clinicopathological parameters, although AGO1 alone in univariate analysis was not of any prognostic value, which was in contrast with Drosha. The significance in the univariate analysis means that the variable can differentiate the lower and higher probability of survival on its own, but the multivariate Cox regression will provide the quality of the variable compared with other (known) patient parameters. According to the Reporting Recommendations for Tumor Marker Prognostic Studies (REMARK), which have been further explained in 2012 [20], we included all variables available in multivariate analysis. Frequently, significant univariate variables lack independence in the multivariate analysis, such as Drosha in our analysis, but there also are variables which only show their quality in multivariate comparison, such as AGO1 in our study. We could confirm the significance of AGO1 in the inclusion model in a backward Likelihood model with the same parameters as in Table S1 ($p = 0.018$). We believe that the value of AGO1 as a prognostic marker should be further evaluated.

Interestingly, in bladder tissue, we found that Drosha was not only present in nuclei, but also in the cytoplasm, which seems contrary to its functional role in nuclear miRNA maturation regulation. However, there are several reports on other tumor entities in which Drosha was observed in both compartments, such as smooth muscle tumors, melanoma, esophageal and breast cancer [21–24]. The data on localization of Drosha and AGO1 in bladder tissue have been lacking until now because Zhang et al. [13] did not present any in their study. We could confirm mainly the cytoplasmic expression of AGO2 described by Yang et al. [12] but added some details on staining for all three targets, such as the expression in endothelial cells or for AGO2 in lymphocytes, which should be taken into consideration by certain measures, such as Western blot analyses.

As the antibodies used were different from ours (AGO2, [12]), or were not exactly described [13], the difference in the results could have risen from different affinities or specificities, which accentuate the limitations of immunohistochemical studies. Our antibodies were selected according to the literature and were evaluated by an experienced pathologist (E.K.) to avoid artifacts. Another aspect is the difference between our tissue and scoring system (tissue microarray, scoring by intensity) and those of the other groups (full section per case, scoring by intensity and area) [12,13]; both have advantages and disadvantages. For our microarray, we wanted to avoid any bias in an area score for little spots. In histological tissue analysis, the quality of processed formalin-fixed and paraffin-embedded archival material may also influence the staining intensity. In our explorative study, the number of events analyzed was limited because of the limited number of investigated patients for whom comprehensive data were available. This seems to be the main restriction of our work. Further studies are necessary to elucidate the role of Drosha and AGOs in bladder cancer due to the shortcomings of the existing contradictory data.

4. Materials and Methods

4.1. Tissue Sample Selection

A TMA composed of 112 human urothelial carcinomas of the bladder was used for our retrospective study. Appropriate tissue was selected in accordance to availability and follow-up data of the cases. The study was approved by the Ethics Committee of the HELIOS Hospital in Bad Saarow, Germany (HRC-006913, 21, March, 2012), where all bladder cancer patients underwent radical cystectomy (RTX) or transurethral resection (TUR-B) between 1999 and 2010. Written informed consent was given according to the Declaration of Helsinki. In total, 85 TUR-B and 27 RTX were carried out and none of the patients received any chemotherapy or radiation prior to surgery. For each patient, the following clinical and pathological information was recorded: sex, age, tumor staging according to the International Union Against Cancer, histological grading in accordance with the WHO/ISUP criteria of 2016 and overall survival time in the months after surgery. An overview of patient clinicopathological characteristics is given in Table 1.

The surgical specimens of normal adjacent urothelial and urothelial tumor tissue were fixed in 4% buffered formaldehyde and embedded in paraffin. Histological diagnosis was established on standard hematoxylin and eosin-stained sections by a pathologist. Tumor tissue samples were subdivided into 62 NMIBC (pTa = 42 and pT1 = 20) and 50 MIBC tissue samples (pT2 = 26, pT3 = 18 and pT4 = 6) according to the European Association of Urology guidelines, 2011 [25] (Table 1). Additionally, the adjacent normal bladder tissues of 35 bladder tumor cases without any evidence for reactive histology were included. Patients with carcinoma in situ or metastasis were excluded.

4.2. Construction of Tissue Microarray

The areas of bladder carcinoma and adjacent normal tissue were marked on 3-µm hematoxylin/eosin (HE) stained sections of formalin-fixed paraffin-embedded tissue by a pathologist (A.E.) at Charité-Universitätsmedizin Berlin, Germany. Of the corresponding blocks, cores were punched out with a tissue arrayer (1.0 mm diameter; Beecher Instruments, Woodland, CA, USA) according to the previously marked areas, which were subsequently embedded into a new paraffin block as a TMA with maximal 125 cores per block and a tissue of at least 2 mm diameter. Histological conformation was established on HE stained sections (A.E.) according to tumor staging and WHO grading system of 2016.

4.3. Immunohistochemistry

Immunostaining was done as described previously [26]. The optimal concentration of the primary antibody was determined in a dilution series on test sections of larger urothelial cancer and corresponding adjacent normal tissue. Finally, the primary antibody against AGO1 (rabbit monoclonal antibody, cat. no. 5053 [clone D84G10]; Cell Signaling Technology, Inc.; Boston, MA, USA) was used at a dilution of 1:50 and incubated overnight at 4 °C. AGO2 (rabbit polyclonal antibody, cat. no. ab32381; Abcam, Cambridge, UK) was used at a dilution of 1:50 and incubated for 1 h at room temperature, while Drosha (rabbit polyclonal antibody, cat. no. ab12286, Abcam) was used at a dilution of 1:250 and incubated for 1 h at room temperature in a humid chamber. Detection was performed by conventional labeled streptavidin-biotin method with alkaline phosphatase as the reporting enzyme. Fast-Red TR/Naphthol AS-MX (cat. no. F4648; Sigma-Aldrich, Munich, Germany) was used as the chromogen. Finally, the TMA was counterstained with hematoxylin and fixed in an aqueous embedding medium. Antibody diluent solution without the application of respective primary antibodies was used as the negative control. Antibodies were checked by Western blotting using the human urinary bladder carcinoma cell lines RT-4 and RT-112 (Figure S1). Immunostainings were evaluated by a pathologist (E.K.) of Charité–Universitätsmedizin Berlin, who was blinded to the clinicopathological data. Immunohistochemical expression of AGO1, AGO2 and Drosha was classified in a binary manner from 0 to 1 according to the following assessment: 0 being no immunoreactivity; and 1 being positive immunoreactivity with staining intensities including cytoplasmic and nuclear staining. The number of assessable cases differed slightly between the three targets, because a few tissue spots disappeared during the staining procedure.

4.4. Statistics

Statistical analyses were carried out with SPSS 21.0 (IBM Corp., Somers, NY, USA). Fisher's exact test, Chi-square test according to Pearson and McNemar test were applied to determine the relationship between AGO1, AGO2 or Drosha immunostaining and clinicopathological characteristics. Univariate analyses for the overall survival time as a function of AGO1, AGO2 or Drosha expression were executed as Kaplan-Meier analyses using the log-rank test. The overall survival time as the primary clinical endpoint was defined as the months elapsed between TUR-B or RTX and either death or the last follow-up date. Multivariate analyses were calculated according to Cox regression. Two-sided p-values < 0.05 were considered to be statistically significant in all cases.

5. Conclusions

In our study, the altered expressions of AGO1, AGO2, and Drosha were investigated immunohistochemically in bladder cancer to evaluate their diagnostic and prognostic potential in non-invasive and invasive bladder carcinoma. The upregulation of the targets and differentiation of NMIBC and MIBC cases could improve diagnostics; additionally, AGO1 seems to hold prognostic potential for bladder cancer. However, our results stress the need for further research to bridge the gap of prognostic markers in urothelial carcinomas of the bladder. Based on our results, we suggest that Drosha and AGOs are important factors in the tumor biology of bladder cancer.

Supplementary Materials: Supplementary materials can be found at http://www.mdpi.com/1422-0067/19/6/1622/s1.

Author Contributions: N.R., K.J. and T.H.E. contributed to conception and design of the study. Acquisition of data was done by A.R., N.R., A.E., T.H.E and E.K., A.R., N.R. and K.J. analyzed and interpreted data. A.R., N.R. and A.H. wrote the manuscript. A.R. and K.J. revised the manuscript. All authors read and approved the final manuscript.

Acknowledgments: A.R., N.R. and K.J. were supported by the Foundation for Urologic Research. We acknowledge support from the German Research Foundation (DFG) and the Open Access Publication Fund of Charité-Universitätsmedizin Berlin. The authors thank Siegrun Blauhut and Bettina Ergün for excellent technical assistance.

Conflicts of Interest: The authors declare no conflict of interest.

References

1. Antoni, S.; Ferlay, J.; Soerjomataram, I.; Znaor, A.; Jemal, A.; Bray, F. Bladder Cancer Incidence and Mortality: A Global Overview and Recent Trends. *Eur. Urol.* **2017**, *71*, 96–108. [CrossRef] [PubMed]
2. Zhao, M.; He, X.L.; Teng, X.D. Understanding the molecular pathogenesis and prognostics of bladder cancer: An overview. *Chin. J. Cancer Res.* **2016**, *28*, 92–98. [PubMed]
3. Mohammed, A.A.; El-Tanni, H.; El-Khatib, H.M.; Mirza, A.A.; Mirza, A.A.; Alturaifi, T.H. Urinary Bladder Cancer: Biomarkers and Target Therapy, New Era for More Attention. *Oncol. Rev.* **2016**, *10*. [CrossRef] [PubMed]
4. Bartel, D.P. MicroRNAs: Genomics, biogenesis, mechanism, and function. *Cell* **2004**, *116*, 281–297. [CrossRef]
5. Calin, G.A.; Croce, C.M. MicroRNA signatures in human cancers. *Nat. Rev. Cancer* **2006**, *6*, 857–866. [CrossRef] [PubMed]
6. Dong, F.; Xu, T.; Shen, Y.; Zhong, S.; Chen, S.; Ding, Q.; Shen, Z. Dysregulation of miRNAs in bladder cancer: Altered expression with aberrant biogenesis procedure. *Oncotarget* **2017**, *8*, 27547–27568. [CrossRef] [PubMed]
7. Mitash, N.; Tiwari, S.; Agnihotri, S.; Mandhani, A. Bladder cancer: Micro RNAs as biomolecules for prognostication and surveillance. *Indian J. Urol.* **2017**, *33*, 127–133. [PubMed]
8. Hata, A.; Kashima, R. Dysregulation of microRNA biogenesis machinery in cancer. *Crit. Rev. Biochem. Mol. Biol.* **2016**, *51*, 121–134. [CrossRef] [PubMed]
9. Cheloufi, S.; Dos Santos, C.O.; Chong, M.M.; Hannon, G.J. A dicer-independent miRNA biogenesis pathway that requires Ago catalysis. *Nature* **2010**, *465*, 584–589. [CrossRef] [PubMed]
10. Li, W.; Liu, M.; Feng, Y.; Xu, Y.F.; Che, J.P.; Wang, G.C.; Zheng, J.H.; Gao, H.J. Evaluation of Argonaute protein as a predictive marker for human clear cell renal cell carcinoma. *Int. J. Clin. Exp. Pathol.* **2013**, *6*, 1086–1094. [PubMed]
11. Bian, X.J.; Zhang, G.M.; Gu, C.Y.; Cai, Y.; Wang, C.F.; Shen, Y.J.; Zhu, Y.; Zhang, H.L.; Dai, B.; Ye, D.W. Down-regulation of Dicer and Ago2 is associated with cell proliferation and apoptosis in prostate cancer. *Tumor Biol.* **2014**, *35*, 11571–11578. [CrossRef] [PubMed]
12. Yang, F.Q.; Huang, J.H.; Liu, M.; Yang, F.P.; Li, W.; Wang, G.C.; Che, J.P.; Zheng, J.H. Argonaute 2 is up-regulated in tissues of urothelial carcinoma of bladder. *Int. J. Clin. Exp. Pathol.* **2014**, *7*, 340–347. [PubMed]
13. Zhang, Z.; Zhang, G.; Kong, C.; Bi, J.; Gong, D.; Yu, X.; Shi, D.; Zhan, B.; Ye, P. EIF2C, Dicer, and Drosha are up-regulated along tumor progression and associated with poor prognosis in bladder carcinoma. *Tumor Biol.* **2015**, *36*, 5071–5079. [CrossRef] [PubMed]
14. Sand, M.; Skrygan, M.; Georgas, D.; Arenz, C.; Gambichler, T.; Sand, D.; Altmeyer, P.; Bechara, F.G. Expression levels of the microRNA maturing microprocessor complex component DGCR8 and the RNA-induced silencing complex (RISC) components argonaute-1, argonaute-2, PACT, TARBP1, and TARBP2 in epithelial skin cancer. *Mol. Carcinog.* **2012**, *51*, 916–922. [CrossRef] [PubMed]

15. Vaksman, O.; Hetland, T.E.; Trope, C.G.; Reich, R.; Davidson, B. Argonaute, Dicer, and Drosha are up-regulated along tumor progression in serous ovarian carcinoma. *Hum. Pathol.* **2012**, *43*, 2062–2069. [CrossRef] [PubMed]
16. Adams, B.D.; Claffey, K.P.; White, B.A. Argonaute-2 expression is regulated by epidermal growth factor receptor and mitogen-activated protein kinase signaling and correlates with a transformed phenotype in breast cancer cells. *Endocrinology* **2009**, *150*, 14–23. [CrossRef] [PubMed]
17. Yoo, N.J.; Hur, S.Y.; Kim, M.S.; Lee, J.Y.; Lee, S.H. Immunohistochemical analysis of RNA-induced silencing complex-related proteins AGO2 and TNRC6A in prostate and esophageal cancers. *APMIS* **2010**, *118*, 271–276. [CrossRef] [PubMed]
18. Zhou, Y.; Chen, L.; Barlogie, B.; Stephens, O.; Wu, X.; Williams, D.R.; Cartron, M.A.; van, R.F.; Nair, B.; Waheed, S.; et al. High-risk myeloma is associated with global elevation of miRNAs and overexpression of EIF2C2/AGO2. *Proc. Natl. Acad. Sci. USA* **2010**, *107*, 7904–7909. [CrossRef] [PubMed]
19. Pop-Bica, C.; Gulei, D.; Cojocneanu-Petric, R.; Braicu, C.; Petrut, B.; Berindan-Neagoe, I. Understanding the Role of Non-Coding RNAs in Bladder Cancer: From Dark Matter to Valuable Therapeutic Targets. *Int. J. Mol. Sci.* **2017**, *18*, 1514. [CrossRef] [PubMed]
20. Altman, D.G.; McShane, L.M.; Sauerbrei, W.; Taube, S.E. Reporting Recommendations for Tumor Marker Prognostic Studies (REMARK): Explanation and elaboration. *PLoS. Med.* **2012**, *9*, e1001216. [CrossRef] [PubMed]
21. Jafarnejad, S.M.; Sjoestroem, C.; Martinka, M.; Li, G. Expression of the RNase III enzyme DROSHA is reduced during progression of human cutaneous melanoma. *Mod. Pathol.* **2013**, *26*, 902–910. [CrossRef] [PubMed]
22. Papachristou, D.J.; Sklirou, E.; Corradi, D.; Grassani, C.; Kontogeorgakos, V.; Rao, U.N. Immunohistochemical analysis of the endoribonucleases Drosha, Dicer and Ago2 in smooth muscle tumours of soft tissues. *Histopathology* **2012**, *60*, E28–E36. [CrossRef] [PubMed]
23. Passon, N.; Gerometta, A.; Puppin, C.; Lavarone, E.; Puglisi, F.; Tell, G.; Di, L.C.; Damante, G. Expression of Dicer and Drosha in triple-negative breast cancer. *J. Clin. Pathol.* **2012**, *65*, 320–326. [CrossRef] [PubMed]
24. Sugito, N.; Ishiguro, H.; Kuwabara, Y.; Kimura, M.; Mitsui, A.; Kurehara, H.; Ando, T.; Mori, R.; Takashima, N.; Ogawa, R.; et al. RNASEN regulates cell proliferation and affects survival in esophageal cancer patients. *Clin. Cancer Res.* **2006**, *12*, 7322–7328. [CrossRef] [PubMed]
25. Babjuk, M.; Oosterlinck, W.; Sylvester, R.; Kaasinen, E.; Bohle, A.; Palou-Redorta, J.; Roupret, M. EAU guidelines on non-muscle-invasive urothelial carcinoma of the bladder, the 2011 update. *Eur. Urol.* **2011**, *59*, 997–1008. [CrossRef] [PubMed]
26. Xu, C.; Jung, M.; Burkhardt, M.; Stephan, C.; Schnorr, D.; Loening, S.; Jung, K.; Dietel, M.; Kristiansen, G. Increased CD59 protein expression predicts a PSA relapse in patients after radical prostatectomy. *Prostate* **2005**, *62*, 224–232. [CrossRef] [PubMed]

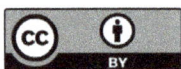

© 2018 by the authors. Licensee MDPI, Basel, Switzerland. This article is an open access article distributed under the terms and conditions of the Creative Commons Attribution (CC BY) license (http://creativecommons.org/licenses/by/4.0/).

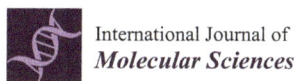

Article

Evaluation of a New Survivin ELISA and UBC® *Rapid* for the Detection of Bladder Cancer in Urine

Jan Gleichenhagen [1,*], Christian Arndt [2], Swaantje Casjens [1], Carmen Meinig [1], Holger Gerullis [3], Irina Raiko [1], Thomas Brüning [1], Thorsten Ecke [4] and Georg Johnen [1]

[1] Institute for Prevention and Occupational Medicine of the German Social Accident Insurance, Institute of the Ruhr-University Bochum (IPA), 44789 Bochum, Germany; casjens@ipa-dguv.de (S.C.); meinig@ipa-dguv.de (C.M.); raiko@ipa-dguv.de (I.R.); bruening@ipa-dguv.de (T.B.); johnen@ipa-dguv.de (G.J.)
[2] Department of Urology, Lukaskrankenhaus Neuss, 41464 Neuss, Germany; CArndt@lukasneuss.de
[3] University Hospital for Urology, Klinikum Oldenburg, 26133 Oldenburg, Germany; holger.gerullis@gmx.net
[4] Department of Urology, HELIOS Hospital, 15526 Bad Saarow, Germany; thorsten.ecke@helios-gesundheit.de
* Correspondence: Gleichenhagen@ipa-dguv.de; Tel.: +49-234-302-4747

Received: 9 November 2017; Accepted: 8 January 2018; Published: 11 January 2018

Abstract: Urine-based biomarkers for non-invasive diagnosis of bladder cancer are urgently needed. No single marker with sufficient sensitivity and specificity has been described so far. Thus, a combination of markers appears to be a promising approach. The aim of this case-control study was to evaluate the performance of an in-house developed enzyme-linked immunosorbent assay (ELISA) for survivin, the UBC® *Rapid* test, and the combination of both assays. A total of 290 patients were recruited. Due to prior bladder cancer, 46 patients were excluded. Urine samples were available from 111 patients with bladder cancer and 133 clinical controls without urologic diseases. Antibodies generated from recombinant survivin were utilized to develop a sandwich ELISA. The ELISA and the UBC® *Rapid* test were applied to all urine samples. Receiver operating characteristic (ROC) analysis was used to evaluate marker performance. The survivin ELISA exhibited a sensitivity of 35% with a specificity of 98%. The UBC® *Rapid* test showed a sensitivity of 56% and a specificity of 96%. Combination of both assays increased the sensitivity to 66% with a specificity of 95%. For high-grade tumors, the combination showed a sensitivity of 82% and a specificity of 95%. The new survivin ELISA and the UBC® *Rapid* test are both able to detect bladder cancer, especially high-grade tumors. However, the performance of each individual marker is moderate and efforts to improve the survivin assay should be pursued. A combination of both assays confirmed the benefit of using marker panels. The results need further testing in a prospective study and with a high-risk population.

Keywords: survivin; UBC® *Rapid*; bladder cancer; urine; biomarker combination; non-invasive

1. Introduction

Bladder cancer is the most common cancer of the urinary tract and ranks fifth among cancers in men in western countries [1]. It is typically diagnosed by cystoscopy followed by pathological examination of suspicious tissue. Cystoscopy is a time-consuming method that requires an experienced urologist to perform and can be painful for the patients. Thus, there is a need for an easier and non-invasive diagnostic method. Being minimally- or non-invasive is a key characteristic of biomarkers, facilitating the use of easily accessible body fluids instead of tissue, which requires invasive sampling. Because of its close proximity to the target organ, it is of general acceptance that urine might be a good source for bladder cancer-specific biomarkers [2].

Based on urine or urinary cells, only a few molecular markers have been approved by the federal Food and Drug Administration (FDA) so far. In addition, these markers are designated merely as supporting tools for monitoring bladder cancer patients instead of replacing cystoscopy [3,4]. The nuclear mitotic apparatus protein 1 (NUMA1) can be quantitated by the commercial NMP22® test or detected by the BladderChek® test [5]. The reported sensitivities of the NMP22 assays in case-control studies vary between 47% and 100%, while the specificities range from 58% to 91% [6,7]. In contrast to the results from case-control studies, in a prospective study (UroScreen), the assay reached a sensitivity of 97% and a specificity of 29% in prediagnostic samples [7]. The performance of NMP22 was limited by a relative high number of false-positive test results, which can be caused, for example, by hematuria or infections [5,7]. Using fluorescence in situ hybridization (FISH), the UroVysion test is applied to detect chromosomal copy number variations in exfoliated urothelial cells sedimented from urine samples. In a pooled analysis of FISH-based assays, the average sensitivity was 76% (65–84%) and the specificity 85% (78–92%) [8], another pooled analysis yielded 72% and 83%, respectively [9]. In the prospective study UroScreen, the UroVysion test reached a sensitivity of 45% at a specificity of 97% [10]. While UroVysion is relatively specific, it only showed a moderately increased sensitivity compared to the much cheaper classical cytology. It is also restricted by the requirement of special equipment and a time-consuming, expert-dependent procedure [11,12].

The limited performance of individual markers can be improved by combining two or more markers in a panel. For example, in the prospective study UroScreen, a combination of UroVysion and NMP22 reached a sensitivity of 67% and a specificity of 95% [11]. However, there is still a lack of easy to apply and cost-effective assays with adequate performance that would qualify as candidates for a biomarker panel.

In order to evaluate additional assays of urinary biomarkers, we focused on two candidates, UBC® *Rapid* and survivin, and tested their ability to detect bladder cancer. UBC® *Rapid* is a commercially available point-of-care test measuring cytokeratin fragments 8 and 18 in urine. Affordability and ease of use are factors that would support its implementation in routine diagnostics. Survivin is a well-known protein biomarker and detectable in almost every cancer [13,14], including bladder cancer [15,16]. Detailed information about biological function is discussed in several reviews [13,17] as well as its potential as a therapeutic target [18–20]. Most studies analyzing the expression of survivin used invasively obtained tissue samples or rely on the detection of survivin mRNA in sedimented cells from urine [21–23]. Because of our previous experience with the practical problems associated with the limited stability of mRNA, we decided to focus on the more stable survivin protein. A well-established method for the measurement of proteins in laboratory diagnostics is the enzyme-linked immunosorbent assay (ELISA). ELISAs for the detection of survivin are commercially available, but often lack sufficient performance, particularly when using urine as a sample matrix [24].

The aim of this study was to develop a new ELISA for the quantification of survivin in urine samples and to evaluate the performance of the ELISA in combination with UBC® *Rapid* for urine-based detection of bladder cancer, especially high-grade tumors.

2. Results

2.1. Survivin Production and ELISA Development

Cloning, expression, and affinity purification yielded about 2.5 mg of His_{10}-survivin fusion protein suitable for antibody generation in rabbits (Figure 1a).

Antibodies were purified and partially biotinylated for application in a sandwich ELISA. No cross-reactivity was observed for anti-survivin antibodies. The best signal-to-noise ratio was obtained with a dilution of 1:5000 for the capture antibody and a dilution of 1:10,000 for the detection antibody. The resulting sigmoidal curve could be interpolated within the range of 0.025–5 ng/mL, with a limit of detection (LoD) of about 0.033 ng/mL for the new survivin ELISA (Figure 1b). We compared our ELISA with the commercially available survivin ELISA kits of R&D and Enzo

Life Sciences by performing four-parameter logistic curve-fits for the reference curves. The standard curve of our ELISA was comparable to those of the commercial ELISA kits (Figure S1).

Reproducibility of the new survivin ELISA was investigated by measuring three defined samples of low, medium, and high survivin concentrations multiple times ($n = 24$). The resulting coefficients of variation (CVs) were 7.2% for the low, 4.6% for the medium, and 6.5% for the high concentration sample. In addition, we tested the repeatability with two different samples of medium survivin concentration at different time points. The resulting CVs were 8.8% and 19.4%. Additionally, matrix effects were investigated by spike-in experiments. Defined recombinant survivin concentrations were spiked into survivin-free urine samples. The recovery rate ranged from 74.8 to 88.9%.

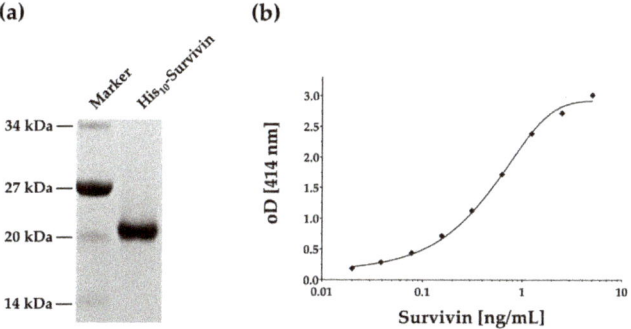

Figure 1. SDS-PAGE and ELISA reference curve. (**a**) Coomassie-blue stained SDS-PAGE of recombinant purified His_{10}-survivin; (**b**) representative four-parameter logistic curve fit for the survivin ELISA.

2.2. Study Group

Table 1 depicts the characteristics of the 244 participants, divided into tumor cases ($n = 111$), and clinical controls ($n = 133$). Most of the participants were men ($n = 175$). The median age of the tumor group and clinical controls was similar (74 vs. 71 years).

Table 1. Characteristics of the study population and patients.

Characteristics	All ($n = 244$)			Tumor ($n = 111$)			Clinical Controls ($n = 133$)		
Gender	Male		Female	Male		Female	Male		Female
n	175		69	83		28	92		41
	n	Median	IQR	n	Median	IQR	n	Median	IQR
Age (years)	244	73	63–80	111	74	65–80	133	71	60–79
Body mass index	244	26.5	24.0–29.8	111	26.9	24.3–30.4	133	26.3	23.6–29.6
Urine volume (mL)	244	30	16–40	111	20	14–40	133	35	20–50
Urine retention within bladder (h)	236	2.0	1.0–3.0	106	1.75	1.0–2.5	130	2.0	1.0–3.5
Specific gravity (g/L)	240	240	1015	109	1015	1015–1020	131	1020	1015–1020
pH	240	5	5.0–6.5	109	5	5–6.5	131	5	5–6.5
Survivin (ng/mL)				111	0.014 *	0–0.528	133	0	0–0.249
UBC® *Rapid* (mg/L)				111	16.3	5–300	133	5	5–28.2

IQR = interquartile range; * extrapolated value.

Among all groups, median volume of urine was 30 mL with a retention time of about 2 h within the bladder before voiding. The median pH of urinary samples was 5.0 in all groups. Additional details regarding the tumor group are listed in Table 2.

Table 2. Characteristics of the tumor group.

Characteristic	Status	(n)
Tumor Stage	Ta	61
	T1	14
	T2	23
	T3	9
	Carcinoma in situ	3
	Missing	1
Histological grade	Low	55
	High	55
	Missing	1
Recurrent	Yes	52
	No	58
	Missing	1
Gross hematuria	Yes	66
	No	45
Dysuria	Yes	33
	No	78
Frequent urination	Yes	51
	No	60
Bladder Stones	Yes	12
	No	99
Diabetes mellitus type II	Yes	12
	No	99
Smoking	Never	23
	Former	51
	Actual	35
	Missing	2

2.3. Survivin in Urine of Bladder Cancer Patients

Initially, we tested voided urine, supernatant, and urinary pellet for measurable amounts of survivin. Only urinary pellet exhibited detectable amounts of survivin. Therefore, all herein presented survivin-related data refer to the urinary pellet.

The distributions of survivin concentrations in tumor and control groups are shown in Figure 2a.

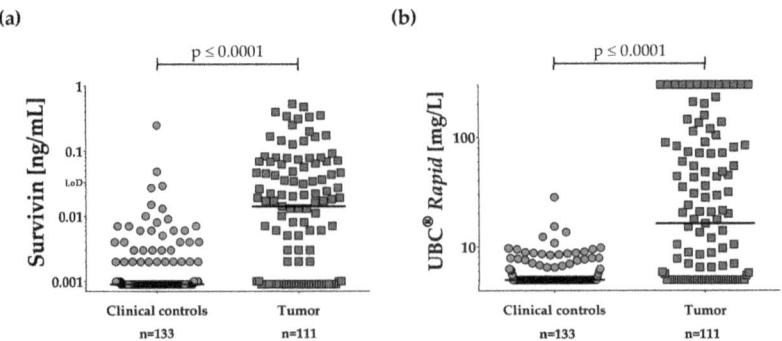

Figure 2. Dot plots of marker results in urine. Comparison of marker concentrations in urinary samples from clinical controls and bladder tumor patients. (**a**) Survivin and (**b**) UBC® Rapid. Lines depict the median for each group. *p*-Values were obtained from the Wilcoxon signed-rank test.

The median survivin concentration was below the LoD (<0.033 ng/mL) in both groups. Normalization by creatinine or amount of total protein was therefore not attempted. However, the median survivin concentration differed between tumor group and clinical controls ($p < 0.0001$). Survivin levels were not influenced by obtained volume of urine, retention time within the bladder, or gender. Using a cut-off of 0.033 ng/mL, our survivin ELISA showed a sensitivity of 35% (39/111 tumors true-positive) and a specificity of 98%, when comparing tumor group and clinical controls. Tumor grade had an influence on the marker performance. The survivin ELISA detected 51% (28/55) of the high-grade tumors but only 18% (10/55) of the low-grade tumors (Table 3, Figure S2a). Grading data was missing for one case. The area under the curve (AUC) was 0.77 for the ROC curve analysis of tumor versus clinical controls (Figure 3).

Table 3. Performance of survivin, UBC® *Rapid*, and combination based on single-marker cut-off for the detection of bladder cancer.

Groups	Cut-Off	Sensitivity (%)	Specificity (%)	True-Positive (n)	True-Negative (n)	False-Positive (n)	False-Negative (n)
			Survivin ELISA				
Tumor vs. Controls		35	98	39	131	2	72
High-grade tumor vs. Controls	0.033 ng/mL	51	98	28	131	2	27
Low-grade tumor vs. Controls		18	98	10	131	2	45
			UBC® *Rapid*				
Tumor vs. Controls		56	96	62	128	5	49
High-grade tumor vs. Controls	10.0 mg/L	73	96	40	128	5	15
Low-grade tumor vs. Controls		40	96	22	128	5	33
			Combination				
Tumor vs. Controls		66	95	73	127	6	38
High-grade tumor vs. Controls	>Survivin or >UBC® *Rapid*	82	95	45	127	6	10
Low-grade tumor vs. Controls		49	95	27	127	6	28

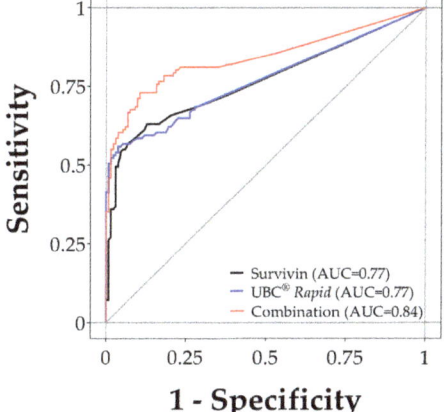

Figure 3. ROC analyses of survivin and UBC® *Rapid*. ROC curves for survivin (AUC = 0.77), UBC® *Rapid* (AUC = 0.77), and the combination of both assays (AUC = 0.84) based on comparing tumor and clinical control group.

2.4. Performance of UBC® Rapid

The distribution of the UBC® *Rapid* results for the clinical controls and the tumor group are depicted as dot plots in Figure 2b. The median UBC® *Rapid* value was <5.0 mg/L for clinical controls and 16.3 mg/L for the tumor group. The difference between the tumor group and the control group was statistically significant ($p < 0.0001$). Using the cut-off (10 mg/L) recommended by the supplier, the UBC® *Rapid* assay reached a sensitivity of 56% (62/111) at a specificity of 96%. As seen with survivin, the sensitivity of the assay increased (to 73%) in high-grade tumors in comparison to controls (Table 3, Figure S2b). ROC curves and AUC values for the UBC® Rapid test were similar to those of the survivin assay and are shown in Figure 3.

2.5. Combination of Survivin and UBC® Rapid

Because of the generally limited performance of individual biomarker assays, we also looked at the possible benefits of a combination of biomarkers. To our knowledge, this is the first approach exploring survivin and UBC® Rapid as a panel. The results of the combination of the survivin ELISA and the UBC® Rapid test are shown in Table 3 and depicted in Figure 3. A scatter plot of the values of the tumor samples indicates a moderate correlation between both assays (Spearman's r_s = 0.38; Figure S3). Further analysis by Venn-diagrams (Figure 4) revealed that, in addition to 28 tumors detected by both assays, 45 tumors were solely detected by either UBC® Rapid (34 tumors) or survivin (11 tumors). From the ROC analysis, an AUC of 0.84, a sensitivity of 66% and a specificity of 95% could be derived for the combination. The difference between each single marker AUC and AUC of the combination is statistically significant (combination vs. survivin: p = 0.0025; combination vs. UBC® Rapid: p = 0.0005). Comparing high-grade tumors with controls revealed an AUC of 0.91, a sensitivity of 82%, and a specificity of 95% (Table 3, Figures S4 and S5). Here, the difference between single marker AUC and combination AUC was not significant (combination vs. survivin: p = 0.1826; combination vs. UBC® Rapid: p = 0.0685).

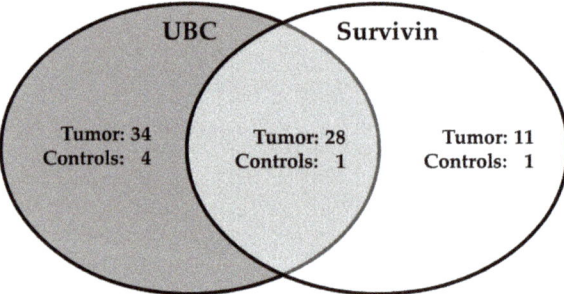

Figure 4. Venn diagrams of all positive test results. The cut-off for UBC® Rapid was >10 mg/L (**left**) and for survivin >0.033 ng/mL (**right**).

2.6. Possible Influence of Microhematuria

Microhematuria could be a possible influencing factor of biomarker performance. We therefore investigated the effect of microhematuria in the control group. Of the 133 controls, 28 had erythrocytes (between 5 and 250 cells [25]) in their urine. Median marker concentrations in controls with and without microhematuria did not show significant differences for both markers (p = 0.4511 for survivin and p = 0.4121 for UBC® Rapid).

3. Discussion

Bladder cancer is one of the most common cancers worldwide [26]. The current gold standard for bladder cancer detection is cystoscopy and cytology. Those methods are routinely applied in patients with hematuria or other symptoms suggestive of bladder cancer [8]. Clinical symptoms are more likely to occur at later stages of tumor development. Biomarkers have the potential to detect cancer at earlier stages, facilitating an earlier and therefore more curative therapy that ideally results in decreased mortality or chance of recurrence, while potentially reducing the number of invasive diagnostic procedures [27]. Urine is apparently an ideal source for non-invasive biomarkers for detection or monitoring urothelial bladder cancer [2]. Screening for bladder cancer is medically reasonable for high-risk groups, e.g., persons with a high recurrence rate or a previous exposure to bladder cancer carcinogens [4,11,15,28]. For instance, in Germany, workers with a previous occupational exposure to aromatic amines are offered free medical exams to screen for bladder cancer [11].

Examples for urine-based biomarkers that have been suggested for screening are UroVysion, uCyt+, or NMP22. However, the markers had some drawbacks, including observer bias, time-consuming procedures, confounders, and/or large variations in reported performance [5,11,29,30]. Survivin is another possible target for biomarker development that has been well published [21]. Unfortunately, most studies relied on immunohistochemistry of tissue samples or mRNA-based approaches [21–23,30]. ELISA-based techniques are an easy-to-use assay format frequently used in routine applications for protein quantification, but less commonly applied to urinary samples [24]. To overcome the limitations associated with survivin mRNA [22], we investigated a newly developed ELISA to detect survivin at the protein level. The ELISA featured a LoD (0.033 ng/mL) and detection range comparable to commercially available ELISAs. We performed a four-parameter curve fit for the calibration curve because this procedure is commonly recommended and appears to be more reliable for values close to the LoD [31].

We could not observe detectable amounts of survivin in urinary supernatant or unprocessed voided urine using the new ELISA. We did not attempt to detect survivin in concentrated urine [32]. Instead, we based our survivin determination on measurements in sedimented cells from urine to avoid matrix effects that might influence the assay. Urine is a dynamic and heterogenic fluid comprising varying salt concentrations and pH values [33–36]. Those parameters are important factors for antibody–antigen interaction [37]. A secretion of survivin from tumor cells via exosomes has been reported recently [38]. An enrichment of exosomes from urine for the subsequent determination of survivin is an interesting approach that should be attempted in the future but may require a more sensitive assay. Currently, we are investigating an improved version of our assay based on a solid-phase proximity ligation assay. This technique replaces the enzymatic reaction of an ELISA with quantitative PCR by transferring the original protein signal to an amplifiable DNA signal [39,40].

The presented case-control study revealed a sensitivity of 35%, a specificity of 98%, and an AUC of 0.77 for our survivin ELISA. The results are in good agreement with the reported sensitivity and specificity by Ohsawa et al. [41]. In comparison, Li et al., Eissa et al., and Srivastava et al. reported a somewhat higher performance with AUC values of 0.85, 0.87, and 0.88, respectively [32,42,43]. The composition of the study populations—e.g., variations in grade and stage of the tumors and variations in the control group—might have contributed to these differences. As seen before with immunohistochemistry and mRNA-based assays, the survivin ELISA was more sensitive for high-grade tumors [22,23,30]. This is also plausible in view of the mechanistic role of survivin, which is involved in suppression of apoptosis as well as regulation of mitosis [13,16,17,44,45].

Parallel to survivin, we examined the commercial point-of-care test UBC® *Rapid*. Compared to other commercially available tests like UroVysion or uCyt+, it is affordable, simple to use and not observer-biased. In our study group, the UBC® *Rapid* test reached an AUC of 0.77 and a sensitivity of 56% at a specificity of 96%, using the recommended cut-off of 10 mg/L. This is in accordance with other reports showing sensitivities in the range of 53–64% and specificities in the range of 63–91% [46–51]. Similar to survivin, UBC® *Rapid* also has a higher sensitivity for high-grade tumors [46,50–52] in comparison to low-grade tumors, indicating that the UBC® *Rapid* test may be more useful for this subgroup. The test may be influenced by urinary tract infections as has been shown before [53].

Screening, even in high-risk populations, requires a high specificity in order to avoid unnecessary invasive diagnostic procedures and psychological burden for the patients, which can be a consequence of false-positive test results [52,54]. As has been reported before, no single marker has reproducibly shown a sufficiently high sensitivity in conjunction with the required high specificity to detect bladder cancer early [2,11]. This was also true for the two biomarkers we investigated in the present study. Both survivin and UBC® *Rapid* had relatively good specificities but moderate sensitivities at the given cut-offs. However, lower sensitivities can be compensated by the use of several biomarkers in a panel. Indeed, the combination of both markers increased the sensitivity to 66% at a specificity of 95%. For the subgroup of high-grade tumors, the sensitivity even increased to 82%. Due to the fact that high-grade tumors have a higher rate of progression and/or recurrence, it is helpful to focus on markers exhibiting a higher sensitivity for this particular subgroup.

A limitation of the markers that has been reported before is the reduced performance associated with other urologic diseases, confounders that would also be expected in a typical clinical setting [45,50,55,56]. Microhematuria apparently does not affect the survivin ELISA or UBC® *Rapid*. Another possible confounder for biomarker assays can be a urinary infection. A typical example is the protein marker NMP22 [5,7]. Because expression of survivin has been reported in some cases of inflammation [56] and links between inflammation pathways and cancer development are generally known [56,57], bladder infections could also influence urinary survivin concentrations. Therefore, a combination with other markers like UroVysion, which are less affected by confounders, and different algorithms to combine the markers may be interesting options. In addition, the aforementioned efforts to refine the survivin assay could lead to a higher sensitivity. An advantage of the survivin ELISA and UBC® *Rapid* is their affordability and ease of use, factors that are important for a future application in screening or surveillance programs. The case-control design and the selection of the control group are limitations of our study, which was intended as an initial assessment of a new assay. Thus, before an application in screening is possible, the markers have to be validated in a prospective study with an independent and larger study population. The establishment of a suitable cohort is currently under way, but the process requires time and some effort.

4. Materials and Methods

4.1. Study Population

Between January 2014 and July 2015, a total of 290 patients were recruited at the Lukaskrankenhaus (Neuss, Germany). Because of a prior bladder cancer diagnosis, 46 patients were excluded. The remaining 244 participants included 111 patients suffering from bladder cancer and 133 control patients visiting for other reasons than bladder cancer or urologic disease. The initial diagnosis of bladder cancer was based on cystoscopy and confirmed by histological and immunohistochemical examination of resected tissue. Tumors have been assigned as low- or high-grade tumors according to the 2004 WHO classification [58]. Urine was collected before transurethral resection. Tumor patients and controls were matched for age and gender. The study was approved by the ethics committee of the Landesärztekammer Brandenburg No. AS 147(bB)/2013 (17 November 2013).

4.2. Urine Sample Collection

Midstream urine samples were collected at the Urology department of the Lukaskrankenhaus Neuss, Germany. Urinary samples were processed immediately or stored at +4 °C for a maximum of 4 h. Urine status was assayed by routine dipstick analysis. For the UBC® *Rapid* assay, three drops of fresh urine were used prior to further processing of a urine sample. After taking a 2-mL aliquot, remaining urine was centrifuged at $1500 \times g$ for 10 min at +10 °C in a swinging bucket rotor. Resulting supernatant was aliquoted (4×2 mL) and the pellet was resuspended in 1 mL of PBS. All samples were stored at -20 °C until further analyses were carried out. For further analysis, the samples were shipped on dry ice to the IPA in Bochum.

4.3. UBC® Rapid Test

The UBC® *Rapid* test (Concile GmbH, Freiburg/Breisgau, Germany) was performed according to the manufacturers' instructions as previously described [46]. The test cartridges were read out by the photometric point-of-care (POC) system Concile® Ω100 reader (Concile GmbH) according to the manufacturers' instructions, allowing a quantitative analysis of the test results.

4.4. Expression and Purification of Recombinant Survivin

Template cDNA of survivin (BIRC5) was obtained from Sino Biologicals, Beijing, China. The standard PCR protocol included the primers p1 (5′-GTATACCATATGGGTGCCCGG-3′) and p2 (5′-CGGATCCTCAATCCATGGCAGC-3′). The PCR product was cut with NdeI and BamHI (New England Biolabs, Ipswich, MA, USA) for an in-frame ligation of the survivin coding sequence into pET16b (Merck Millipore Novagen, Darmstadt, Germany), which provides the coding sequence for an N-terminal polyhistidine-tag. Cloning products were confirmed by sequencing. The resulting pET16b_His-Survivin plasmid was transformed into *E. coli* BL 21 CodonPlus RIPL (Agilent Technologies, Santa Clara, CA, USA) cells for heterologous protein expression. The cells of a 1 L culture were harvested and lysed by urea denaturation in 20 mM Hepes, 100 mM NaCl (pH 8). Purification of the His_{10}-Survivin fusion protein was performed as described elsewhere [59]. Briefly, cell lysate was centrifuged to remove cell debris. Soluble supernatant was applied to an affinity chromatography column (HisTrap HP, GE Healthcare Life Science, Freiburg, Germany). After washing, the purified protein was eluted with elution buffer (20 mM Hepes, 100 mM NaCl, 8 M Urea, 250 mM imidazole, pH 8). Eluted affinity-purified His_{10}-Survivin showed high purity and was further processed on a size-exclusion chromatography column (SuperdexTM 75, Amersham Bioscience, Little Chalfont, Buckinghamshire, UK) for protein refolding. Final proteins in PBS was stored at −20 °C and used for immunization of rabbits for the generation of polyclonal antibodies.

4.5. Immunization and Antibody Purification

Immunization with His_{10}-Survivin was performed at Charles River (Charles River Laboratories, Chatillon-sur-Chalaronne, France) following standard immunization protocols. After 70 days, 90 mL final sera were received and 20 mL of these were further processed for antibody purification. For this purpose, sera were loaded onto a Profinity Protein A column (Bio-Rad, Munich, Germany) linked to a Next Generation Chromatography System (Bio-Rad). The column was washed with PBS and the purified antibodies were eluted with 100 mM glycine (pH 2.8). Purified anti-survivin antibodies were immediately dialyzed against PBS yielding a final IgG concentration of 2.87 mg/mL (15 mL) as determined by absorption at 280 nm.

4.6. Biotinylation of Anti-Survivin Antibody

For ELISA development, the purified survivin antibody was partly biotinylated. Briefly, purified antibody was mixed with 33× molar excess of NHS-Biotin (Thermo Fisher, Waltham, MA, USA) in 10 mM $NaHCO_3$ (pH 8.4), incubated for 3 h at room temperature and finally dialyzed against PBS. The final concentration of biotinylated antibody was 2.18 mg/mL (5 mL).

4.7. Survivin ELISA

In the experiments, 250 µL urinary cell pellet was centrifuged with 1500× *g* for 5 min at +4 °C to remove the storage solution. Afterwards, the pellet was completely dissolved in 500 µL CytoBuster (Merck Millipore, Darmstadt, Germany) and concentrated by using Vivaspin 500 spin columns (Sartorius, Stonehouse, Gloucestershire, UK) to 50 µL. To this solution, 150 µL of PBST (PBS with 0.05% Tween-20) was added and used as sample for measurement. Residual CytoBuster was tested to have no influence on antibody binding. Microtiter plates (Thermo Scientific, Roskilde, Denmark) were coated with purified polyclonal antibodies (100 µL/well, diluted 1:5000 in 100 mM carbonate/bicarbonate buffer, pH 9.6) and allowed to adhere overnight at +4 °C. They were then blocked with 1.5% casein, washed, and incubated with dilutions of the standard and samples for 1 h at room temperature. A stock solution of survivin was diluted in PBST to give standard concentrations between 5 and 0.02 ng/mL. Next, plates were washed three times with PBST and incubated for 1 h with biotinylated polyclonal antibodies (100 µL/well, dilution 1:10,000). After washing, 100 µL/well of 1:20,000 diluted horseradish-peroxidase-streptavidin conjugate (Fitzgerald Industries International, Concord, MA,

USA) was added. After 1 h, plates were washed with PBST and 100 μL H_2O_2-activated ABTS substrate solution was added to each well. The enzyme reaction was stopped by addition of 100 μL 0.32% NaF and absorbance was read at 414 nm.

The dose–response curves for standards were obtained by 4-parameter curve fitting using SoftMax Pro 4.7.1 from Molecular Devices (Sunnyvale, CA, USA). The lower detection limit of the assay was defined by adding 0.05 OD units (2-fold mean of the background standard deviation of 20 plates) to the background value of each plate. Samples were considered as positive for survivin if the measured concentration was above the cut-off. The cut-off was defined as the limit of detection. Reproducibility experiments were performed with samples containing low (0.168 ng/mL), medium (0.667 ng/mL) and high (2.240 ng/mL) survivin concentrations.

4.8. Statistics

Statistical analyses were performed with SAS/STAT and SAS/IML software version 9.4 (SAS Institute Inc., Cary, NC, USA) or Prism 5 (GraphPad Software, Inc., San Diego, CA, USA). Plots were generated with Prism 5. Median and inter-quartile ranges (IQR) were used to describe the distribution of continuous variables. Groups were compared using the non-parametric Wilcoxon signed-rank test. Spearman's correlation coefficients (r_s) and 95% confidence intervals were used to describe rank correlations between variables. The performance of the individual biomarkers and their combination was evaluated by receiver operating characteristic (ROC) analysis. For the panel, an 'or' combination of both markers was used. ROC curves were compared with a non-parametric approach [60].

5. Conclusions

In summary, a new ELISA to quantitate survivin in urine samples has been developed and evaluated alongside the UBC® *Rapid* test in a case-control study. Both assays detected bladder cancer, preferably high-grade tumors, but each with relatively low sensitivity. For the first time, survivin and UBC® *Rapid* have been tested as a panel, demonstrating an increase in sensitivity. However, the results require further testing of the assays with other control groups, like patients at suspicion for bladder cancer, and finally validation in a prospective study using a high-risk cohort.

Supplementary Materials: Supplementary materials can be found at www.mdpi.com/1422-0067/19/1/226/s1.

Acknowledgments: We thank Hans-Peter Rihs for kindly providing survivin coding sequence and Beate Pesch for constructive discussion on study design. We acknowledge support by the Open Access Publication Funds of the Ruhr-University Bochum.

Author Contributions: Jan Gleichenhagen designed and performed survivin experiments, participated in the immunoassay development and data collection, and drafted the manuscript. Christian Arndt carried out the UBC® *Rapid* experiments, participated in recruitment and coordination. Swaantje Casjens performed the statistical analyses and helped to draft the manuscript. Carmen Meinig carried out immunoassays and participated in data collection. Holger Gerullis participated in recruitment and coordination. Irina Raiko carried out initial immunoassay analysis and development. Thomas Brüning participated in the study design and coordination. Thorsten Ecke participated in the study design and coordination, and helped to draft the manuscript. Georg Johnen conceived the study, participated in its design and coordination, and helped to draft the manuscript.

Conflicts of Interest: The authors declare no conflict of interest.

Abbreviations

AUC	Area under the curve
CV	Coefficient of variation
LoD	Limit of detection
ELISA	Enzyme-linked immunosorbent assay
IQR	Interquartile range
ROC	Receiver operating characteristic

References

1. Knowles, M.A.; Hurst, C.D. Molecular biology of bladder cancer: New insights into pathogenesis and clinical diversity. *Nat. Rev. Cancer* **2015**, *15*, 25–41. [CrossRef] [PubMed]
2. Schmitz-Drager, B.J.; Droller, M.; Lokeshwar, V.B.; Lotan, Y.; Hudson, M.L.A.; van Rhijn, B.W.; Marberger, M.J.; Fradet, Y.; Hemstreet, G.P.; Malmstrom, P.-U.; et al. Molecular markers for bladder cancer screening, early diagnosis, and surveillance: The WHO/ICUD consensus. *Urol. Int.* **2015**, *94*, 1–24. [CrossRef] [PubMed]
3. Tilki, D.; Burger, M.; Dalbagni, G.; Grossman, H.B.; Hakenberg, O.W.; Palou, J.; Reich, O.; Roupret, M.; Shariat, S.F.; Zlotta, A.R. Urine markers for detection and surveillance of non-muscle-invasive bladder cancer. *Eur. Urol.* **2011**, *60*, 484–492. [CrossRef] [PubMed]
4. Smith, Z.L.; Guzzo, T.J. Urinary markers for bladder cancer. *F1000prime Rep.* **2013**, *5*, 21. [CrossRef] [PubMed]
5. Miyake, M.; Goodison, S.; Giacoia, E.G.; Rizwani, W.; Ross, S.; Rosser, C.J. Influencing factors on the NMP-22 urine assay: An experimental model. *BMC Urol.* **2012**, *12*, 23. [CrossRef] [PubMed]
6. Chou, R.; Gore, J.L.; Buckley, D.; Fu, R.; Gustafson, K.; Griffin, J.C.; Grusing, S.; Selph, S. Urinary Biomarkers for Diagnosis of Bladder Cancer: A Systematic Review and Meta-analysis. *Ann. Intern. Med.* **2015**, *163*, 922–931. [CrossRef] [PubMed]
7. Huber, S.; Schwentner, C.; Taeger, D.; Pesch, B.; Nasterlack, M.; Leng, G.; Mayer, T.; Gawrych, K.; Bonberg, N.; Pelster, M.; et al. Nuclear matrix protein-22: A prospective evaluation in a population at risk for bladder cancer. Results from the UroScreen study. *BJU Int.* **2012**, *110*, 699–708. [CrossRef] [PubMed]
8. Mowatt, G.; Zhu, S.; Kilonzo, M.; Boachie, C.; Fraser, C.; Griffiths, T.R.L.; N'Dow, J.; Nabi, G.; Cook, J.; Vale, L. Systematic review of the clinical effectiveness and cost-effectiveness of photodynamic diagnosis and urine biomarkers (FISH, ImmunoCyt, NMP22) and cytology for the detection and follow-up of bladder cancer. *Health Technol. Assess.* **2010**, *14*, 1–331. [CrossRef] [PubMed]
9. Hajdinjak, T. UroVysion FISH test for detecting urothelial cancers: Meta-analysis of diagnostic accuracy and comparison with urinary cytology testing. *Urol. Oncol.* **2008**, *26*, 646–651. [CrossRef] [PubMed]
10. Banek, S.; Schwentner, C.; Täger, D.; Pesch, B.; Nasterlack, M.; Leng, G.; Gawrych, K.; Bonberg, N.; Johnen, G.; Kluckert, M.; et al. Prospective evaluation of fluorescence-in situ-hybridization to detect bladder cancer: Results from the UroScreen-Study. *Urol. Oncol.* **2013**, *31*, 1656–1662. [CrossRef] [PubMed]
11. Pesch, B.; Taeger, D.; Johnen, G.; Gawrych, K.; Bonberg, N.; Schwentner, C.; Wellhausser, H.; Kluckert, M.; Leng, G.; Nasterlack, M.; et al. Screening for bladder cancer with urinary tumor markers in chemical workers with exposure to aromatic amines. *Int. Arch. Occup. Environ. Health* **2014**, *87*, 715–724. [CrossRef] [PubMed]
12. Bonberg, N.; Taeger, D.; Gawrych, K.; Johnen, G.; Banek, S.; Schwentner, C.; Sievert, K.-D.; Wellhäußer, H.; Kluckert, M.; Leng, G.; et al. Chromosomal instability and bladder cancer: The UroVysion(TM) test in the UroScreen study. *BJU Int.* **2013**, *112*, E372–E382. [CrossRef] [PubMed]
13. Unruhe, B.; Schroder, E.; Wunsch, D.; Knauer, S.K. An Old Flame Never Dies: Survivin in Cancer and Cellular Senescence. *Gerontology* **2016**, *62*, 173–181. [CrossRef] [PubMed]
14. Jaiswal, P.K.; Goel, A.; Mittal, R.D. Survivin: A molecular biomarker in cancer. *Indian J. Med. Res.* **2015**, *141*, 389–397. [PubMed]
15. Akhtar, M.; Gallagher, L.; Rohan, S. Survivin: Role in diagnosis, prognosis, and treatment of bladder cancer. *Adv. Anat. Pathol.* **2006**, *13*, 122–126. [CrossRef] [PubMed]
16. Shariat, S.F.; Casella, R.; Khoddami, S.M.; Hernandez, G.; Sulser, T.; Gasser, T.C.; Lerner, S.P. Urine detection of survivin is a sensitive marker for the noninvasive diagnosis of bladder cancer. *J. Urol.* **2004**, *171*, 626–630. [CrossRef] [PubMed]
17. Altieri, D.C. Survivin—The inconvenient IAP. *Semin. Cell Dev. Boil.* **2015**, *39*, 91–96. [CrossRef] [PubMed]
18. Groner, B.; Weiss, A. Targeting survivin in cancer: Novel drug development approaches. *BioDrugs* **2014**, *28*, 27–39. [CrossRef] [PubMed]
19. Altieri, D.C. Targeting survivin in cancer. *Cancer Lett.* **2013**, *332*, 225–228. [CrossRef] [PubMed]
20. Chen, X.; Duan, N.; Zhang, C.; Zhang, W. Survivin and Tumorigenesis: Molecular Mechanisms and Therapeutic Strategies. *J. Cancer* **2016**, *7*, 314–323. [CrossRef] [PubMed]
21. Ku, J.H.; Godoy, G.; Amiel, G.E.; Lerner, S.P. Urine survivin as a diagnostic biomarker for bladder cancer: A systematic review. *BJU Int.* **2012**, *110*, 630–636. [CrossRef] [PubMed]

22. Johnen, G.; Gawrych, K.; Bontrup, H.; Pesch, B.; Taeger, D.; Banek, S.; Kluckert, M.; Wellhausser, H.; Eberle, F.; Nasterlack, M.; et al. Performance of survivin mRNA as a biomarker for bladder cancer in the prospective study UroScreen. *PLoS ONE* **2012**, *7*, e35363. [CrossRef] [PubMed]
23. Jeon, C.; Kim, M.; Kwak, C.; Kim, H.H.; Ku, J.H. Prognostic role of survivin in bladder cancer: A systematic review and meta-analysis. *PLoS ONE* **2013**, *8*, e76719. [CrossRef] [PubMed]
24. Chatziharalambous, D.; Lygirou, V.; Latosinska, A.; Stravodimos, K.; Vlahou, A.; Jankowski, V.; Zoidakis, J. Analytical Performance of ELISA Assays in Urine: One More Bottleneck towards Biomarker Validation and Clinical Implementation. *PLoS ONE* **2016**, *11*, e0149471. [CrossRef] [PubMed]
25. Pesch, B.; Nasterlack, M.; Eberle, F.; Bonberg, N.; Taeger, D.; Leng, G.; Feil, G.; Johnen, G.; Ickstadt, K.; Kluckert, M.; et al. The role of hematuria in bladder cancer screening among men with former occupational exposure to aromatic amines. *BJU Int.* **2011**, *108*, 546–552. [CrossRef] [PubMed]
26. Li, H.-T.; Duymich, C.E.; Weisenberger, D.J.; Liang, G. Genetic and Epigenetic Alterations in Bladder Cancer. *Int. Neurourol. J.* **2016**, *20*, S84–S94. [CrossRef] [PubMed]
27. Di Meo, A.; Bartlett, J.; Cheng, Y.; Pasic, M.D.; Yousef, G.M. Liquid biopsy: A step forward towards precision medicine in urologic malignancies. *Mol. Cancer* **2017**, *16*, 80. [CrossRef] [PubMed]
28. Burger, M.; Catto, J.W.F.; Dalbagni, G.; Grossman, H.B.; Herr, H.; Karakiewicz, P.; Kassouf, W.; Kiemeney, L.A.; la Vecchia, C.; Shariat, S.; et al. Epidemiology and risk factors of urothelial bladder cancer. *Eur. Urol.* **2013**, *63*, 234–241. [CrossRef] [PubMed]
29. Öge, Ö.; Kozaci, D.; Gemalmaz, H. The BTA Stat Test is Nonspecific for Hematuria: An Experimental Hematuria Model. *J. Urol.* **2002**, *167*, 1318–1320. [CrossRef]
30. Shariat, S.F.; Karam, J.A.; Lotan, Y.; Karakiewizc, P.I. Critical evaluation of urinary markers for bladder cancer detection and monitoring. *Rev. Urol.* **2008**, *10*, 120–135. [PubMed]
31. Findlay, J.W.A.; Dillard, R.F. Appropriate calibration curve fitting in ligand binding assays. *AAPS J.* **2007**, *9*, E260–E267. [CrossRef] [PubMed]
32. Srivastava, A.K.; Singh, P.K.; Srivastava, K.; Singh, D.; Dalela, D.; Rath, S.K.; Goel, M.M.; Bhatt, M.L.B. Diagnostic Role of Survivin in Urinary Bladder Cancer. *Asian Pac. J. Cancer Prev.* **2013**, *14*, 81–85. [CrossRef] [PubMed]
33. Fichorova, R.N.; Richardson-Harman, N.; Alfano, M.; Belec, L.; Carbonneil, C.; Chen, S.; Cosentino, L.; Curtis, K.; Dezzutti, C.S.; Donoval, B.; et al. Biological and technical variables affecting immunoassay recovery of cytokines from human serum and simulated vaginal fluid: A multicenter study. *Anal. Chem.* **2008**, *80*, 4741–4751. [CrossRef] [PubMed]
34. Wu, J.; Chen, Y.-D.; Gu, W. Urinary proteomics as a novel tool for biomarker discovery in kidney diseases. *J. Zhejiang Univ. Sci. B* **2010**, *11*, 227–237. [CrossRef] [PubMed]
35. Zoidakis, J.; Makridakis, M.; Zerefos, P.G.; Bitsika, V.; Esteban, S.; Frantzi, M.; Stravodimos, K.; Anagnou, N.P.; Roubelakis, M.G.; Sanchez-Carbayo, M.; et al. Profilin 1 is a potential biomarker for bladder cancer aggressiveness. *Mol. Cell. Proteom.* **2012**, *11*. [CrossRef] [PubMed]
36. Adachi, J.; Kumar, C.; Zhang, Y.; Olsen, J.V.; Mann, M. The human urinary proteome contains more than 1500 proteins, including a large proportion of membrane proteins. *Genome Biol.* **2006**, *7*, R80. [CrossRef] [PubMed]
37. Reverberi, R.; Reverberi, L. Factors affecting the antigen-antibody reaction. *Blood Transfus.* **2007**, *5*, 227–240. [PubMed]
38. Khan, S.; Bennit, H.F.; Wall, N.R. The emerging role of exosomes in survivin secretion. *Histol. Histopathol.* **2015**, *30*, 43–50. [PubMed]
39. Nong, R.Y.; Di, W.; Yan, J.; Hammond, M.; Gu, G.J.; Kamali-Moghaddam, M.; Landegren, U.; Darmanis, S. Solid-phase proximity ligation assays for individual or parallel protein analyses with readout via real-time PCR or sequencing. *Nat. Protoc.* **2013**, *8*, 1234–1248. [CrossRef] [PubMed]
40. Darmanis, S.; Nong, R.Y.; Hammond, M.; Gu, J.; Alderborn, A.; Vanelid, J.; Siegbahn, A.; Gustafsdottir, S.; Ericsson, O.; Landegren, U.; et al. Sensitive plasma protein analysis by microparticle-based proximity ligation assays. *Mol. Cell. Proteom.* **2010**, *9*, 327–335. [CrossRef] [PubMed]
41. Ohsawa, I.; Nishimura, T.; Kondo, Y.; Kimura, G.; Satoh, M.; Matsuzawa, I.; Hamasaki, T.; Ohta, S. Detection of urine survivin in 40 patients with bladder cancer. *J. Nippon Med. Sch.* **2004**, *71*, 379–383. [CrossRef] [PubMed]
42. Li, X.; Wang, Y.; Xu, J.; Zhang, Q. Sandwich ELISA for detecting urinary Survivin in bladder cancer. *Chin. J. Cancer Res.* **2013**, *25*, 375–381. [PubMed]

43. Eissa, S.; Badr, S.; Barakat, M.; Zaghloul, A.; Mohanad, M. The Diagnostic Efficacy of Urinary Survivin and Hyaluronidase mRNA as Urine Markers in Patients with Bladder Cancer. *Clin. Lab.* **2013**, *59*, 893–900. [CrossRef] [PubMed]
44. Garg, M. Urothelial cancer stem cells and epithelial plasticity: Current concepts and therapeutic implications in bladder cancer. *Cancer Metastasis Rev.* **2015**, *34*, 691–701. [CrossRef] [PubMed]
45. Adamowicz, J.; Pokrywczynska, M.; Tworkiewicz, J.; Wolski, Z.; Drewa, T. The relationship of cancer stem cells in urological cancers. *Cent. Eur. J. Urol.* **2013**, *66*, 273–280. [CrossRef] [PubMed]
46. Ecke, T.; Arndt, C.; Stephan, C.; Hallmann, S.; Lux, O.; Otto, T.; Ruttloff, J.; Gerullis, H. Preliminary Results of a Multicentre Study of the UBC® Rapid Test for Detection of Urinary Bladder Cancer. *Anticancer Res.* **2015**, *2015*, 2651–2656.
47. D'Costa, J.J.; Goldsmith, J.C.; Wilson, J.S.; Bryan, R.T.; Ward, D.G. A Systematic Review of the Diagnostic and Prognostic Value of Urinary Protein Biomarkers in Urothelial Bladder Cancer. *Bladder Cancer* **2016**, *2*, 301–317. [CrossRef] [PubMed]
48. Ritter, R.; Hennenlotter, J.; Kuhs, U.; Hofmann, U.; Aufderklamm, S.; Blutbacher, P.; Deja, A.; Hohneder, A.; Gerber, V.; Gakis, G.; et al. Evaluation of a new quantitative point-of-care test platform for urine-based detection of bladder cancer. *Urol. Oncol.* **2014**, *32*, 337–344. [CrossRef] [PubMed]
49. Hakenberg, O.W.; Fuessel, S.; Richter, K.; Froehner, M.; Oehlschlaeger, S.; Rathert, P.; Meye, A.; Wirth, M.P. Qualitative and quantitative assessment of urinary cytokeratin 8 and 18 fragments compared with voided urine cytology in diagnosis of bladder carcinoma. *Urology* **2004**, *64*, 1121–1126. [CrossRef] [PubMed]
50. Styrke, J.; Henriksson, H.; Ljungberg, B.; Hasan, M.; Silfverberg, I.; Einarsson, R.; Malmström, P.-U.; Sherif, A. Evaluation of the diagnostic accuracy of UBC® Rapid in bladder cancer: A Swedish multicentre study. *Scand. J. Urol.* **2017**, *51*, 293–300. [CrossRef] [PubMed]
51. Ecke, T.H.; Weiß, S.; Stephan, C.; Hallmann, S.; Barski, D.; Otto, T.; Gerullis, H. UBC® Rapid Test for detection of carcinoma in situ for bladder cancer. *Tumour Biol.* **2017**, *39*. [CrossRef] [PubMed]
52. Pesch, B.; Bruning, T.; Johnen, G.; Casjens, S.; Bonberg, N.; Taeger, D.; Muller, A.; Weber, D.G.; Behrens, T. Biomarker research with prospective study designs for the early detection of cancer. *Biochim. Biophys. Acta* **2014**, *1844*, 874–883. [CrossRef] [PubMed]
53. Sánchez-Carbayo, M.; Herrero, E.; Megias, J.; Mira, A.; Espasa, A.; Chinchilla, V.; Soria, F. Initial evaluation of the diagnostic performance of the new urinary bladder cancer antigen test as a tumor marker for transitional cell carcinoma of the bladder. *J. Urol.* **1999**, *161*, 1110–1115. [CrossRef]
54. Larré, S.; Catto, J.W.F.; Cookson, M.S.; Messing, E.M.; Shariat, S.F.; Soloway, M.S.; Svatek, R.S.; Lotan, Y.; Zlotta, A.R.; Grossman, H.B. Screening for bladder cancer: Rationale, limitations, whom to target, and perspectives. *Eur. Urol.* **2013**, *63*, 1049–1058. [CrossRef] [PubMed]
55. Altznauer, F.; Martinelli, S.; Yousefi, S.; Thurig, C.; Schmid, I.; Conway, E.M.; Schoni, M.H.; Vogt, P.; Mueller, C.; Fey, M.F.; et al. Inflammation-associated cell cycle-independent block of apoptosis by survivin in terminally differentiated neutrophils. *J. Exp. Med.* **2004**, *199*, 1343–1354. [CrossRef] [PubMed]
56. Atsumi, T.; Singh, R.; Sabharwal, L.; Bando, H.; Meng, J.; Arima, Y.; Yamada, M.; Harada, M.; Jiang, J.-J.; Kamimura, D.; et al. Inflammation amplifier, a new paradigm in cancer biology. *Cancer Res.* **2014**, *74*, 8–14. [CrossRef] [PubMed]
57. Guven Maiorov, E.; Keskin, O.; Gursoy, A.; Nussinov, R. The structural network of inflammation and cancer: Merits and challenges. *Semin. Cancer Biol.* **2013**, *23*, 243–251. [CrossRef] [PubMed]
58. Sauter, G.; Eble, J.N.; Epstein, J.I.; Sesterhenn, I.A. (Eds.) *World Health Organization Classification of Tumours. Pathology and Genetics of Tumours of the Urinary System and Male Genital Organs*; IARC Press: Lyon, France, 2004; Volume 6.
59. Shen, C.; Liu, W.; Buck, A.K.; Reske, S.N. Pro-apoptosis and anti-proliferation effects of a recombinant dominant-negative survivin-T34A in human cancer cells. *Anticancer Res.* **2009**, *29*, 1423–1428. [PubMed]
60. DeLong, E.R.; DeLong, D.M.; Clarke-Pearson, D.L. Comparing the Areas under Two or More Correlated Receiver Operating Characteristic Curves: A Nonparametric Approach. *Biometrics* **1988**, *44*, 837–845. [CrossRef] [PubMed]

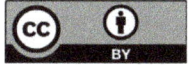

© 2018 by the authors. Licensee MDPI, Basel, Switzerland. This article is an open access article distributed under the terms and conditions of the Creative Commons Attribution (CC BY) license (http://creativecommons.org/licenses/by/4.0/).

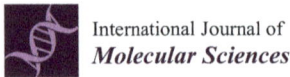

Article

Aberrant *N*-Glycosylation Profile of Serum Immunoglobulins is a Diagnostic Biomarker of Urothelial Carcinomas

Toshikazu Tanaka [1], Tohru Yoneyama [2,*], Daisuke Noro [1], Kengo Imanishi [1], Yuta Kojima [1], Shingo Hatakeyama [1], Yuki Tobisawa [1], Kazuyuki Mori [1], Hayato Yamamoto [1], Atsushi Imai [1], Takahiro Yoneyama [1], Yasuhiro Hashimoto [2], Takuya Koie [1], Masakazu Tanaka [3], Shin-Ichiro Nishimura [3], Shizuka Kurauchi [4], Ippei Takahashi [4] and Chikara Ohyama [1,2]

1. Department of Urology, Hirosaki University Graduate School of Medicine, Hirosaki 036-8562, Japan; yosage1205@yahoo.co.jp (T.T.); noro.daisuke@camel.plala.or.jp (D.N.); born_2b_snower@yahoo.co.jp (K.I.); y_kojima0319@yahoo.co.jp (Y.K.); shingoh@hirosaki-u.ac.jp (S.H.); tobisawa@hirosaki-u.ac.jp (Y.T.); moribio@hirosaki-u.ac.jp (K.M.); yamahaya10@yahoo.co.jp (H.Y.); tsushi.imai@gmail.com (A.I.); uroyone@hirosaki-u.ac.jp (T.Y.); goodwin@hirosaki-u.ac.jp (T.K.); coyama@hirosaki-u.ac.jp (C.O.)
2. Department of Advanced Transplant and Regenerative Medicine, Hirosaki University Graduate School of Medicine, Hirosaki 036-8562, Japan; bikkuri@opal.plala.or.jp
3. Graduate School of Life Science, Frontier Research Centre for Advanced Material and Life Science, Hokkaido University, Sapporo 060-0810, Japan; tanaka@soyaku.co.jp (M.T.); shin@sci.hokudai.ac.jp (S.-I.N.)
4. Department of Social Medicine, Hirosaki University Graduate School of Medicine, Hirosaki 036-8562, Japan; k-shizu@hirosaki-u.ac.jp (S.K.); ippei@hirosaki-u.ac.jp (I.T.)
* Correspondence: tohruyon@hirosaki-u.ac.jp; Tel.: +81-172-39-5091

Received: 21 November 2017; Accepted: 2 December 2017; Published: 6 December 2017

Abstract: The aim of this study to determine whether the aberrant *N*-glycosylated serum immunoglobulins (Igs) can be applied as a diagnostic marker of urothelial carcinoma (UC). Between 2009 and 2016, we randomly obtained serum available from 237 UC and also 96 prostate cancer as other cancer controls from our serum bank and also obtained—from 339 healthy volunteers (HV)—controls obtained from community-dwelling volunteers in Iwaki Health Promotion Project. A total of 32 types of *N*-glycan levels on Igs were determined by high-throughput *N*-glycomics and analyzed by multivariable discriminant analysis. We found five UC-associated aberrant *N*-glycans changes on Igs and also found that asialo-bisecting GlcNAc type *N*-glycan on Igs were significantly accumulated in UC patients. The diagnostic *N*-glycan Score (dNGScore) established by combination of five *N*-glycans on Igs discriminated UC patients from HV and prostate cancer (PC) patients with 92.8% sensitivity and 97.2% specificity. The area under the curve (AUC) for of the dNGScore was 0.969 for UC detection that was much superior to that of urine cytology (AUC, 0.707) and hematuria (AUC, 0.892). Furthermore, dNGScore can detect hematuria and urine cytology negative patients. The dNGscore based on aberrant *N*-glycosylation signatures of Igs were found to be promising diagnostic biomarkers of UCs.

Keywords: diagnostic biomarker; urothelial carcinoma of the bladder; upper urinary tract urothelial carcinoma; *N*-glycomics; immunogloburins; aberrant *N*-glycosylation

1. Introduction

Urothelial carcinomas (UCs) are the eighth-most lethal cancer in men in the United States [1]. The majority of UCs originate from bladder, called UC of the bladder (UCB), and between 5% and 10% of UCs originate from the ureter or renal pelvis [2,3], which are collectively called upper urinary tract UCs (UTUCs), with a worse prognosis than that of UCB. The most common symptom is visible- or non-visible hematuria (70–80%) [4,5] and then the standard examinations are performed, involving urine cytology, urinary tract imaging and cystoscopy, which are powerful diagnostic tools for UCs. However, 60% of UTUCs are invasive at time of diagnosis [6,7]. Urine cytology is not reliable in patients with early stage UCs, including UTUC, and it is difficult to visualise small tumors via imaging modalities, such as ultrasound or computed tomography. Several diagnostic urine-based biomarkers are reported such as bladder tumor antigen (BTA), nuclear matrix protein number 22 (NMP22) and UroVysion [8–10]. Although sensitivities can be better for BTA (50–80%), NMP22 (68.5–88.5%) and UroVysion (58–96%) over urine cytology (50–67%), the specificities are quite low. Because those tests are soluble antigen test or cellular assay depending on the amount of tumor cells, they are not suitable for the detection of low-grade and low-stage tumors. Furthermore, the prevalence of urinary markers of only about 30% is not enough to complement urine cytology and other invasive tests. Thus, more sensitive and non-invasive biomarkers, such as serum-based biomarkers, to avoid under-detection in patients at high risk of UCs is required.

Glycosylation is a common post-translational modification that has an important role in various biological functions. Previously, our group demonstrated that high-throughput, comprehensive and quantitative N-glycomics based on the glycoblotting method combined with mass spectrometry is a promising way to screen glycans for use as diagnostic and prognostic markers of several cancer [11–15]. Recently, the evaluation of glycosylation profile is an innovative topic in different cancer types, especially in immunotherapeutic targets, as like as PD-L1 [16–18]. Most recently, our group reported that a combination of several serum N-glycans (N-glycan score, NGScore) is a novel serum marker for UCs including UTUC that detected 93% of UC patients and is therefore far more specific than classic urine cytology [19]. We hypothesized that these serum aberrant N-glycan change is derived from serum major N-glycosylated proteins, such as immunoglobulins (Igs). Although differences in Ig glycosylation are mainly described in immune system-related diseases [20–23], there are several papers describing aberrant glycosylation of IgG in cancer such as prostate cancer, gastric cancer and colorectal cancer [24–27]. In addition, aberrant N-glycosylation of immunoglobulins in UC has not been reported elsewhere. Thus, in the present study, we performed N-glycomics of serum Igs fractions between healthy volunteers (HVs), prostate cancer (PC) and UCs patients to identify the UC-specific aberrant N-glycosylated Igs. Furthermore, for clinical applications, we established a diagnostic NGScore (dNGScore) based on a combination of five N-glycans of Igs associated with detection of UCs.

2. Results

2.1. Downregulation of Asialo Biantennary Type N-Glycans and Accumulation of Asialo-Bisecting GlcNAc with Core Fucosylated N-Glycan on Igs May Occur as a UC-Associated Aberrant N-Glycosylation of Igs

SDS-PAGE analysis between whole serum (Figure A1b, lanes 1–4) and Igs fractions (Figure A1b, lanes 5–8) revealed that non-Igs proteins were effectively eliminated from whole serum by Melon Gel chromatography. N-glycomics of the Igs fraction (Figure A1a–e) identified 32 types of BOA-labelled N-glycans on Igs (Table A1, Figure A1f). Patient characteristics in the non-UC (HV and PC) and UC groups are shown in Table 1. There were no statistically significant differences in age, history of smoking, benign prostatic hyperplasia (BPH) and stone former between both non-UC group and UC group.

To detect UC, we performed multivariable discriminant analysis by inputting UCs event as an explanatory variable and the N-glycan level of Igs as objective variables and selected candidate N-glycans (complex biantennary type: m/z 1606, 1769, 2074; core fucosylated bisecting GlcNAc type: m/z 2118, 2423) that formed the most sensitive and specific combination for detection of UCs (Figure 1a–c and Table 2).

Table 1. Patients' demographics in each cohort.

	Non-UC [a]		UC [b]	p Value a vs. b
	HV n, (%)	PC n, (%)	n, (%)	
Total patients (n)	339	96	237	
Sex (Male, %)	122 (36.0)	96 (100)	191 (80.6)	<0.001
Median age (IQR [1])	68.0 (63–73)	74.0 (68–78)	70.0 (62–75)	0.700
Former or current smoker	75 (22.1)	18 (18.8)	71 (29.9)	0.101
Stone former	4 (1.2)	0 (0)	0 (0)	0.184
BPH [2]	7 (2.1)	0 (0)	0 (0)	0.145
HSPC [3]	0 (0)	96 (100)	0 (0)	<0.001
hematuria+	0 (0)	0 (0)	186 (78.5)	<0.001
Urine Cytology Class				
I, II			81 (34.2)	
III			58 (24.5)	
IV			16 (6.7)	
V			82 (34.6)	
Tumor Location of UC				
Bladder			177 (67.6)	
Renal pelvis			27 (11.4)	
Ureter			28 (11.8)	
Multiple			4 (1.7)	
Tumor Grade of UC				
Low grade noninvasive			68 (28.7)	
High grade noninvasive			43 (18.1)	
Muscle invasive			109 (45.9)	
Lymph node stage N1		0 (0.0)	20 (8.4)	0.115
Metastatic disease		4 (4.2)	47 (19.8)	0.010

[1] IQR, Interquartile range; [2] BPH, benign prostatic hyperplasia; [3] HSPC, hormone sensitive prostate cancer; HV: healthy volunteers; PC: prostate cancer. [a] non-urothelial carcinoma, non-UC; [b] urothelial carcinoma, UC.

Table 2. Multivariable discriminant analysis for prediction of UCs.

Variables	Wilks' Lambda	F Value	ODF [1]	TDF [2]	p Value	Discriminant Function
m/z 1606	0.9742	17.72	1	670	<0.001	0.1925
m/z 1769	0.9707	20.24	1	670	<0.001	0.4932
m/z 2074	0.9377	44.54	1	670	<0.001	0.4941
m/z 2118	0.5894	466.73	1	670	<0.001	-3.2460
m/z 2423	0.9984	1.04	1	670	<0.001	0.6179
				Constant term		-0.4905

[1] ODF, one degree of freedom; [2] TDF, two degrees of freedom.

The asialo biantennary type N-glycans (m/z 1606 and 2074) on Igs were significantly downregulated in the UC group compared with the levels in the HV and PC groups ($p = 0.0001$). Only the asialo biantennary type N-glycan (m/z 1769) on Igs was significantly downregulated in the PC group compared with the level in the UC and HV groups ($p = 0.0001$). The monosialyl bisecting GlcNAc with core fucosylated bisecting GlcNAc N-glycan (m/z 2423) was not significantly changed between UC and HV group, but significantly decreased in PC and UTUC group ($p = 0.0001$). Especially the asialo bisecting GlcNAc with core fucosylated N-glycan (m/z 2118) on Igs was significantly upregulated in UC group ($p = 0.0001$) but not detectable in HV and PC groups. However, total Igs level in UC patients was significantly lower than HV and PC patients (Figure 2a–d).

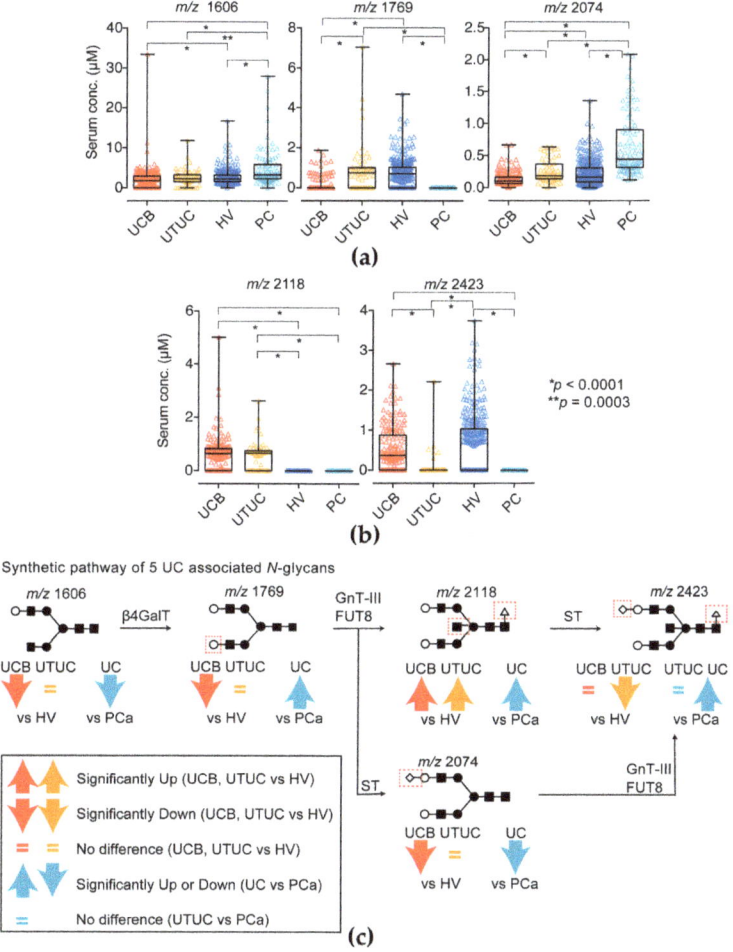

Figure 1. Five UC-associated *N*-glycan levels of immunoglobulins (Igs) fractions. (**a**) Complex biantennary-type *N*-glycan (*m*/*z* 1606, 1769 and 2074) levels and (**b**) fucosylated bisecting GlcNAc-type *N*-glycan (*m*/*z* 2118 and 2423) of the Ig fractions in the UC, HV and PC groups. The results shown are representative of three independent experiments. Intergroup differences were statistically compared using the Mann–Whitney *U*-test for non-normally distributed models; (**c**) Synthetic pathway of candidate *N*-glycans in the present study. Red up- and downward arrows indicates significantly changed in UC compare with HV group. Cyan up- and downward arrows indicates significantly changed in UC compare with PC group. The equals mark indicates that it did not significantly change. *N*-glycan structures are indicated by monosaccharide symbols: white circles, galactose (Gal); black circles, mannose (Man); black squares, *N*-acetylglucosamine (GlcNAc); black triangle, fucose (Fuc) and black diamonds, sialic acid. β4GalT: β1,4-galactosyltransferase, GnT-III: *N*-acetylglucosaminyltransferase-III, FUT8: fucosyltransferase 8, ST: sialyltransferase.

According to the synthetic pathway of *N*-glycans shown in Figure 1b and the above results, a downregulation of asialo biantennary type *N*-glycans and accumulation of asialo-bisecting GlcNAc with core fucosylated *N*-glycan on Igs may occur as a UC-associated aberrant *N*-glycosylation of Igs.

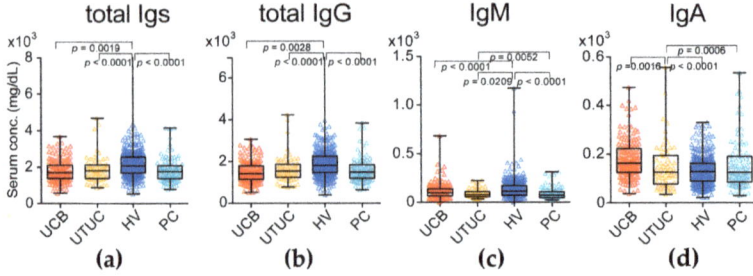

Figure 2. Serum immunoglobulin (Ig) levels in UC (UC of the bladder (UCB) and upper urinary tract UC (UTUC)) patients and healthy volunteers (HVs) and prostate cancer (PC). (**a**) Serum total Igs (sum of IgG1-4, IgM and IgA) levels in the UC, HV and PC groups; (**b**) Serum total IgG (IgG1-4) levels in the UC, HV and PC groups; (**c**) Serum IgM levels in the UC, HV and PC groups; (**d**) Serum IgA levels in the UC, HV and PC groups. The results shown are representative of three independent experiments. Intergroup differences were statistically compared using the Mann–Whitney U-test for non-normally distributed models.

2.2. UC Diagnostic N-Glycan Score Based on Aberrant N-Glycosylation of Igs Was Far Superior to Classic Urine Cytology and Hematuria Status

To apply these candidate aberrant N-glycosylation profile on Igs for UC detection, we established the UC diagnostic N-glycan score (dNGScore) that was calculated according to the following formula:

$$\text{dNGScore} = (\text{serum level of } m/z\ 1606 \times 0.1925) + (\text{serum level of } m/z\ 1769 \times 0.4932) \\ + (\text{serum level of } m/z\ 2074 \times 0.4941) + (\text{serum level of } m/z\ 2118 \times -3.2460) + (\text{serum level of } m/z\ 2423 \times 0.6179) + (-0.4905) \quad (1)$$

The dNGScore was significantly lower in the UC (UCB and UTUC) patients than in the non-UC group including HVs and PC (Mann–Whitney U-test: $p = 0.0001$, permutation test: $p = 0.001$) (Figure 3a,c). The dNGScore of UCB was significantly lower than those of HV (Mann–Whitney U-test: $p = 0.0001$, permutation test: $p = 0.012$) and PC (Mann–Whitney U-test: $p = 0.0001$, permutation test: $p = 0.0017$) (Figure 3a). The dNGScore of UTUC was also significantly lower than those of HV (Mann–Whitney U-test: $p = 0.0001$, permutation test: $p = 0.014$) and PC (Mann–Whitney U-test: $p = 0.0001$, permutation test: $p = 0.0021$) (Figure 3a). The AUC of dNGScore for prediction of UCs (for UCs, 0.969, for UCB, 0.993, for UTUC, 0.907, respectively) was much higher than that of hematuria (AUC, 0.892) and urine cytology (AUC, 0.707) (Figure 3b and Table 3). At the cut-off dNGScore (−0.0955 points) for prediction of UCs, the negative predictive value (NPV) was 96.1%, which was much higher than the NPV of urine cytology (75.8%) and hematuria (89.5%). The dNGScore was not significantly associated with hematuria status and class of urine cytology (Figure 3d,e), but significantly associated with invasiveness of UCB (Figure 3f).

Table 3. Comparing diagnostic performance of UCs on each test.

Variables	AUC	95% CI	Sensitivity (%)	Specificity (%)	PPV (%)	NPV (%)
Hematuria	0.892	0.861–0.924	78.5	100.0	100.0	89.5
Urine cytology	0.707	0.661–0.753	41.4	100.0	100.0	75.8
dNGScore [1] for UC	0.969	0.952–0.986	92.8	97.2	94.8	96.1
dNGScore for UCB	0.993	0.982–0.100	98.3	97.2	93.5	99.3
dNGScore for UTUC	0.907	0.854–0.959	77.1	97.2	79.7	96.8

[1] dNGScore, diagnostic N-glycan score.

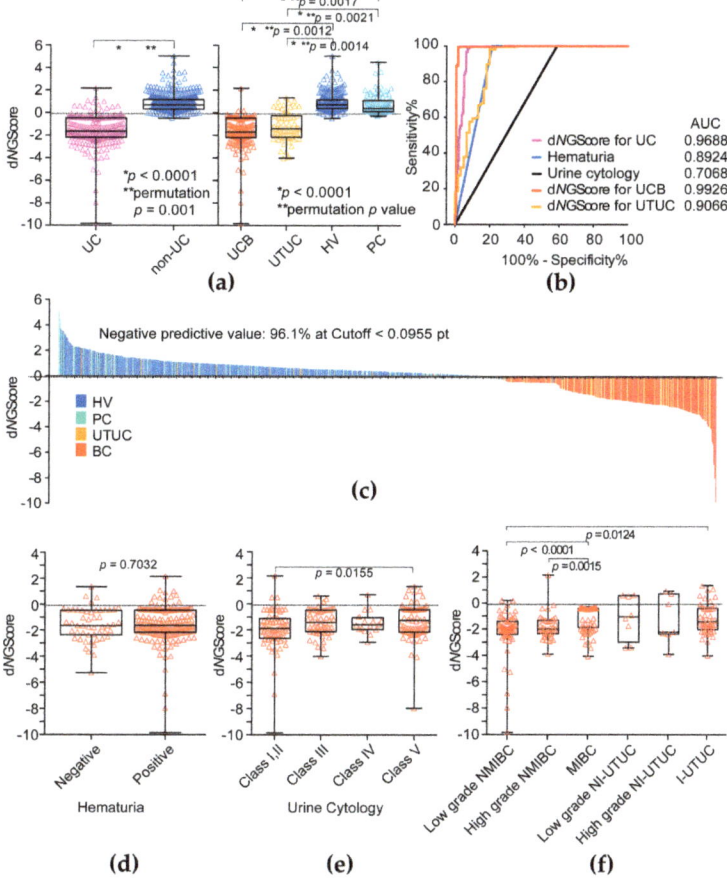

Figure 3. Clinical significance of diagnostic *N*-glycan score. (**a**) The diagnostic *N*-glycan score (d*N*GScore) level was significantly higher in the UC (UCB and UTUC) group than in the HV and PC group; (**b**) ROC curve analysis of d*N*GScore, hematuria and urine cytological results for detection of UC (UCB and UTUC); (**c**) Waterfall plot of d*N*GScore; (**d**) Association between d*N*GScore level and hematuria status; (**e**) Association between d*N*GScore level and urine cytology; (**f**) Association between d*N*GScore level and tumor invasiveness. NMIBC: non-muscle invasive bladder cancer, MIBC: muscle invasive bladder cancer, NI-UTUC: noninvasive UTUC, I-UTUC: invasive UTUC. Intergroup differences were statistically compared using the Mann–Whitney *U*-test for non-normally distributed models and performed permutation test.

3. Discussion

Several studies have shown that differences in serum *N*-glycan profiles between diseased and benign states analyzing high-throughput, comprehensive and quantitative *N*-glycomics may be useful in the diagnosis or prognosis of diseases [11–14,19]. A few studies have investigated the use of serum *N*-glycans as diagnostic markers for UC, including UTUC [13,19]. Although these reports showed that the levels of highly branched sialylated *N*-glycans (*m*/*z* 2890, 3560, 3865) were increased in the sera of patients with bladder cancer [13,19], they did not identify carrier proteins of aberrant *N*-glycosylation. Furthermore, these highly branched sialylated *N*-glycans in serum were also significantly upregulated in plural cancer, such as prostate or kidney cancer [11,12]. To identify which carrier protein is aberrantly glycosylated, in the present study, we focused on N-glycomics of serum major N-glycosylated protein such as Igs. We showed that, in total, five types of N-glycans, including bisecting GlcNAc-, biantennary-type N-glycans with or without core fucose in serum Igs fractions, were associated with UC detection (Figure 1). According to the biosynthetic pathway of N-glycans (Figure 1c), bisecting GlcNAc N-glycans were synthesized from biantennary-type N-glycan by β1,4-N-acetylglucosaminyltransferase (GnT-III) and then modified terminal galactosylation and/or sialylation by galactosyltransferase and sialyltransferase. In this study, we found asialo biantennary- (m/z 1606 and 1769) and monosialyl biantennary-typed N-glycan (m/z 2074) and monosialyl bisecting GlcNAc-typed N-glycans (m/z 2423) were significantly decreased in UC patients and upregulated only asialo bisecting GlcNAc typed N-glycan (m/z 2118) on Igs in UC patients. Thus, we hypothesize asialo biantennary typed N-glycan on Igs was transformed to asialo bisecting type N-glycan on Igs by GnT-III activity and less sialyltransferase activity in UC patients and resulted in a decrease of biantennary and sialyl bisecting GlcNAc type N-glycan on Igs in UC patients. In addition, in the UTUC case, the level of monosialyl bisecting GlcNAc-typed N-glycans (m/z 2423) on Igs was significantly lower than that of UCB group. Thus, accumulation of asialo bisecting GlcNAc typed N-glycan (m/z 2118) was more of a UTUC-specific phenomenon than that of UCB. This suggests that aberrant N-glycosylation profile UTUC was little different from that of UCB. This difference may reflect the difference of tumor environment between bladder and urinary/renal pelvis, and/or may reflect different embryonic background of tumor origin. On the other hand, in PC case, upregulation of monosialyl biantennary-typed N-glycan (m/z 2074) and down-regulation of monosialyl bisecting GlcNAc-typed N-glycans (m/z 2423) is observed. This suggests that monosialyl biantennary-typed N-glycan (m/z 2074) on Igs is significantly accumulated in PC patients and might be the candidate aberrant glycosylation of prostate cancer detection. These aberrant N-glycosylation profiles of Igs were different from the whole serum aberrant N-glycosylation profiles obtained in previous studies [13,19]. Thus, asialo bisecting type N-glycosylated Igs can be applied as a promising UC-specific diagnostic biomarker. To the best of our knowledge, this is the first report to demonstrate the clinical significance of aberrant N-glycosylated Igs as diagnostic biomarkers of UCs. It is well known that glycosylation of Igs has a critical role in the development of diseases. Wuhrer et al. reported that asialo bisecting type N-glycosylated IgG induced anti-inflammatory response and agalactosyl bisecting type N-glycosylated IgG induced pro-inflammatory response in cerebrospinal fluid [20]. Overproduction of aberrantly glycosylated IgA1 has a key role in the development of IgA nephropathy [21]. A recent report suggested that antibody-mediated rejection after kidney transplantation is closely associated with the levels of immunomodulatory sialylated IgG antibodies [22]. Furthermore, Kazuno et al. reported that α2,6-sialylated IgG was significantly decreased in prostate cancer immunoreactions [24]. Rademacher et al. reported that agalactosyl bisecting GlcNAc type N-glycoslated IgG was increased in rheumatoid arthritis patient and related autoimmune disease [23]. From these observations, aberrant glycosylated Igs appear to change their glycans because of disease-associated immunoreactions. In a future study, we will examine N-glycosylation profile of Igs between benign disease and UC patients to address the UC associated aberrant glycosylation on Igs are part of inflammatory response.

In the present study, the dNGScore, combination of 5 N-glycans including biantennary and bisecting GlcNAc, clearly discriminate UC from healthy controls and prostate cancer patients with 92.8% sensitivity and 97.2% specificity. Our results also suggested that the level of dNGScore was not related to urine cytological classifications and hematuria (Figure 3d,e), which suggested a higher predictive value for urine cytology-negative (<Class IV) cases and hematuria negative cases. In addition, dNGScore can discriminate both low- and high-grade non-muscle invasive bladder cancer as well as muscle invasive bladder cancer. This suggests that the dNGScore may be useful for early diagnosis of UCB.

The limitations of the present study were its small sample size, retrospective nature, selection bias, lack of independent validation group and non-clinical setting. Therefore, the results obtained in this study have to be regarded as preliminary and need further validation study. Because urine cytological results are not reliable in patients with early stage UCs, including UTUC, a large-scale prospective validation study in a natural cohort of patients with hematuria is required. In addition, the usefulness of regular follow-up for detecting recurrence after surgery remains unclear; furthermore, a large-scale prospective follow-up study after surgery was also needed. In addition, this study did not include patients with benign diseases or infections such as calculi, UTI, cystitis, prostatitis. Despite these limitations, the strength of the present study was that it is the largest to assess the implications of aberrant N-glycosyleted Igs for UCs detection. Our findings may be useful for detection of UC patients and identification of patients at urine cytology negative UC. Furthermore, to apply the routine clinical practice, we now developed lectin-sandwich immunoassay system to detect aberrant asialo bisecting GlcNAc type N-glycosylated Igs as described previously [28].

4. Materials and Methods

4.1. Serum Samples

The present study was conducted in accordance with the ethical standards of the Declaration of Helsinki and approved by the institutional review board of Hirosaki University School of Medicine ("study about carbohydrate structure change in urological disease"; approval number: 2014-195, approval date: 22 December 2014). Written or verbal informed consent was obtained from all serum donors. Between 2009 and 2016, we randomly selected serum available 237 patients with UC and also 96 patients with prostate cancer as other cancer controls from our serum bank. Serum from any clinical treated patients were excluded. We also obtained from 339 healthy controls selected from community-dwelling volunteers in the health maintenance programme of Iwaki Health Promotion Project [19,29]. All serum samples were collected at the first visit and stored at $-80\ °C$ until use. All tumors were staged according to the 2017 tumor-node-metastasis classification, 8th edition [30]. Histological classification of UC was performed according to the World Health Organization 1973 and 2004 grading systems [31]. Urine cytology classification was performed according to guideline of The Paris System working group [32]. Patient demographics are shown in Table 1.

4.2. Purification and Quantification of the Igs Fraction from Serum

Each serum sample (100 µL) was applied to the center of the Zeba™ Spin desalting resin plate (Thermo Fisher Scientific, Waltham, MA, USA) equilibrated with phosphate-buffered saline and centrifuged at $1000\times g$ for 2 min. The flow-through was collected as buffer-exchanged serum (100 µL). Purification of Igs fraction performed by using Melon™ Gel Spin Purification Kit (Thermo Fisher Scientific) according to the instructions. Buffer-exchanged serum (100 µL) was applied to the center of the Melon Gel resin equilibrated with purification buffer. After 5 min incubation, the Melon Gel resin was centrifuged at $1000\times g$ for 2 min and the flow-through was collected as a purified Igs fraction. A 10-µL aliquot of the Igs fraction was subjected to N-glycomics. To confirm the purity of the Igs fraction, the Melon Gel flow-through Igs fraction was subjected to SDS-PAGE and stained with CBB. Igs (total IgG, IgM and IgA) levels of purified Igs fraction were measured by using a Bio-plex Pro Human Isotyping 6-plex kit (Bio-Rad Laboratories, Hercules, CA, USA) according to the instructions.

4.3. Serum N-Glycomics of Igs Performed by Using the Glycoblotting Method and Mass Spectorometric Analysis

N-glycomics was performed as described previously. A 10-µL aliquot of the purified Igs fractions were analyzed using the glycoblotting method [11,12,15,33] on a Sweetblot instrument (System Instruments, Hachioji, Tokyo, Japan). Then, the resulting benzyloxiamine (BOA)-labelled glycans were detected by matrix-assisted laser desorption time-of-flight (MALDI-TOF) mass spectrometry (Ultraflex 3 TOF/TOF mass spectrometer; Bruker Daltonics, Bremen, Germany) (Figure A1a–f). Composition and structures of the glycans were predicted using the GlycoMod Tool (available online:

http://web.expasy.org/glycomod/) (Table A1). Quantitative reproducibility test of each N-glycans levels were then evaluated as described previously [19].

4.4. Statistical Analysis

Statistical analyses of clinical data were performed using SPSS v.22.0 (IBM Corporation, Armonk, NY, USA) and GraphPad Prism v.6.03 (GraphPad Software, San Diego, CA, USA). Categorical variables were reported as percentages and compared using the Fisher exact test. Age data were expressed as medians with 25th and 75th quartiles (Q1, Q3). Differences between the groups were statistically compared using the Student *t*-test for normally distributed data or the Mann–Whitney *U*-test for non-normally distributed data. Multivariable discriminant analysis for detection of UCs was performed by inputting UC event as an explanatory variable and N-glycan level as an objective variable. The diagnostic N-glycan score was calculated by multiplying candidate N-glycan levels by each discriminant function value. The diagnostic performance of N-glycan scores was evaluated using receiver operating characteristic (ROC) curve analysis developed using the library "rms" in R (available online: http://www.r-project.org/), and statistical differences between area under the curves (AUCs) were calculated using the same programme [34]. In order to assess the significant difference among two group of subjects we implemented a permutation tests and calculate permutation p value [35]. Differences with $p < 0.05$ were considered statistically significant.

5. Conclusions

In conclusion, aberrant N-glycosylation profiles of Igs determined by N-glycomics may be useful as diagnostic biomarkers for identifying UC patients. Future large-scale prospective validation studies are of vital importance.

Acknowledgments: The authors thank Satomi Sakamoto, Shoko Nagata and Yukie Nishizawa for their invaluable help with patient data management. This work was supported by Grants-in-Aid for Scientific Research (Nos. 15H02563 15K15579, 25220206, 17K11118, 17K11119, 17K16768, 17K16770 and 17K16771) from the Japan Society for the Promotion of Science.

Author Contributions: Toshikazu Tanaka and Tohru Yoneyama performed the bulk of the experiments. Shingo Hatakeyama, Kazuyuki Mori, Yuki Tobisawa, Shizuka Kurauchi and Ippei Takahashi provided serum samples and provided the patients' clinical information from healthy volunteers and urothelial carcinoma and prostate cancer patients. Daisuke Noro, Kengo Imanishi, Yuta Kojima, Shingo Hatakeyama, Hayato Yamamoto, Atsushi Imai, Takahiro Yoneyama, Yasuhiro Hashimoto, Takuya Koie and Chikara Ohyama diagnosed urothelial carcinoma and prostate cancer patients. Masakazu Tanaka and Shin-Ichiro Nishimura performed MALDI-TOF MS analysis. Yasuhiro Hashimoto performed pathological analyses. Chikara Ohyama and Tohru Yoneyama designed all the experiments, interpreted the data and wrote the manuscript.

Conflicts of Interest: Japanese patent application number 2017-207525. This patent application is a domestic priority application from Japanese patent application number 2017-076018.

Abbreviations

UC	Urothelial carcinoma
UCB	Urothelial carcinoma of the bladder
UTUC	Upper urinary tract urothelial carcinoma
HV	Healthy volunteers
PC	Prostate cancer
BPH	Beneign prostatic hyperplasia
HSPC	Hormone sensitive prostate cancer
NMIBC	Nonmuscle invasive bladder cancer
MIBC	Muscle invasive bladder cancer
NI-UTUC	Noninvasive UTUC
I-UTUC	Invasive UTUC
Igs	Immunogloblins
dNGScore	Diagnostic N-glycan Score

AUC	Area under the curve
ROC	Receiver operating characteristic curves
BTA	Bladder tumor antigen
NMP22	Nuclear matrix protein number 22
IQR	Interquartile range
NPV	Negative predictive value
PPV	Positive predictive value
UTI	Urinary tract infection
MALDI-TOF	Matrix-assisted laser desorption time-of-flight
Man	Mannose
Gal	Galactose
GlcNAc	N-acetylglucosamine
Fuc	Fucose
Sia	N-acetylneuraminic acid
CBB	Coomassie brilliant blue

Appendix A

Table A1. Thirty-two types of N-glycans that showed good quantitative reproducibility in all Igs fraction samples and could be analyzed statistically.

#	m/z	Composition
1	1362.5	(Hex)2 + (Man)3(GlcNAc)2
2	1524.5	(Hex)3 + (Man)3(GlcNAc)2
3	1565.5	(Hex)5 + (HexNAc)3
4	1590.6	(HexNAc)2(dHex)1 + (Man)3(GlcNAc)2
5	1606.6	(Hex)1(HexNAc)2 + (Man)3(GlcNAc)2
6	1647.6	(HexNAc)3 + (Man)3(GlcNAc)2
7	1686.6	(Hex)4 + (Man)3(GlcNAc)2
8	1708.6	(Hex)1(HexNAc)1(NeuAc)1 + (Man)3(GlcNAc)2
9	1752.6	(Hex)1(HexNAc)2(dHex)1 + (Man)3(GlcNAc)2
10	1768.6	(Hex)2(HexNAc)2 + (Man)3(GlcNAc)2
11	1793.7	(HexNAc)3(dHex)1 + (Man)3(GlcNAc)2
12	1809.7	(Hex)1(HexNAc)3 + (Man)3(GlcNAc)2
13	1848.6	(Hex)5 + (Man)3(GlcNAc)2
14	1870.7	(Hex)2(HexNAc)1(NeuAc)1 + (Man)3(GlcNAc)2
15	1914.7	(Hex)2(HexNAc)2(dHex)1 + (Man)3(GlcNAc)2
16	1955.7	(Hex)1(HexNAc)3(dHex)1 + (Man)3(GlcNAc)2
17	2010.7	(Hex)6 + (Man)3(GlcNAc)2
18	2032.7	(Hex)3(HexNac)1(NeuAc)1 + (Man)3(GlcNAc)2
19	2057.8	(Hex)1(HexNAc)2(dHex)1(NeuAc)1 + (Man)3(GlcNAc)2
20	2073.8	(Hex)2(HexNAc)2(NeuAc)1 + (Man)3(GlcNAc)2
21	2117.8	(Hex)2(HexNAc)3(dHex)1 + (Man)3(GlcNAc)2
22	2219.8	(Hex)2(HexNAc)2(dHex)1(NeuAc)1 + (Man)3(GlcNAc)2
23	2336.9	(Hex)3(HexNAc)4 + (Man)3(GlcNAc)2
IS	2348.9 [1]	Internal standard (BOA-labeled A2 amide)
24	2378.9	(Hex)2(HexNAc)2(NeuAc)2 + (Man)3(GlcNAc)2
25	2422.9	(Hex)2(HexNAc)3(dHex)1(NeuAc)1 + (Man)3(GlcNAc)2
26	2524.9	(Hex)2(HexNAc)2(dHex)1(NeuAc)2 + (Man)3(GlcNAc)2
27	2727.9	(Hex)2(HexNAc)3(dHex)1(NeuAc)2 + (Man)3(GlcNAc)2
28	2743.9	(Hex)3(HexNAc)3(NeuAc)2 + (Man)3(GlcNAc)2
29	2890.1	(Hex)3(HexNAc)3(dHex)1(NeuAc)2 + (Man)3(GlcNAc)2
30	3049.1	(Hex)3(HexNAc)3(NeuAc)3 + (Man)3(GlcNAc)2
31	3195.2	(Hex)3(HexNAc)3(dHex)1(NeuAc)3 + (Man)3(GlcNAc)2
32	3341.2	(Hex)3 (HexNAc)3 (Deoxyhexose)2 (NeuAc)3 + (Man)3(GlcNAc)2

[1] m/z 2348.9 is the internal standard, disialo-galactosylated biantennary N-glycan, which contains amidated sialic acid residues (A2 amide glycans). Compositional annotations and putative structures are represented by the following abbreviations. Hex: hexose, HexNAc: N-acetylhexosamine, dHex: deoxyhexose.

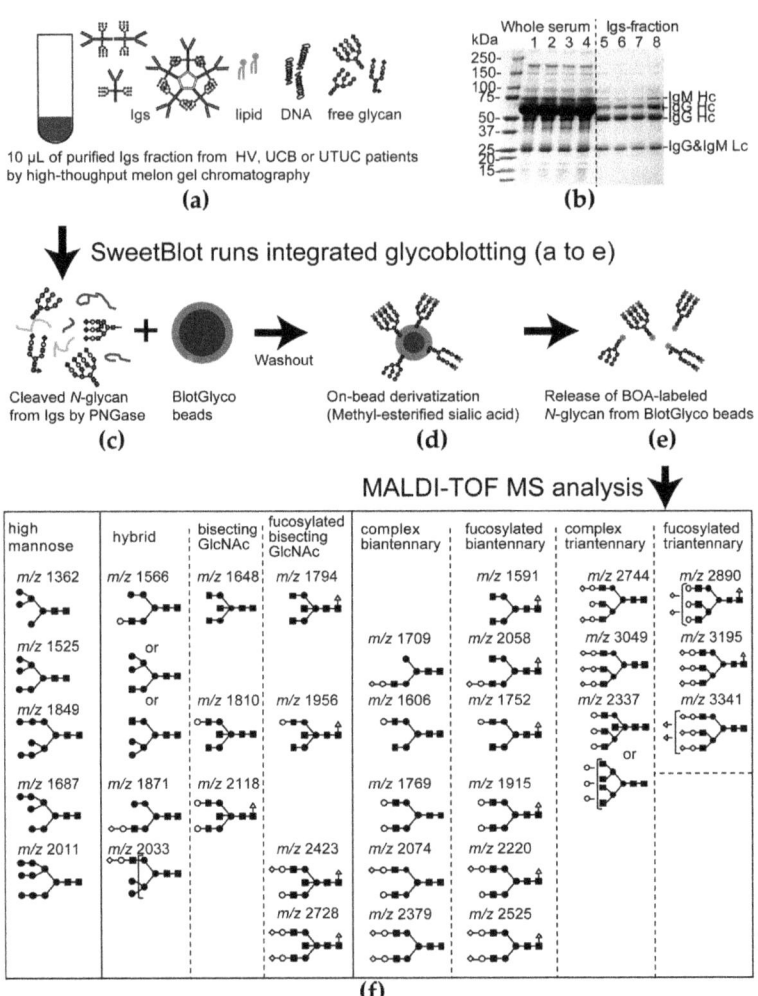

Figure A1. The general protocol for the integrated glycoblotting technique and workflow for glycoblotting-based high-throughput clinical glycan analysis. (**a**) Ten-microliter serum Ig fraction samples were applied to SweetBlot™ (System Instruments, Hachioji, Japan) for glycoblotting; (**b**) Coomassie brilliant blue (CBB)-stained band patterns on a sodium dodecyl sulfate-polyacrylamide gel for representative whole serum and purified Ig fraction samples; (**c**) After enzymatic N-glycan cleavage from Ig proteins, the total N-glycans released into the digestion mixture were directly mixed with BlotGlyco H beads (Sumitomo Bakelite, Co., Tokyo, Japan) to capture N-glycans; (**d**) After the beads were separated from other molecules by washing, sialic acid was methyl esterified; (**e**) These processed N-glycans were then labelled with benzyloxyamine (BOA) and released from BlotGlyco H beads; (**f**) Mass spectra of BOA-labelled N-glycans from Ig fractions were acquired using an Ultraflex III instrument (Bruker Daltonics, Germany). Total 32 type of N-glycans were identified in Igs fraction. Identified N-glycan structures are indicated by monosaccharide symbols: white circles, galactose (Gal); black circles, mannose (Man); black squares, N-acetylglucosamine (GlcNAc); black triangle, fucose (Fuc) and black diamonds, sialic acid.

References

1. Park, J.C.; Hahn, N.M. Bladder cancer: A disease ripe for major advances. *Clin. Adv. Hematol. Oncol.* **2014**, *12*, 838–845. [PubMed]
2. Munoz, J.J.; Ellison, L.M. Upper tract urothelial neoplasms: Incidence and survival during the last 2 decades. *J. Urol.* **2000**, *164*, 1523–1525. [CrossRef]
3. Siegel, R.; Naishadham, D.; Jemal, A. Cancer statistics, 2012. *CA Cancer J. Clin.* **2012**, *62*, 10–29. [CrossRef] [PubMed]
4. Inman, B.A.; Tran, V.T.; Fradet, Y.; Lacombe, L. Carcinoma of the upper urinary tract: Predictors of survival and competing causes of mortality. *Cancer* **2009**, *115*, 2853–2862. [CrossRef] [PubMed]
5. Cowan, N.C. CT urography for hematuria. *Nat. Rev. Urol.* **2012**, *9*, 218–226. [CrossRef] [PubMed]
6. Babjuk, M.; Bohle, A.; Burger, M.; Capoun, O.; Cohen, D.; Comperat, E.M.; Hernandez, V.; Kaasinen, E.; Palou, J.; Roupret, M.; et al. EAU Guidelines on Non-Muscle-invasive Urothelial Carcinoma of the Bladder: Update 2016. *Eur. Urol.* **2016**, *71*, 447–461. [CrossRef] [PubMed]
7. Margulis, V.; Shariat, S.F.; Matin, S.F.; Kamat, A.M.; Zigeuner, R.; Kikuchi, E.; Lotan, Y.; Weizer, A.; Raman, J.D.; Wood, C.G. Outcomes of radical nephroureterectomy: A series from the Upper Tract Urothelial Carcinoma Collaboration. *Cancer* **2009**, *115*, 1224–1233. [CrossRef] [PubMed]
8. Ramakumar, S.; Bhuiyan, J.; Besse, J.A.; Roberts, S.G.; Wollan, P.C.; Blute, M.L.; O'Kane, D.J. Comparison of screening methods in the detection of bladder cancer. *J. Urol.* **1999**, *161*, 388–394. [CrossRef]
9. Narayan, V.M.; Adejoro, O.; Schwartz, I.; Ziegelmann, M.; Elliott, S.; Konety, B.R. The Prevalence and Impact of Urinary Marker Testing in Patients with Bladder Cancer. *J. Urol.* **2017**. [CrossRef] [PubMed]
10. Gopalakrishna, A.; Longo, T.A.; Fantony, J.J.; Owusu, R.; Foo, W.C.; Dash, R.; Inman, B.A. The diagnostic accuracy of urine-based tests for bladder cancer varies greatly by patient. *BMC Urol.* **2016**, *16*, 30. [CrossRef] [PubMed]
11. Hatakeyama, S.; Amano, M.; Tobisawa, Y.; Yoneyama, T.; Tsuchiya, N.; Habuchi, T.; Nishimura, S.-I.; Ohyama, C. Serum N-Glycan Alteration Associated with Renal Cell Carcinoma Detected by High Throughput Glycan Analysis. *J. Urol.* **2014**, *191*, 805–813. [CrossRef] [PubMed]
12. Ishibashi, Y.; Tobisawa, Y.; Hatakeyama, S.; Ohashi, T.; Tanaka, M.; Narita, S.; Koie, T.; Habuchi, T.; Nishimura, S.-I.; Ohyama, C.; et al. Serum tri- and tetra-antennary N-glycan is a potential predictive biomarker for castration-resistant prostate cancer. *Prostate* **2014**, *74*, 1521–1529. [CrossRef] [PubMed]
13. Maho Amano, M.T. N- and O-glycome analysis of serum and urine from bladder cancer patients using a high-throughput glycoblotting method. *J. Glycom. Lipidom.* **2013**, *3*, 108. [CrossRef]
14. Narita, T.; Hatakeyama, S.; Yoneyama, T.; Narita, S.; Yamashita, S.; Mitsuzuka, K.; Sakurai, T.; Kawamura, S.; Tochigi, T.; Takahashi, I.; et al. Clinical implications of serum N-glycan profiling as a diagnostic and prognostic biomarker in germ-cell tumors. *Cancer Med.* **2017**, *6*, 739–748. [CrossRef] [PubMed]
15. Nouso, K.; Amano, M.; Ito, Y.M.; Miyahara, K.; Morimoto, Y.; Kato, H.; Tsutsumi, K.; Tomoda, T.; Yamamoto, N.; Nakamura, S.; et al. Clinical utility of high-throughput glycome analysis in patients with pancreatic cancer. *J. Gastroenterol.* **2013**, *48*, 1171–1179. [CrossRef] [PubMed]
16. Kirwan, A.; Utratna, M.; O'Dwyer, M.E.; Joshi, L.; Kilcoyne, M. Glycosylation-Based Serum Biomarkers for Cancer Diagnostics and Prognostics. *Biomed. Res. Int.* **2015**, *2015*, 490531. [CrossRef] [PubMed]
17. Li, C.W.; Lim, S.O.; Xia, W.; Lee, H.H.; Chan, L.C.; Kuo, C.W.; Khoo, K.H.; Chang, S.S.; Cha, J.H.; Kim, T.; et al. Glycosylation and stabilization of programmed death ligand-1 suppresses T-cell activity. *Nat. Commun.* **2016**, *7*, 12632. [CrossRef] [PubMed]
18. Veillon, L.; Fakih, C.; Abou-El-Hassan, H.; Kobeissy, F.; Mechref, Y. Glycosylation Changes in Brain Cancer. *ACS Chem. Neurosci.* **2017**. [CrossRef] [PubMed]
19. Oikawa, M.; Hatakeyama, S.; Yoneyma, T.; Tobisawa, Y.; Narita, T.; Yamamoto, H.; Hashimoto, Y.; Koie, T.; Narita, S.; Sasaki, A.; et al. Significance of Serum N-glycan Profiling as a Diagnostic Biomarker in Urothelial Carcinoma. *Eur. Urol. Focus* **2016**. [CrossRef] [PubMed]
20. Wuhrer, M.; Selman, M.H.; McDonnell, L.A.; Kumpfel, T.; Derfuss, T.; Khademi, M.; Olsson, T.; Hohlfeld, R.; Meinl, E.; Krumbholz, M. Pro-inflammatory pattern of IgG1 Fc glycosylation in multiple sclerosis cerebrospinal fluid. *J. Neuroinflamm.* **2015**, *12*, 235. [CrossRef] [PubMed]

21. Suzuki, Y.; Suzuki, H.; Makita, Y.; Takahata, A.; Takahashi, K.; Muto, M.; Sasaki, Y.; Kelimu, A.; Matsuzaki, K.; Yanagawa, H.; et al. Diagnosis and activity assessment of immunoglobulin A nephropathy: Current perspectives on noninvasive testing with aberrantly glycosylated immunoglobulin A-related biomarkers. *Int. J. Nephrol. Renovasc. Dis.* **2014**, *7*, 409–414. [CrossRef] [PubMed]
22. Malard-Castagnet, S.; Dugast, E.; Degauque, N.; Pallier, A.; Soulillou, J.P.; Cesbron, A.; Giral, M.; Harb, J.; Brouard, S. Sialylation of antibodies in kidney recipients with de novo donor specific antibody, with or without antibody mediated rejection. *Hum. Immunol.* **2015**, *77*, 1076–1083. [CrossRef] [PubMed]
23. Rademacher, T.W.; Parekh, R.B.; Dwek, R.A.; Isenberg, D.; Rook, G.; Axford, J.S.; Roitt, I. The role of IgG glycoforms in the pathogenesis of rheumatoid arthritis. *Springer Semin. Immunopathol.* **1988**, *10*, 231–249. [CrossRef] [PubMed]
24. Kazuno, S.; Furukawa, J.; Shinohara, Y.; Murayama, K.; Fujime, M.; Ueno, T.; Fujimura, T. Glycosylation status of serum immunoglobulin G in patients with prostate diseases. *Cancer Med.* **2016**, *5*, 1137–1146. [CrossRef] [PubMed]
25. Ruhaak, L.R.; Barkauskas, D.A.; Torres, J.; Cooke, C.L.; Wu, L.D.; Stroble, C.; Ozcan, S.; Williams, C.C.; Camorlinga, M.; Rocke, D.M.; et al. The Serum Immunoglobulin G Glycosylation Signature of Gastric Cancer. *EuPA Open Proteom.* **2015**, *6*, 1–9. [CrossRef] [PubMed]
26. Theodoratou, E.; Thaci, K.; Agakov, F.; Timofeeva, M.N.; Stambuk, J.; Pucic-Bakovic, M.; Vuckovic, F.; Orchard, P.; Agakova, A.; Din, F.V.; et al. Glycosylation of plasma IgG in colorectal cancer prognosis. *Sci. Rep.* **2016**, *6*, 28098. [CrossRef] [PubMed]
27. Zhang, D.; Chen, B.; Wang, Y.; Xia, P.; He, C.; Liu, Y.; Zhang, R.; Zhang, M.; Li, Z. Disease-specific IgG Fc N-glycosylation as personalized biomarkers to differentiate gastric cancer from benign gastric diseases. *Sci. Rep.* **2016**, *6*, 25957. [CrossRef] [PubMed]
28. Hagiwara, K.; Tobisawa, Y.; Kaya, T.; Kaneko, T.; Hatakeyama, S.; Mori, K.; Hashimoto, Y.; Koie, T.; Suda, Y.; Ohyama, C.; et al. Wisteria floribunda Agglutinin and Its Reactive-Glycan-Carrying Prostate-Specific Antigen as a Novel Diagnostic and Prognostic Marker of Prostate Cancer. *Int. J. Mol. Sci.* **2017**, *18*, 261. [CrossRef] [PubMed]
29. Tanaka, T.; Hatakeyama, S.; Yamamoto, H.; Narita, T.; Hamano, I.; Matsumoto, T.; Soma, O.; Tobisawa, Y.; Yoneyama, T.; Yoneyama, T.; et al. Clinical relevance of aortic calcification in urolithiasis patients. *BMC Urol.* **2017**, *17*, 25. [CrossRef] [PubMed]
30. James, D.B.; Gospodarowicz, M.K.; Wittekind, C. *TNM Classification of Malignant Tumours*, 8th ed.; Wiley-Blackwell: Oxford, UK, 2016; p. 272.
31. Humphrey, P.A.; Moch, H.; Cubilla, A.L.; Ulbright, T.M.; Reuter, V.E. The 2016 WHO Classification of Tumours of the Urinary System and Male Genital Organs-Part B: Prostate and Bladder Tumours. *Eur. Urol.* **2016**, *70*, 106–119. [CrossRef] [PubMed]
32. Barkan, G.A.; Wojcik, E.M.; Nayar, R.; Savic-Prince, S.; Quek, M.L.; Kurtycz, D.F.; Rosenthal, D.L. The Paris System for Reporting Urinary Cytology: The Quest to Develop a Standardized Terminology. *Adv. Anat. Pathol.* **2016**, *23*, 193–201. [CrossRef] [PubMed]
33. Hatakeyama, S.; Amano, M.; Tobisawa, Y.; Yoneyama, T.; Tsushima, M.; Hirose, K.; Yoneyama, T.; Hashimoto, Y.; Koie, T.; Saitoh, H.; et al. Serum N-Glycan Profiling Predicts Prognosis in Patients Undergoing Hemodialysis. *Sci. World J.* **2013**, *2013*, 268407. [CrossRef] [PubMed]
34. Harrell, F.E., Jr.; Lee, K.L.; Mark, D.B. Multivariable prognostic models: Issues in developing models, evaluating assumptions and adequacy, and measuring and reducing errors. *Stat. Med.* **1996**, *15*, 361–387. [CrossRef]
35. Christie, D. Resampling with Excel. *Teach. Stat.* **2004**, *26*, 9–14. [CrossRef]

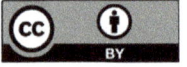

© 2017 by the authors. Licensee MDPI, Basel, Switzerland. This article is an open access article distributed under the terms and conditions of the Creative Commons Attribution (CC BY) license (http://creativecommons.org/licenses/by/4.0/).

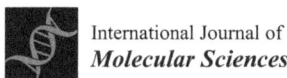

Article

Regulatory T Cells and Tumor-Associated Macrophages in the Tumor Microenvironment in Non-Muscle Invasive Bladder Cancer Treated with Intravesical Bacille Calmette-Guérin: A Long-Term Follow-Up Study of a Japanese Cohort

Makito Miyake [1,*], Yoshihiro Tatsumi [1,2], Daisuke Gotoh [1], Sayuri Ohnishi [1], Takuya Owari [1], Kota Iida [1], Kenta Ohnishi [1], Shunta Hori [1], Yosuke Morizawa [1], Yoshitaka Itami [1], Yasushi Nakai [1], Takeshi Inoue [1], Satoshi Anai [1], Kazumasa Torimoto [1], Katsuya Aoki [1], Keiji Shimada [3], Noboru Konishi [2], Nobumichi Tanaka [1] and Kiyohide Fujimoto [1]

1. Department of Urology, Nara Medical University, 840 Shijo-cho, Kashihara-shi, Nara 634-8522, Japan; takuro.birds.nest@gmail.com (Y.T.); dgotou@gmail.com (D.G.); sayuri3@naramed-u.ac.jp (S.O.); tintherye@gmail.com (T.O.); kota1006ida@yahoo.co.jp (K.I.); kenzmedico0912@yahoo.co.jp (K.O.); horimaus@gmail.com (S.H.); tigers.yosuke@gmail.com (Y.M.); y.itami.324@gmail.com (Y.I.); nakaiyasusiuro@live.jp (Y.N.); you1513tt@yahoo.co.jp (T.I.); sanai@naramed-u.ac.jp (S.A.); torimoto@nmu-gw.naramed-u.ac.jp (K.T.); aokik@naramed-u.ac.jp (K.A.); sendo@naramed-u.ac.jp (N.T.); kiyokun@naramed-u.ac.jp (K.F.)
2. Department of Pathology, Nara Medical University, 840 Shijo-cho, Kashihara-shi, Nara 634-8522, Japan; n-konishi@takai-hp.com
3. Department of Pathology, Nara City Hospital, 1501 Higashi kidera-cho, Nara-shi, Nara 630-8305, Japan; k-shimada@nara-jadecom.jp
* Correspondence: makitomiyake@naramed-u.ac.jp; Tel.: +81-744-223-051 (ext. 2338); Fax: +81-744-22-9282

Received: 23 September 2017; Accepted: 17 October 2017; Published: 19 October 2017

Abstract: The clinical significance of regulatory T cells (Treg) and tumor-associated macrophages (TAM) in the tumor microenvironment of human bladder cancer remains unclear. The aim of this study is to explore their relevance to oncological features in non-muscle invasive bladder cancer (NMIBC). We carried out immunohistochemical analysis of forkhead box P3 (FOXP3, Treg maker), CD204 (TAM marker), and interleukin-6 (IL6) using surgical specimens obtained from 154 NMIBC patients. The Treg and TAM counts surrounding the cancer lesion and IL6-positive cancer cell counts were evaluated against clinicopathological variables. We focused on the ability of the Treg and TAM counts around the cancer lesion to predict outcomes after adjuvant intravesical Bacille Calmette–Guérin (BCG) treatment. High Treg counts were associated with female patients, older age, T1 category, and high tumor grade. TAM count was significantly correlated with Treg count and with IL6-positive cancer cell count. In our analysis of 71 patients treated with BCG, high counts of Treg and TAM were associated with shorter recurrence-free survival, and the former was an independent predictor of recurrence. Poor response to intravesical BCG was associated with Treg and TAM in the tumor microenvironment. Disrupting the immune network can be a supplementary therapeutic approach for NMIBC patients receiving intravesical BCG.

Keywords: regulatory T cell; tumor-associated macrophage; non-muscle invasive bladder cancer; intravesical recurrence; progression; Bacille Calmette–Guérin

1. Introduction

Urothelial carcinoma (UC) of the bladder is a heterogeneous disease in terms of its clinical and biological aspects [1]. Among non-muscle invasive bladder cancer (NMIBC) patients, several factors such as age, T category, tumor grade, tumor size, and multiplicity are recognized to predict the risk of intravesical recurrence and progression after transurethral resection of bladder tumor (TURBT) [2,3]. Despite advancements in detection technologies, surgical techniques, and adjuvant intravesical treatment, clinical management of high-risk diseases remains challenging [4,5].

Intravesical administration of Bacille Calmette–Guérin (BCG) is a standard treatment for carcinoma in situ (CIS) and an adjuvant option for T1 and high-risk Ta tumors following TURBT [6]. However, a delay in radical cystectomy (RC) leads to shortened cancer-specific survival as compared to immediate RC at the time of NMIBC [7]. Thus, there is an urgent need for biomarkers to identify patients who will benefit from intravesical BCG or should undergo immediate RC. Although possible mechanisms underlying BCG-induced antitumor activity and relevant molecules have been studied [8–10], they are not fully understood. Briefly, BCG is internalized into urothelial cells through the formation of a complex with fibronectin, followed by antigen presentation to BCG-specific CD4+ T-cells by antigen-presenting cells. Pro-inflammatory cytokines such as interleukin-6 (IL6) and interferon-γ are secreted to recruit a Th1-induced immunoreaction with the recognition of cancer cells through the activation of macrophages, CD8+ T-cells, and natural killer cells.

Several previous studies have demonstrated that the pre-BCG baseline status of Th1/Th2 balance, regulatory T cell (Treg) recruitment, and tumor-associated macrophage (TAM) polarization in the tumor microenvironment could influence the clinical response to BCG [10–12]. In light of the sparse data on the clinical significance of Treg/TAM and their relevance to oncological outcomes of NMIBC treated with intravesical BCG—especially in Japanese patients—this study was conducted with the goal of improving patient care.

2. Results

2.1. Association of Treg and TAM in the Cancerous Area with Baseline Characteristics

Treg and TAM significantly differed in their localization patterns (Figure 1A). Most of the Treg cells localized in the stroma around the cancer lesion regardless of tumor stage and grade, whereas TAM had a tendency to infiltrate into the tumor area in high-grade tumors compared to low-grade tumors. In an analysis of 154 tumors, the median counts per high power field (HPF) of Treg and TAM were eight (interquartile range [IQR], 3–15) and 23 (IQR 16–33), respectively. The appropriate cutoff points of Treg and TAM count have not been established yet, especially in bladder UC. The cutoff values for separating low counts and high counts for Treg and TAM were set as 10 and 25 respectively, based on the median values. With these thresholds, high counts of Treg and TAM were found in 68 (44%) and 62 (41%) out of 154 tumors, respectively. The clinicopathological variables and their association with Treg and TAM in 154 patients with NMIBC are outlined in Table 1. High Treg count was associated with female patients ($p = 0.001$), older age ($p = 0.024$), T1 category ($p < 0.001$), high tumor grade ($p < 0.001$), and the presence of CIS ($p = 0.011$), whereas the count of TAM was not associated with any variable (Table 1).

Table 1. Clinicopathologic variables and association with Treg and TAM in primary NMIBC.

Variables	N	Treg (FOXP3+ Cell)			TAM (CD204+ Cell)		
		Low	High	p Value	Low	High	p Value
Total	154 (100%)	86 (56%)	68 (44%)	—	92 (59%)	62 (41%)	—
Sex				0.0012			0.45
Male	137 (89%)	83 (61%)	54 (39%)		78 (57%)	59 (43%)	
Female	17 (11%)	3 (18%)	14 (82%)		8 (47%)	9 (53%)	
Age at initial TURBT categorical				0.056			0.75

Table 1. Cont.

Variables	N	Treg (FOXP3+ Cell)			TAM (CD204+ Cell)		
		Low	High	p Value	Low	High	p Value
<60	18 (12%)	15 (83%)	3 (17%)		11 (61%)	7 (39%)	
60 to 70	55 (36%)	34 (62%)	21 (38%)		32 (58%)	23 (42%)	
>70	81 (52%)	43 (53%)	38 (47%)		43 (53%)	38 (47%)	
Continuous median (IQR)	71 (65–76)	69 (63–76)	73 (69–79)	0.024	71 (64–76)	71 (68–77)	0.22
T category				<0.001			0.25
Ta	68 (44%)	52 (76%)	16 (24%)		41 (60%)	27 (40%)	
T1	73 (47%)	30 (41%)	43 (59%)		36 (49%)	37 (51%)	
Tis	13 (9%)	10 (77%)	3 (23%)		9 (69%)	4 (31%)	
Tumor grade				<0.001			0.16
Low	71 (46%)	53 (75%)	18 (25%)		44 (62%)	27 (38%)	
High	83 (54%)	39 (47%)	44 (53%)		42 (51%)	41 (49%)	
Tumor architecture				0.98			0.69
Papillary	134 (87%)	80 (60%)	54 (40%)		74 (55%)	60 (45%)	
Non-papillary	20 (13%)	12 (60%)	8 (40%)		12 (60%)	8 (40%)	
Multiplicity				0.64			0.71
Single	88 (57%)	54 (61%)	34 (39%)		48 (55%)	40 (45%)	
Multiple	66 (43%)	38 (58%)	28 (42%)		38 (58%)	28 (42%)	
Tumor size				0.45			0.99
Less than 3 cm	119 (77%)	73 (61%)	46 (39%)		69 (58%)	50 (42%)	
3 cm or more	35 (23%)	19 (54%)	16 (46%)		17 (49%)	18 (51%)	
CIS				0.011			0.29
No	91 (59%)	62 (68%)	29 (32%)		54 (59%)	37 (41%)	
Yes	63 (41%)	30 (48%)	33 (52%)		32 (51%)	31 (49%)	
LVI (in T1 tumor, n = 73)				0.66			0.93
Negative	49 (67%)	21 (43%)	28 (57%)		24 (49%)	25 (51%)	
Positive	24 (33%)	9 (38%)	15 (62%)		12 (50%)	12 (50%)	
Intravesical adjuvant therapy				0.65			0.37
No	64 (42%)	41 (64%)	23 (36%)		40 (62%)	24 (38%)	
BCG	71 (46%)	40 (56%)	31 (44%)		36 (51%)	35 (49%)	
Chemotherapy	19 (12%)	11 (58%)	8 (42%)		10 (53%)	9 (47%)	

Treg, regulatory T cell; TAM, Tumor-associated macrophage; NMIBC, non-muscle invasive bladder cancer; TURBT, transurethral resection of bladder tumor; IQR, interquartile range; CIS, Carcinoma in situ; LVI, lymphovascular invasion; BCG, Bacillus Calmette-Guerin.

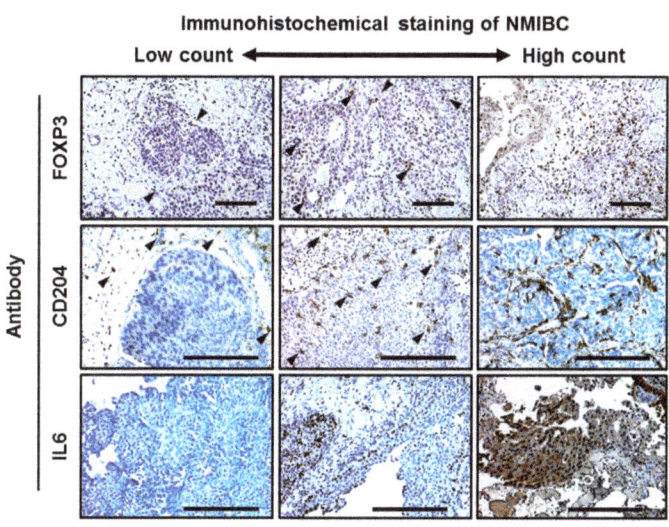

Figure 1. Cont.

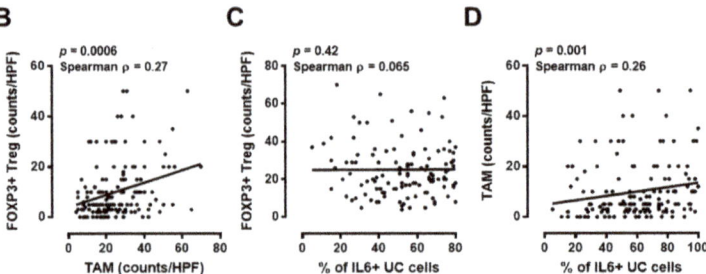

Figure 1. Immunohistochemical quantification of regulatory T cells, tumor-associated macrophages, and IL6-positive urothelial carcinoma cells. (**A**) Representative expression status of FOXP3, CD204, and IL6 in human bladder cancer tissues. Images were captured at 100× (FOXP3) or 200× (CD204 and IL6) magnification. Black arrowheads in the FOXP3 and CD204 images indicate positive-stained immune cells that exist in the stroma near the cancer cells or filtrate to the tumors. Scale bars, 200 μm. The interrelationship between (**B**) the Treg counts and TAM counts, (**C**) the Treg counts and the percentage of IL6$^+$ cancer cells, and (**D**) the TAM counts and the percentage of IL6+ cancer cells were examined using Spearman's correlation. HPF, high power field; Treg, regulatory T cell; TAM, tumor-associated macrophage; UC, urothelial carcinoma.

2.2. Correlation among Treg, TAM, and IL6 in the Bladder Tumor Microenvironment

IL6 is one of the major pro-inflammatory cytokines in the tumor microenvironment, and promotes cancer progression and therapeutic resistance [13]. To investigate the correlation between Treg, TAM, and IL6+ UC cells, the Spearman correlation coefficient was analyzed among the three markers. There was a weak positive correlation between the counts of Treg and TAM ($p < 0.001$, Figure 1B). The count of TAM, but not Treg ($p = 0.42$, Figure 1C), positively correlated with counts of IL6+ cancer cells ($p = 0.001$, Figure 1D).

2.3. Prognostic Role of Baseline Treg and TAM in NMIBC Treated with Intravesical BCG

In the analysis of 71 patients treated with intravesical BCG, 40 (56%) had recurrence and 17 (24%) developed progression after a median follow-up period of 83 (IQR 61–115) months. To examine the relevance of the studied variables and prognosis, we performed univariate and multivariate analyses for recurrence-free survival (RFS) and progression-free survival (PFS) (Table 2). High counts of Treg and TAM and low tumor grade were associated with shorter recurrence-free survival in the univariate analysis (Figure 2A,B,D,E), while high count of Treg ($p = 0.001$, hazard ratio (HR) = 3.07, vs. low count) and low tumor grade ($p = 0.01$, HR = 0.27, vs. high tumor grade) were identified as independent predictors for recurrence. An additional analysis revealed that a high count of Treg was an independent predictor for progression ($p = 0.021$, HR = 3.43, vs. low count), whereas high counts of TAM showed marginal association with short PFS in the univariate analysis ($p = 0.052$, HR = 3.35, vs. low count). When patients were stratified into three groups according to the counts of Treg and TAM, 26 (37%) patients exhibited low counts of both, 24 (34%) exhibited a high count of either Treg or TAM, and the remaining 21 (29%) exhibited high counts of both. Both RFS and PFS decreased dramatically as the number of high counts of immune cells increased (Figure 2C,F).

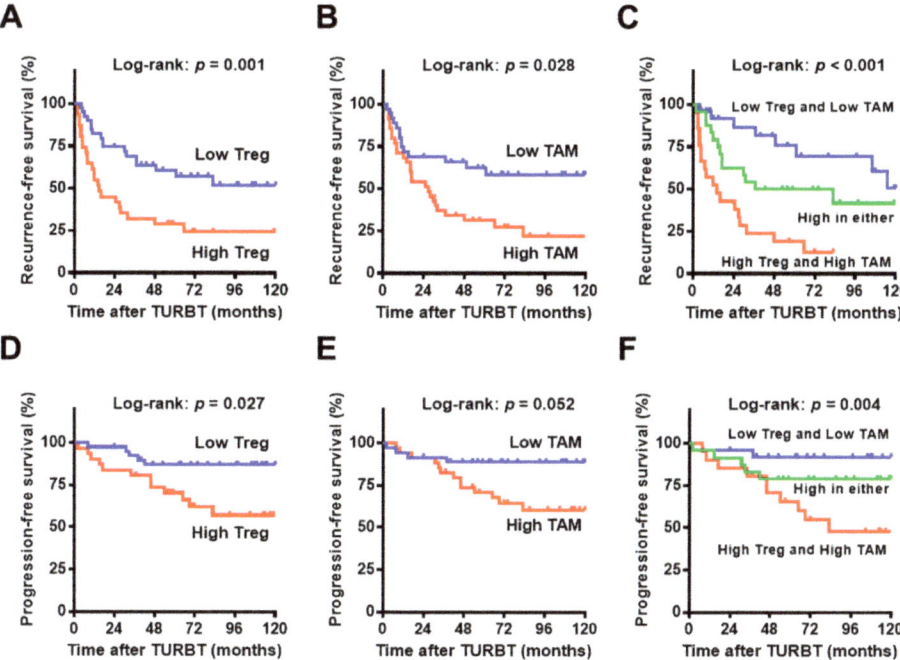

Figure 2. Kaplan–Meier plots for 71 patients treated with intravesical BCG. Intravesical recurrence-free survival (**A–C**) and progression-free survival (**D–F**) after initial TURBT are plotted. (**A,D**) Survival curves according to the Treg count, low (<10 cells/HPF) vs. high (≥10 cells/HPF); (**B,E**) survival curves according to the TAM count, low (<25 cells/HPF) vs. high (≥25 cells/HPF); (**C,F**) survival curves according to the number of immune cells with high counts (0, blue; 1, green; 2, red). The log-rank test was used for comparison. Treg, regulatory T cell; TAM, tumor-associated macrophage. Author 1, A.B. Title of Thesis. Level of Thesis, Degree-Granting University, Location of University, Date of Completion.

Table 2. The prognostic factors for recurrence and progression in 71 NMIBC patients treated with BCG.

Variables	N	Intravesical Recurrence-Free Survival						Progression-Free Survival					
		Univariate			Multivariate †			Univariate			Multivariate †		
		HR	95% CI	p Value	HR	95% CI	p Value	HR	95% CI	p Value	HR	95% CI	p Value
Sex													
Male	63 (89%)	1						1					
Female	8 (11%)	0.64	0.24–1.72	0.52	NA			1.24	0.25–6.21	0.98	NA		
Age													
≤70	37 (52%)	1						1					
>70	34 (48%)	1.05	0.56–1.97	0.91	NA			1.88	0.73–4.86	0.22	NA		
T stage													
Ta or isolated Tis	30 (42%)	1						1					
T1	41 (58%)	1.20	0.64–2.26	0.69	NA			1.29	0.49–3.40	0.81	NA		
Tumor grade													
Low	13 (18%)	1						1					
High	58 (82%)	0.68	0.26–0.96	0.04	0.81	0.24–1.16	0.10	1.85	0.56–6.09	0.48	NA		
Multiplicity													
Single	38 (54%)	1						1					
Multiple	33 (46%)	0.74	0.39–1.39	0.78	NA			1.20	0.46–3.15	0.46	NA		
Tumor size													
<3 cm	52 (73%)	1						1					
≥3 cm	19 (27%)	0.76	0.38–1.52	0.58	NA			1.05	0.39–2.87	0.89	NA		
Concomitant CIS													
No	22 (31%)	1						1					
Yes	49 (69%)	0.48	0.24–1.06	0.097	NA			2.48	0.91–6.74	0.14	NA		
Treg													
Low	31 (44%)	1						1					
High	40 (56%)	2.53	1.32–4.86	0.001	3.07	1.55–6.07	0.001	3.38	1.29–8.88	0.027	3.43	1.20–9.74	0.021
TAM													
Low	35 (49%)	1						1					
High	36 (51%)	2.31	1.27–4.30	0.029	1.39	0.68–2.84	0.37	3.35	1.29–8.66	0.052	2.50	0.79–8.02	0.12
IL6+ UC cells													
Low	32 (45%)	1						1					
High	39 (55%)	1.36	0.73–2.56	0.22	NA			1.39	0.53–3.61	0.54	NA		

NMIBC, non-muscle invasive bladder cancer; BCG, Bacillus Calmette-Guerin; HR, hazard ratio; CI, confidence interval; CIS, Carcinoma in situ; Treg, regulatory T cell; TAM, Tumor-associated macrophage; UC, urothelial carcinoma; † Multivariate Cox regression analysis; NA, not analyzed.

3. Discussion

This study demonstrates the association between poor responses to intravesical BCG and both Treg and TAM in the tumor microenvironment of human bladder UC. Although it has been decades since intravesical BCG was first introduced for bladder UC treatment in 1976 [14], no molecular biomarkers are available in clinical settings for predicting responses. There is currently little clinical evidence about associations between these tumor-supporting immune cells and resistance to intravesical BCG. A recent report by Pichler et al. investigated the baseline immune environment in NMIBC treated with intravesical BCG by IHC analysis using a total of 10 antibodies. The authors concluded that increased counts of CD4+ and GATA3+ T-cells were associated with prolonged RFS, whereas high counts of TAM and Treg were associated with shortened RFS [10]. Suriano et al. performed detailed population analyses of macrophages in the bladder tumor environment using dual immunofluorescence staining using CD68/iNOS (M1 polarization) and CD68/CD163 (M2 polarization) combinations, suggesting a prognostic value of TAM infiltration for RFS in patients with NMIBC treated with intravesical BCG [12]. One of the major drawbacks in both of these reports is the limited number of patients (only 40 each), which did not allow for multivariate analysis providing reliable prognostic values. Moreover, the topical immune environment, response pattern toward exposure of BCG, and the strains of BCG used can vary among races and countries. Therefore, we conducted the present study to explore the relevance to oncological features in a larger sample size and a Japanese cohort.

Immune cells in the tumor area or in the stroma around the tumor area can influence survival, with either poor or improved prognosis and with either sensitivity or resistance to treatment, depending on their subsets and polarization [10]. Muscle-invasive bladder cancer (MIBC) patients with FOXP3 expression in tumor cells showed shorter survival compared to those with negative cancers [15]. Another report demonstrated that an elevated FOXP3/CD8 ratio in tumor tissues was an independent predictor of poor prognosis after RC [16]. In a multivariate analysis of MIBCs, a high count of CD68+ TAM was correlated with high T category, high-grade cancer [17], and higher risk of cancer-specific death when adjusted for CD3 [18]. Although extensive studies on muscle-invasive bladder cancer have been conducted, there is little information on NMIBC, especially about its response to intravesical BCG. The present study demonstrated that high counts of Treg and TAM acted as a predictor of poor prognosis with a 2.5-fold and 2.3-fold higher risk of recurrence and a 3.38-fold and 3.35-fold higher risk of progression in univariate analysis, respectively (Table 2). These results strongly suggest a possible relationship between resistance to BCG and Treg/TAM in the tumor microenvironment.

Treg plays crucial roles in the evasion of antitumor immunity and escape from response to treatments in various malignancies, leading to poor oncological outcomes [10,19,20]. BCG treatment is known to cause Th1-polarized immunomodulation [21]. Treg can suppress effector mechanisms of the immune response in vaccination models. However, simultaneous inhibition of Th2 polarization and Tregs could promote host-protective immunity [22] and BCG-induced vaccination response using a mouse model through enhanced Th1 polarization [23]. Many studies have demonstrated that TAM cells are markedly present in various malignancies and involved in promoting neoangiogenesis and producing immunoregulatory and immunosuppressive cytokines, culminating in worsened oncological outcomes [24]. Previous studies have stated that the predominant locations of TAM are the stroma and lamina propria [10,25]. However, our analysis showed that a large number of TAM localize in the tumor area in high-grade tumors compared to low-grade tumors. Ayari et al. demonstrated that CD68+ TAM in the stroma or within tumor nests were found to have no predictive value for outcomes after intravesical BCG [26]. Further studies with larger sample sizes are needed to clarify the influence of the predominant location of Treg and TAM on prognostic significance.

IL6 is one of the major pro-inflammatory cytokines in the tumor microenvironment, and exhibits tumor-supporting activities [13,27,28]. In the present study, we examined the correlation between Treg/TAM and IL6 in the bladder tumor microenvironment. There was a positive correlation between the count of TAM and IL6+ UC cells, whereas significant correlation was not observed between the counts of Treg and IL6+ UC cells (Figure 1C,D). This finding is consistent with evidence from previous studies. Hasita et al. investigated the significance of TAM and Treg in patients with intrahepatic cholangiocarcinoma, demonstrating that IL6 production from tumor cells was correlated with the number of infiltrating TAMs, but not with the numbers of Treg cells or vessels [27]. This result supports the idea that IL6 is one of the vital molecules that differentiates macrophages. Another report by Hinz et al. revealed that specific down-regulation of FOXP3 with small interfering RNA in the pancreatic carcinoma cell line Panc89 resulted in the up-regulation of IL6 and IL8 via the activation of nuclear factor-κB (NF-κB), providing evidence for the control of inflammatory cytokine production by FOXP3 [28]. IL8 promotes angiogenesis and growth of cancer cells. However, the biological significance of FOXP3-mediated suppression of IL6 and IL8 production in malignant diseases is not fully understood.

The present study has several limitations. The first is its retrospective nature with potential selection bias; for example, some patients were excluded because of aggressive treatment (immediate radical cystectomy for T1 disease). Second, tumor tissue analysis was performed by immunohistochemistry (IHC) with possible technical biases, for example specimen fixation, antigen retrieval, antibody binding, color development, and quantification, which may affect the interpretation. Third, this study includes 71 patients, which is considered to be a relatively low sample size. Because low sample size constitutes a limitation of the work and to acknowledge this issue, further study including additional tumors and patients is needed to verify our results.

4. Materials and Methods

4.1. Data Collection of the Patients

All subjects gave their informed consent for inclusion before they participated in the study. The study was conducted in accordance with the Declaration of Helsinki, and the protocol was approved by the Ethics Committee of the Nara Medical University (Project identification code: 1630, accepted: 21 August 2017). In total, 154 patients with newly diagnosed NMIBC undergoing TURBT between 2004 and 2013 were enrolled in this study. Clinical information was retrieved from medical charts. All hematoxylin and eosin-stained specimens obtained by initial TURBT were reassessed independently by two experienced uropathologists (Keiji Shimada and Noboru Konishi) to determine T category (2010 American Joint Committee on Cancer TNM Staging system), tumor grade (2004 WHO classification), CIS, and lymphovascular invasion. Follow-up was performed according to our institutional protocol [29].

4.2. Immunohistochemical Staining and Quantification

IHC staining of paraffin-embedded, formalin-fixed tissue blocks was performed using the Histofine SAB-PO kit (Nichirei Co., Tokyo, Japan) as previously described [30,31]. Briefly, the sections were autoclaved for 10 min in 0.01 M citrate buffer (pH 6.0) for antigen retrieval. The primary antibodies were monoclonal mouse anti-FOXP3 (dilution 1/100; Ref. ab20034, Abcam, Cambridge, MA, USA), monoclonal mouse anti-MRS-A (CD204) (dilution 1/2000; Ref. KT022; Trans Genic Inc., Kobe, Japan), and polyclonal rabbit anti-IL6 (dilution 1/500; Ref. sc-1265, Santa Cruz, Dallas, TX, USA).

FOXP3-positive Treg was quantified as previously described [32]. Lymphocytes exhibiting nuclear immunostaining for FOXP3 in the cancerous area were counted in at least five independent HPFs ($400\times$, 0.0625 μm^2). The mean count of each patient was determined by dividing the sum by the number of assessed fields. Similarly, CD204$^-$positive TAM in the cancerous area was counted [30]. To quantify the expression level of IL6 in the UC cells, immunoreactive tumor cells were counted in at least five independent fields, and the percentage of positive cells was calculated by dividing that number by the total counted UC cells (1–100%) [30]. The median values (IQR) of total count cells for the quantification of the FOXP3-positive Treg, CD204-positive TAM, and IL6+ cells were 185 (132–125), 185 (132–125), and 221 (158–291), respectively. Evaluation was carried out by two trained investigators (M.M. and Y.T.) in a blind manner, without knowledge of the patients' outcome or other clinicopathological characteristics.

4.3. Adjuvant Intravesical Therapy for NMIBC after TURBT

TURBT was carried out according to a standardized procedure used by all surgeons at the single institute [29]. Because of the study's retrospective nature, the criteria, dosage, and scheme for adjuvant intravesical therapy were not consistent between patients, and depended on the physician's decision. In general, patients with high-risk NMIBC, such as those positive for concomitant CIS, T1 category, and high-grade tumors, were treated with intravesical BCG. A substantial number of patients were given intravesical BCG as initial adjuvant therapy. The schedule for intravesical BCG consisted of weekly instillations for 6–8 consecutive weeks of Immunobladder (BCG Tokyo 172 strain; Japan BCG Laboratory Tokyo, Japan) or ImmuCyst (Connaught strain; Sanofi, Paris, France; currently not being supplied as of October 2017). A single immediate post-TURBT chemotherapy instillation and/or maintenance chemotherapy instillation using anthracyclines or mitomycin-C was given to a subset of the cohort.

4.4. Statistical Analysis

The clinicopathological characteristics were compared using the Mann–Whitney U test and Fisher's exact test as appropriate. The interrelationships among the studied parameters were examined using the Spearman correlation coefficient and linear regression analysis. RFS and progression-free survival were calculated from the date of TURBT for the initial TURBT to the date of intravesical recurrence and progression, respectively. Progression was defined as recurrent disease when there was invasion into the muscularis propria ($\geq$T2), lymph node involvement, and/or occurrence of distant metastases. Survival rates were analyzed using the Kaplan–Meier method and compared using the log-rank test for univariate analysis. Multivariate analysis was used to identify independent prognostic variables using a stepwise Cox proportional hazards regression model. IBM SPSS version 21 (SPSS, Inc., Chicago, IL, USA) and PRISM software version 7.00 (GraphPad Software, Inc., San Diego, CA, USA) were used for statistical analyses and data plotting, respectively. Statistical significance in this study was set at $p < 0.05$, and all reported p values were two-sided.

5. Conclusions

We explored the clinical significance of Treg and TAM in the bladder tumor environment, suggesting that the immunological response to intravesical BCG is a complicated mechanism involving multiple subpopulations of immune cells. Moreover, IL6 production from UC cells might play a key role in the induction of TAM and the protection of the cancer cells from BCG treatment. Therefore, disrupting the recruitment of Treg and TAM, in combination with conventional intravesical BCG could be a potential therapeutic approach. Randomized control trials are required to determine the true clinical benefit.

Acknowledgments: We would like to thank Editage (www.editage.jp) for English language editing.

Author Contributions: Makito Miyake, Daisuke Gotoh, Takuya Owari, and Kiyohide Fujimoto contributed to conception and design, and acquisition of patients' data, and analysis and interpretation of data. Yoshihiro Tatsumi, Sayuri Ohnishi, Kenta Ohnishi, Kota Iida, Shunta Hori, Yosuke Morizawa, and Yoshitaka Itami contributed to acquisition of data and interpretation of data. Yasushi Nakai, Takeshi Inoue, Satoshi Anai, Kazumasa Torimoto, and Katsuya Aoki contributed to analysis and interpretation of data. Keiji Shimada, Noboru Konishi, and Nobumichi Tanaka contributed to conception and design and review of pathologic diagnosis of surgical specimens.

Conflicts of Interest: The authors declare no conflicts of interest.

Abbreviations

BCG	Bacille Calmette–Guérin
CIS	Carcinoma in situ
FR	Hazard ratio
FOXP3	Forkhead box P3
HPF	High-power microscopic fields
IHC	Immunohistochemistry
IL6	Interleukin-6
LVI	Lymphovascular invasion
MIBC	Muscle-invasive bladder cancer
NF-κB	Nuclear factor-κB
NMIBC	Non-muscle invasive bladder cancer
PFS	Progression-free survival
RC	Radical cystectomy
RFS	Recurrence-free survival
TAM	Tumor-associated macrophage
TURBT	Transurethral resection of bladder tumor
Treg	Regulatory T cell
UC	Urothelial carcinoma

References

1. Miyake, M.; Fujimoto, K.; Hirao, Y. Active surveillance for nonmuscle invasive bladder cancer. *Investig. Clin. Urol.* **2016**, *57* (Suppl. S1), S4–S13. [CrossRef] [PubMed]
2. Fernandez-Gomez, J.; Madero, R.; Solsona, E. Predicting nonmuscle invasive bladder cancer recurrence and progression in patients treated with bacillus Calmette-Guerin: The CUETO scoring model. *J. Urol.* **2009**, *182*, 2195–2203. [CrossRef] [PubMed]
3. Sylvester, R.J.; van der Meijden, A.P.; Oosterlinck, W. Predicting recurrence and progression in individual patients with stage Ta T1 bladder cancer using EORTC risk tables: A combined analysis of 2596 patients from seven EORTC trials. *Eur. Urol.* **2006**, *49*, 466–477. [CrossRef] [PubMed]
4. Witjes, J.A.; Compérat, E.; Cowan, N.C.; De Santis, M.; Gakis, G.; Lebret, T.; Ribal, M.J.; Van der Heijden, A.G.; Sherif, A.; European Association of Urology. EAU guidelines on muscle-invasive and metastatic bladder cancer: Summary of the 2013 guidelines. *Eur. Urol.* **2014**, *65*, 778–792. [CrossRef] [PubMed]
5. Reis, L.O.; Moro, J.C.; Ribeiro, L.F.; Voris, B.R.; Sadi, M.V. Are we following the guidelines on non-muscle invasive bladder cancer? *Int. Braz. J. Urol.* **2016**, *42*, 22–28. [CrossRef] [PubMed]
6. Lamm, D.L.; Blumenstein, B.A.; Crawford, E.D. A randomized trial of intravesical doxorubicin and immunotherapy with bacilli Calmette-Guerin for transitional-cell carcinoma of the bladder. *N. Engl. J. Med.* **1991**, *325*, 1205–1209. [CrossRef] [PubMed]
7. Raj, G.V.; Herr, H.; Serio, A.M.; Donat, S.M.; Bochner, B.H.; Vickers, A.J.; Dalbagni, G. Treatment paradigm shift may improve survival of patients with high risk superficial bladder cancer. *J. Urol.* **2007**, *177*, 1283–1286. [CrossRef] [PubMed]
8. Kitamura, H.; Tsukamoto, T. Immunotherapy for urothelial carcinoma: Current status and perspectives. *Cancers* **2011**, *3*, 3055–3071. [CrossRef] [PubMed]
9. Abebe, F. Is interferon-gamma the right marker for bacilli Calmette-Guérin-induced immune protection? The missing link in our understanding of tuberculosis immunology. *Clin. Exp. Immunol.* **2012**, *169*, 213–219. [CrossRef] [PubMed]
10. Pichler, R.; Fritz, J.; Zavadil, C.; Schäfer, G.; Culig, Z.; Brunner, A. Tumor-infiltrating immune cell subpopulations influence the oncologic outcome after intravesical Bacillus Calmette-Guérin therapy in bladder cancer. *Oncotarget* **2016**, *7*, 39916–39930. [CrossRef] [PubMed]
11. Nunez-Nateras, R.; Castle, E.P.; Protheroe, C.A.; Stanton, M.L.; Ocal, T.I.; Ferrigni, E.N.; Ochkur, S.I.; Jacobsen, E.A.; Hou, Y.X.; Andrews, P.E.; et al. Predicting response to bacillus Calmette-Guérin (BCG) in patients with carcinoma in situ of the bladder. *Urol. Oncol.* **2014**, *32*, e23–e30. [CrossRef] [PubMed]

12. Suriano, F.; Santini, D.; Perrone, G.; Amato, M.; Vincenzi, B.; Tonini, G.; Muda, A.; Boggia, S.; Buscarini, M.; Pantano, F. Tumor associated macrophages polarization dictates the efficacy of BCG instillation in non-muscle invasive urothelial bladder cancer. *J. Exp. Clin. Cancer Res.* **2013**, *32*, 87. [CrossRef] [PubMed]
13. Kumari, N.; Dwarakanath, B.S.; Das, A.; Bhatt, A.N. Role of interleukin-6 in cancer progression and therapeutic resistance. *Tumour Biol.* **2016**, *37*, 11553–11572. [CrossRef] [PubMed]
14. Morales, A.; Eidinger, D.; Bruce, A.W. Intracavitary Bacillus Calmette-Guerin in the treatment of superficial bladder tumors. *J. Urol.* **1976**, *116*, 180–183. [CrossRef]
15. Winerdal, M.E.; Marits, P.; Winerdal, M.; Hasan, M.; Rosenblatt, R.; Tolf, A.; Selling, K.; Sherif, A.; Winqvist, O. FOXP3 and survival in urinary bladder cancer. *BJU Int.* **2011**, *108*, 1672–1678. [CrossRef] [PubMed]
16. Horn, T.; Laus, J.; Seitz, A.K.; Maurer, T.; Schmid, S.C.; Wolf, P.; Haller, B.; Winkler, M.; Retz, M.; Nawroth, R.; et al. The prognostic effect of tumour-infiltrating lymphocytic subpopulations in bladder cancer. *World J. Urol.* **2016**, *34*, 181–187. [CrossRef] [PubMed]
17. Boström, M.M.; Irjala, H.; Mirtti, T.; Taimen, P.; Kauko, T.; Ålgars, A.; Jalkanen, S.; Boström, P.J. Tumor-Associated Macrophages Provide Significant Prognostic Information in Urothelial Bladder Cancer. *PLoS ONE* **2015**, *10*, e0133552. [CrossRef] [PubMed]
18. Sjödahl, G.; Lövgren, K.; Lauss, M.; Chebil, G.; Patschan, O.; Gudjonsson, S.; Månsson, W.; Fernö, M.; Leandersson, K.; Lindgren, D.; et al. Infiltration of CD3+ and CD68+ cells in bladder cancer is subtype specific and interacts the outcome of patients with muscle-invasive tumors. *Urol. Oncol.* **2014**, *32*, 791–797. [CrossRef] [PubMed]
19. Mahmoud, S.M.; Paish, E.C.; Powe, D.G.; Macmillan, R.D.; Lee, A.H.; Ellis, I.O.; Green, A.R. An evaluation of the clinical significance of FOXP3+ infiltrating cells in human breast cancer. *Breast Cancer Res. Treat.* **2011**, *127*, 99–108. [CrossRef] [PubMed]
20. Shimizu, K.; Nakata, M.; Hirami, Y.; Yukawa, T.; Maeda, A.; Tanemoto, K. Tumor-infiltrating FOXP3+ regulatory T cells are correlated with cyclooxygenase-2 expression and are associated with recurrence in resected non-small cell lung cancer. *J. Thorac. Oncol.* **2010**, *5*, 585–590. [CrossRef] [PubMed]
21. Ponticiello, A.; Perna, F.; Maione, S.; Stradolini, M.; Testa, G.; Terrazzano, G.; Ruggiero, G.; Malerba, M.; Sanduzzi, A. Analysis of local T lymphocyte subsets upon stimulation with intravesical BCG: A model to study tuberculosis immunity. *Respir. Med.* **2004**, *98*, 509–514. [CrossRef] [PubMed]
22. Bhattacharya, D.; Dwivedi, V.P.; Maiga, M.; Maiga, M.; Van Kaer, L.; Bishai, W.R.; Das, G. Small molecule-directed immunotherapy against recurrent infection by Mycobacterium tuberculosis. *J. Biol. Chem.* **2014**, *289*, 16508–16515. [CrossRef] [PubMed]
23. Bhattacharya, D.; Dwivedi, V.P.; Kumar, S.; Reddy, M.C.; Van Kaer, L.; Moodley, P.; Das, G. Simultaneous inhibition of T helper 2 and T regulatory cell differentiation by small molecules enhances Bacillus Calmette-Guerin vaccine efficacy against tuberculosis. *J. Biol. Chem.* **2014**, *289*, 33404–33411. [CrossRef] [PubMed]
24. Pollard, J.W. Tumour-educated macrophages promote tumour progression and metastasis. *Nat. Rev. Cancer* **2004**, *4*, 71–78. [CrossRef] [PubMed]
25. Takayama, H.; Nishimura, K.; Tsujimura, A.; Nakai, Y.; Nakayama, M.; Aozasa, K.; Okuyama, A.; Nonomura, N. Increased infiltration of tumor associated macrophages is associated with poor prognosis of bladder carcinoma in situ after intravesical bacillus Calmette-Guerin instillation. *J. Urol.* **2009**, *181*, 1894–1900. [CrossRef] [PubMed]
26. Ayari, C.; LaRue, H.; Hovington, H.; Decobert, M.; Harel, F.; Bergeron, A.; Têtu, B.; Lacombe, L.; Fradet, Y. Bladder tumor infiltrating mature dendritic cells and macrophages as predictors of response to bacillus Calmette-Guérin immunotherapy. *Eur. Urol.* **2009**, *55*, 1386–1395. [CrossRef] [PubMed]
27. Hasita, H.; Komohara, Y.; Okabe, H.; Masuda, T.; Ohnishi, K.; Lei, X.F.; Beppu, T.; Baba, H.; Takeya, M. Significance of alternatively activated macrophages in patients with intrahepatic cholangiocarcinoma. *Cancer Sci.* **2010**, *101*, 1913–1919. [CrossRef] [PubMed]
28. Hinz, S.; Pagerols-Raluy, L.; Oberg, H.H.; Ammerpohl, O.; Grüssel, S.; Sipos, B.; Grützmann, R.; Pilarsky, C.; Ungefroren, H.; Saeger, H.D.; et al. FOXP3 expression in pancreatic carcinoma cells as a novel mechanism of immune evasion in cancer. *Cancer Res.* **2007**, *67*, 8344–8350. [CrossRef] [PubMed]

29. Miyake, M.; Gotoh, D.; Shimada, K.; Tatsumi, Y.; Nakai, Y.; Anai, S.; Torimoto, K.; Aoki, K.; Tanaka, N.; Konishi, N.; et al. Exploration of risk factors predicting outcomes for primary T1 high-grade bladder cancer and validation of the Spanish Urological Club for Oncological Treatment scoring model: Long-term follow-up experience at a single institute. *Int. J. Urol.* **2015**, *22*, 541–547. [CrossRef] [PubMed]
30. Miyake, M.; Hori, S.; Morizawa, Y.; Tatsumi, Y.; Nakai, Y.; Anai, S.; Torimoto, K.; Aoki, K.; Tanaka, N.; Shimada, K.; et al. CXCL1-Mediated Interaction of Cancer Cells with Tumor-Associated Macrophages and Cancer-Associated Fibroblasts Promotes Tumor Progression in Human Bladder Cancer. *Neoplasia* **2016**, *18*, 636–646. [CrossRef] [PubMed]
31. Miyake, M.; Hori, S.; Morizawa, Y.; Tatsumi, Y.; Toritsuka, M.; Ohnishi, S.; Shimada, K.; Furuya, H.; Khadka, V.S.; Deng, Y.; et al. Collagen type IV alpha 1 (COL4A1) and collagen type XIII alpha 1 (COL13A1) produced in cancer cells promote tumor budding at the invasion front in human urothelial carcinoma of the bladder. *Oncotarget* **2017**, *8*, 36099–36114. [CrossRef] [PubMed]
32. Schwarz, S.; Butz, M.; Morsczeck, C.; Reichert, T.E.; Driemel, O. Increased number of CD25+ FOXP3+ regulatory T cells in oral squamous cell carcinomas detected by chromogenic immunohistochemical double staining. *J. Oral Pathol. Med.* **2008**, *37*, 485–489. [CrossRef] [PubMed]

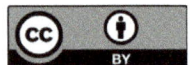

© 2017 by the authors. Licensee MDPI, Basel, Switzerland. This article is an open access article distributed under the terms and conditions of the Creative Commons Attribution (CC BY) license (http://creativecommons.org/licenses/by/4.0/).

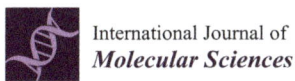

Review

Impact of Sarcopenia as a Prognostic Biomarker of Bladder Cancer

Hiroshi Fukushima, Kosuke Takemura, Hiroaki Suzuki and Fumitaka Koga *

Department of Urology, Tokyo Metropolitan Cancer and Infectious Diseases Center Komagome Hospital, 3-18-22 Honkomagome, Bunkyo-ku, Tokyo 113-8677, Japan; fukuuro@tmd.ac.jp (H.F.); takemura-urol@cick.jp (K.T.); smu.udm@gmail.com (H.S.)
* Correspondence: f-koga@cick.jp; Tel.: +81-3-3823-2101; Fax: +81-3-3823-5433

Received: 26 August 2018; Accepted: 29 September 2018; Published: 1 October 2018

Abstract: Sarcopenia, the degenerative and systemic loss of skeletal muscle mass, indicates patient frailty and impaired physical function. Sarcopenia can be caused by multiple factors, including advanced age, lack of exercise, poor nutritional status, inflammatory diseases, endocrine diseases, and malignancies. In patients with cancer cachexia, anorexia, poor nutrition and systemic inflammation make the metabolic state more catabolic, resulting in sarcopenia. Thus, sarcopenia is considered as one of manifestations of cancer cachexia. Recently, growing evidence has indicated the importance of sarcopenia in the management of patients with various cancers. Sarcopenia is associated with not only higher rates of treatment-related complications but also worse prognosis in cancer-bearing patients. In this article, we summarized metabolic backgrounds of cancer cachexia and sarcopenia and definitions of sarcopenia based on computed tomography (CT) images. We conducted a systematic literature review regarding the significance of sarcopenia as a prognostic biomarker of bladder cancer. We also reviewed recent studies focusing on the prognostic role of changes in skeletal muscle mass during the course of treatment in bladder cancer patients. Lastly, we discussed the impact of nutritional support, medication, and exercise on sarcopenia in cancer-bearing patients.

Keywords: sarcopenia; prognosis; biomarker; bladder cancer; urothelial carcinoma

---

1. Introduction

Bladder cancer is the most common malignancy of the urinary tract in the world, with approximately 430,000 new cases and 165,000 deaths each year [1]. The major histology of bladder cancer is urothelial carcinoma. Based on the pathological depth of tumor invasion, bladder cancer is classified into two groups: non-muscle-invasive bladder cancer (NMIBC) and muscle-invasive bladder cancer (MIBC). NMIBC is treated with bladder-preserving treatments, including transurethral resection of the bladder tumor and intravesical instillation therapy [2]. Patients with MIBC generally require total cystectomy and urinary diversion as a curative treatment [3]. However, approximately half of MIBC patients undergoing total cystectomy die within five years because MIBC is potentially an aggressive disease and frequently progresses to a metastatic disease postoperatively [4]. Once MIBC patients develop distant metastasis, their prognoses are poor despite receiving systemic chemotherapy with a median overall survival (OS) of approximately 15 months [5]. Thus, bladder cancer is still a challenging disease, although the recent advent of immuno-oncology drugs is shifting the paradigm of the management of bladder cancer patients [6]. Pre-therapeutic risk assessment based on prognostic biomarkers can help clinicians to predict their outcomes and counsel patients about treatment options. Therefore, identifying prognostic biomarkers contributes to better management for bladder cancer patients.

Sarcopenia is a syndrome representing the degenerative and systemic loss of skeletal muscle mass [7]. According to recent surveys, the prevalence of sarcopenia is relatively high, ranging from 15% at 65 years to 50% at 80 years [8]. Variations in genes, such as *MSTN*, *VDR*, and *ACE*, determine the variability in skeletal muscle phenotype and the prevalence of sarcopenia in an elderly population [9]. Sarcopenia is associated with lower physical activity, morbidity, and mortality [10,11]. Sarcopenic patients tend to have higher morbidity from infectious diseases [12], metabolic syndrome [13], insulin resistance [14], and cardiovascular diseases [15]. Sarcopenia is pathophysiologically associated with various etiologies, including advanced age, lack of exercise, poor nutritional status, inflammatory diseases, and endocrine diseases [7]. Malignant diseases can also cause sarcopenia [16]. In patients with cancer cachexia, anorexia, poor nutrition, and systemic inflammation make the metabolic state more catabolic, resulting in sarcopenia [17]. Therefore, sarcopenia is considered as one of manifestations of cancer cachexia.

Recent studies have shown the prognostic impact of sarcopenia in various cancers. Sarcopenic patients show significantly worse survival than non-sarcopenic counterparts with lung or gastrointestinal cancer [18,19], hepatic cell carcinoma [20], esophageal cancer [21], lymphoma [22], melanoma [23], or renal cell carcinoma [24,25]. In bladder cancer, the role of sarcopenia in predicting survival has been clarified. In this article, we summarized metabolic backgrounds of cancer cachexia and sarcopenia and definitions of sarcopenia based on computed tomography (CT) images. Moreover, we conducted a systematic literature review on published studies to summarize comprehensively the current clinical evidence on the prognostic role of sarcopenia in bladder cancer patients. We also reviewed recent studies focusing on the prognostic importance of changes in skeletal muscle mass during the course of treatment in bladder cancer patients. Finally, we discussed the impact of nutritional support, medications, and exercise on cancer cachexia and sarcopenia in cancer-bearing patients.

2. Metabolic Background of Cancer Cachexia and Sarcopenia

Cancer cachexia is a multifactorial syndrome characterized by progressive weight loss, which is due to the depletion of adipose tissue and skeletal muscle mass. In the early phase of cancer cachexia, adipose tissue is depleted [26]. Skeletal muscle wasting is promoted after the progression of cancer cachexia [27]. Anorexia, which is caused by cancer itself or treatment for cancer, is frequently observed in patients with cancer cachexia. Moreover, resting energy expenditure increases in patients with cancer cachexia, leading to the progressive loss of body weight [28]. In the process of the progression of cancer cachexia, lipolysis and fatty acid oxidation are activated in skeletal muscle, whereas glycolysis is suppressed [29,30]. Increased oxidative stress caused by up-regulated fatty acid oxidation can contribute to skeletal muscle wasting [30]. Several mechanisms, including epinephrine stimulation and increased secretion of cytokines, are involved in these metabolic changes [31]. Moreover, skeletal muscle depletion is caused by increased protein degradation mainly by the activated ubiquitin-proteasome pathway, in which multiple receptor-mediated signaling pathways are involved [27]. In this section, we summarize the metabolic changes and the mechanisms of the depletion of adipose tissue and skeletal muscle mass during cancer cachexia.

2.1. Adipose Tissue Depletion in Cancer Cachexia

Adipose tissue volume decreases in the early process of cancer cachexia [26]. The breakdown of adipose tissue is caused by lipolysis of triglyceride, which is mediated by adipose triglyceride lipase (ATGL) and hormonal-sensitive lipase (HSL) [32]. In a previous study of ATGL- or HSL-deficient animal models, the absence of ATGL and, to lesser degree, HSL reduces fatty acid mobilization and adipose tissue loss, leading to maintained skeletal muscle mass, suggesting that excessive depletion of adipose tissue may be involved in the progression of skeletal muscle atrophy [29]. Up-regulation of lipolysis is induced by various factors, including enhanced stimulation of β-adrenergic receptor, increased secretion of cytokines such as tumor necrosis factor (TNF)-α, interleukin (IL)-1, IL-6, and IL-8, and increased expression of lipid-mobilizing factors, such as zinc-α2 glycoprotein-1 (AZGP1) [32]. White adipose tissue browning, which is associated with increased expression of uncoupling protein 1 (UCP1), increases thermogenesis and energy expenditure during cancer cachexia [28]. This process is also affected by β-adrenergic receptor stimulation and cytokines such as TNF-α and IL-6 [28].

2.2. Skeletal Muscle Depletion in Cancer Cachexia

Skeletal muscle depletion occurs as a consequence of reduced protein synthesis and increased degradation of proteins in the late phase of cancer cachexia [27]. Reduced protein synthesis can be caused by low nutritional status as a result of anorexia and decreased food intake [27,32]. Skeletal muscle protein degradation is promoted mainly by the ubiquitin-proteasome pathway, which is induced by myostatin, activin A, cytokines such as TNF-α and IL-6, and proteolysis-inducing factor [31,32]. Myostatin and activin A, members of the transforming-growth factor β (TGF-β) family, bind activin type 2 receptor B (ActR2B) and activate Smad2/3 and p38 mitogen-activated protein kinase (MAPK) signaling, resulting in the up-regulation of Atrogin-1 and the muscle ring finger protein 1 (MuRF-1), which are muscle-specific E3 ligases and play roles as key regulators of ubiquitin-driven protein degradation in the skeletal muscle [27,31]. Moreover, the phosphatidylinositol-3 kinase (PI3K)/Akt/mammalian target of rapamycin (mTOR) pathway and forkhead box O (FOXO), which are general regulators of skeletal muscle mass homeostasis, are affected in cancer cachexia [31–33]. TNF-α up-regulates Atrogin-1 by increasing nuclear FOXO4 protein in skeletal muscle [34]. Glucocorticoid receptor regulates the expression of Atrogin-1 and MuRF-1 [27,31]. The binding of insulin-like growth factor-1 (IGF-1) to its receptor causes the activation of PI3K/Akt/mTOR pathway, which down-regulates FOXO3 and results in decreased expression of Atrogin-1 and MuRF-1 [27,31]. Taken together, various signaling pathways are related to the regulation of skeletal muscle protein degradation. Their inhibition may contribute to the prevention of cancer cachexia and sarcopenia.

Oxidative stress promotes skeletal muscle wasting. Fukawa et al. revealed up-regulation of fatty acid oxidation and down-regulation of glycolysis in the skeletal muscle using transcriptomics of human muscle stem cell-based models and human cancer-induced cachexia models in mice [30]. Interestingly, they also showed that increased oxidative stress caused by excessive fatty acid oxidation could impair muscle growth [30]. Therefore, increased oxidative stress can cause sarcopenia through excessive fatty acid oxidation in the process of the progression of cancer cachexia. Inhibiting the process of fatty acid oxidation could be efficacious in preventing cancer cachexia and sarcopenia. In contrast, skeletal muscle mitochondrial oxidative capacities decrease without alteration of adenosine triphosphate (ATP) production efficiency in a rat model of cancer cachexia [35], which appears to be inconsistent with the results reported by Fukawa et al. [30], but this may contribute to lipid droplet accumulation in skeletal muscle mass [36].

3. Evaluation of Sarcopenia Using Computed Tomography (CT) Images

According to the European Working Group of Sarcopenia in Older People (EWGSOP), sarcopenia is determined based on three factors: lower skeletal muscle mass, lower skeletal muscle strength, and lower physical performance [7]. Skeletal muscle strength can be evaluated by upper-limb hand-grip dynamometry and lower-limb extension strength testing. The assessment of physical function is generally based on walking speed. As for skeletal muscle mass, bioimpedance analysis, anthropometry, dual energy X-ray imaging, CT, and magnetic resonance imaging (MRI) are recommended as methods to measure skeletal muscle mass by EWGSOP [7]. In cancer-bearing patients, including bladder cancer patients, CT images are generally used in the evaluation of sarcopenia, since abdominal CT scans are routinely performed for diagnosis, staging, surveillance of recurrence after treatment, and assessment of therapeutic response [37]. Therefore, most of the previous studies on sarcopenia and bladder cancer used CT images to measure skeletal muscle mass and define sarcopenia (Figure 1). In our systematic literature review below, all the articles used CT images.

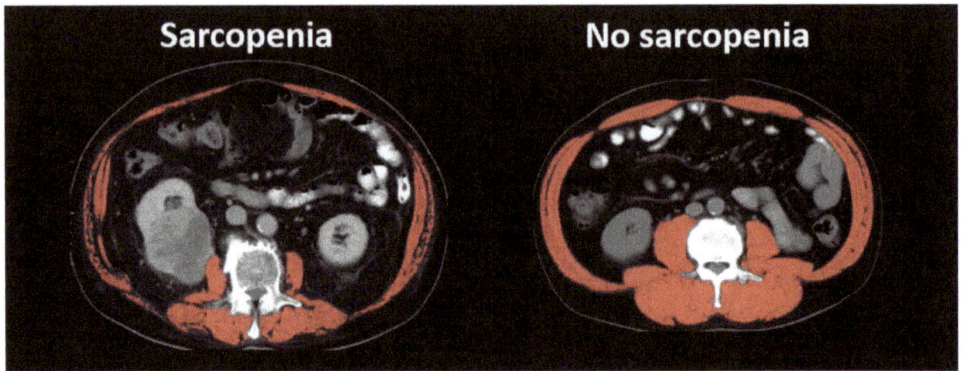

Figure 1. Computed tomography (CT) images of typical sarcopenic and non-sarcopenic cases. Skeletal muscle area is shown in red.

3.1. Measurement of Skeletal Muscle Mass Using CT Images

Axial CT images at the lumbar vertebral level are used to measure skeletal muscle areas because the total lumbar-skeletal muscle cross-sectional area is linearly correlated to the whole-body skeletal muscle mass [38]. The total skeletal muscle area at the third lumbar vertebra, including the psoas, paraspinal muscles (the erector spinae and quadratus lumborum), and abdominal wall muscles (the transversus abdominus, external and internal obliques, and rectus abdominus), is measured using software such as Slice-O-Matic (Tomovision, Montreal, QC, Canada) and OsiriX imaging software (Pixmeo, Geneva, Switzerland). The cross-sectional areas of skeletal muscle are identified using Hounsfield Unit thresholds of -29 to $+150$.

3.2. Skeletal Muscle Index (SMI)

Skeletal muscle index (SMI) is used widely in evaluating sarcopenia in cancer-bearing patients. SMI is calculated by normalizing skeletal muscle area for height in meters squared, as is body mass index (BMI). Two major established definitions of sarcopenia have been proposed so far. First, the International Consensus of Cancer Cachexia (ICCC) proposed cutoff values of SMI as 55 cm^2/m^2 for males and 39 cm^2/m^2 for females [16]. Second, Martin et al., defined BMI-incorporated cutoff values of SMI as <43 cm^2/m^2 for males with BMI < 25 kg/m^2, <53 cm^2/m^2 for males with BMI $\geq$ 25 kg/m^2, and <41 cm^2/m^2 for females [18]. Both of the two definitions were the best cutoffs to predict overall mortality using a cohort of patients with lung or gastrointestinal cancer, and either of them has been used to define sarcopenia in most previous studies on bladder cancer [37].

3.3. Psoas Muscle Index (PMI)

In some previous studies, only the psoas muscle area was measured on axial CT images at the lumbar vertebral level. The psoas muscle index (PMI) is calculated by normalizing the psoas muscle area for height in meters squared. Although a correlation between PMI and whole-body skeletal muscle mass has not yet been evaluated, the strong correlation between PMI and SMI suggests that PMI also represents whole-body skeletal muscle mass [39]. Hamaguchi et al. proposed the cutoff values of PMI to define sarcopenia as 6.36 cm^2/m^2 for males and 3.92 cm^2/m^2 for females, using a cohort of adult donors for living donor liver transplantation [39]. However, because their cohort included only Japanese patients, the use of their values may be limited to Asian populations.

3.4. Skeletal Muscle Density

In addition to the volume of the skeletal muscle, the quality of the skeletal muscle can be evaluated on CT scan. Skeletal muscle density is determined based on the CT density (Hounsfield unit) of the skeletal muscle [40]. Lower skeletal muscle density reflects more fat infiltration in skeletal muscle mass, which is related to lower function of the skeletal muscle and lower physical performance. Moreover, increased fat infiltration in skeletal muscle mass is involved in insulin resistance [41], which decreases glucose uptake in skeletal muscles and can eventually contribute to skeletal muscle atrophy. Because increased fat infiltration in the skeletal muscle is one of the characteristics of cancer cachexia, lower skeletal muscle density is considered as an indicator of the progression of cancer cachexia [40].

4. Hybrid Nature of Sarcopenia as a Prognostic Biomarker

Prognostic tumor biomarkers generally reflect tumor aggressiveness, including tumor stage, histological grade, lymphovascular invasion, and patient survival. Several prognostic biomarkers are related to the general condition of the host; e.g., age, sex, performance status, BMI, anemia, etc. Notably, sarcopenia reflects both tumor and host factors (Figure 2). Because sarcopenia develops as a consequence of tumor progression, tumor-induced systemic inflammation, or metabolic aberration, its presence indicates tumor aggressiveness. In addition, sarcopenic patients are characterized by poor general health and physical performance, which can contribute to worse prognosis of cancer-bearing patients. High prognostic performance of sarcopenia could be explained by its hybrid nature, which is a unique feature as a prognostic biomarker.

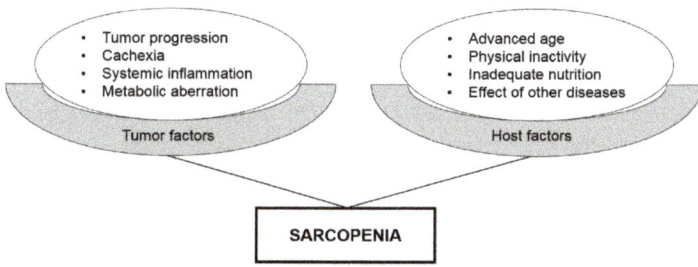

Figure 2. Hybrid nature of sarcopenia.

5. Systematic Literature Review

A systematic literature review was performed to search for studies investigating the prognostic role of sarcopenia in bladder cancer patients according to the PRISMA guidelines [42]. The search was restricted to articles written in English and performed using PubMed, Medline, and Cochrane Libraries by entering the terms "sarcopenia and urothelial carcinoma" and "sarcopenia and bladder cancer". Twenty-nine articles published from June 2014 to April 2018 were identified on 1 April 2018. There was no literature before June 2014 according to our literature search. Two independent investigators (H.F. and K.T.) conducted the literature search and selection of articles. Potential discrepancies were resolved by open discussion. Details of the search and article selection are summarized in the flow diagram (Figure 3). Studies were included if they were published as original articles investigating the prognostic role of sarcopenia in bladder cancer patients. Review articles, case reports, editorial comments, letters, meeting abstracts, and studies not meeting our inclusion criteria in their content were excluded. Our systematic literature review has several limitations. First, 12 articles were included in our systematic review, all of which were retrospective, and no study of level 1 evidence was included, indicating possible high risks of bias. Second, several different methods and definitions were used to evaluate sarcopenia using CT images in included studies.

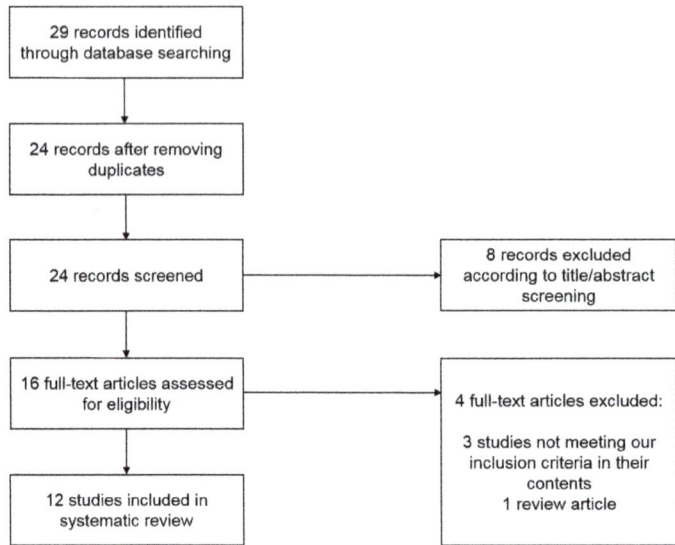

Figure 3. Flow diagram of systematic literature search.

6. Prognostic Role of Sarcopenia in Bladder Cancer

Table 1 lists published studies on the prognostic role of sarcopenia in bladder cancer patients. Most studies reported that sarcopenia was associated with worse prognosis. A systematic literature review identified six studies involving patients undergoing a radical cystectomy (due to high-risk NMIBC or MIBC) and four studies involving patients with inoperable locoregionally advanced and/or metastatic diseases. No studies investigated the association between sarcopenia and survival in low- or intermediate-risk NMIBC patients. Nine of the 10 studies used either SMI or PMI to define sarcopenia.

6.1. Survival after a Radical Cystectomy

Although a radical cystectomy with pelvic lymph node dissection is the standard of care for high-risk NMIBC and MIBC patients, its main problems include high incidences of perioperative complications [3]. In the contemporary radical cystectomy series, the incidence of major complications of Clavien–Dindo classification grade 3 or greater ranges from 5 to 26%, with a mortality rate of 0–3.9% [43]. Several studies showed that sarcopenia is significantly associated with higher rates of perioperative complications of a radical cystectomy [44,45].

Table 1. Reported series of the prognostic role of sarcopenia in bladder cancer cancers.

Study (Year)	Country	No. of Total Patients	No. of Sarcopenic Patients	Cancer Type	Therapeutic Interventions	Definition of Sarcopenia	Main Findings	Ref.
Smith et al. (2014)	United States	200	77 (39%)	Bladder cancer	Radical cystectomy	TPA [†] < 653 cm^2/m^2 for males and <523 cm^2/m^2 for females	The Kaplan–Meier curves showed no significant association between OS and sarcopenia ($p = 0.36$).	[45]
Psutka et al. (2014)	United States	205	141 (69%)	Bladder cancer	Radical cystectomy	SMI < 55 cm^2/m^2 for males and <39 cm^2/m^2 for females	Sarcopenia was an independent poor prognostic factor with HR 2.14 for CSS ($p = 0.007$) and 1.93 for OS ($p = 0.004$).	[46]
Hirasawa et al. (2016)	Japan	136	65 (48%)	Bladder cancer	Radical cystectomy	SMI < 43 cm^2/m^2 for males with BMI < 25 cm^2/m^2, <53 cm^2/m^2 for males with BMI ≥ 25 cm^2/m^2, and <41 cm^2/m^2 for females	Sarcopenia was an independent poor prognostic factor with HR 2.3 for CSS ($p = 0.015$).	[47]
Miyake et al. (2017)	Japan	89	22 (25%)	Bladder cancer	Radical cystectomy	SMI < 43 cm^2/m^2 for males with BMI < 25 cm^2/m^2, <53 cm^2/m^2 for males with BMI ≥ 25 cm^2/m^2, and <41 cm^2/m^2 for females	Sarcopenia was an independent poor prognostic factor with HR 2.2 for OS ($p = 0.03$).	[48]
Saitoh-Maeda et al. (2018)	Japan	63 (male only)	141 (69%)	Bladder cancer	Radical cystectomy	PMI < 400 cm^2/m^2	In male patients, non-sarcopenic patients had a significantly better OS than sarcopenic counterparts (2,889 vs. 2,109 days; $p = 0.023$).	[49]
Mayr et al. (2018)	Germany	500	189 (38%)	Bladder cancer	Radical cystectomy	SMI < 43 cm^2/m^2 for males with BMI < 25 cm^2/m^2, <53 cm^2/m^2 for males with BMI ≥ 25 cm^2/m^2, and <41 cm^2/m^2 for females	Sarcopenia was an independent poor prognostic factor with HR 1.42 for CSS ($p = 0.048$) and 1.43 for OS ($p = 0.01$).	[50]
Fukushima et al. (2015)	Japan	88	67 (76%)	Advanced urothelial carcinoma	Miscellaneous	SMI < 43 cm^2/m^2 for males with BMI < 25 cm^2/m^2, <53 cm^2/m^2 for males with BMI ≥ 25 cm^2/m^2, and <41 cm^2/m^2 for females	Sarcopenia was an independent poor prognostic factor with HR 3.36 for OS ($p < 0.001$).	[51]
Taguchi et al. (2015)	Japan	100	Not reported	Metastatic urothelial carcinoma	Systemic chemotherapy	SMI < 55 cm^2/m^2 for males and <39 cm^2/m^2 for females	Sarcopenia was an independent poor prognostic factor with HR 2.07 for CSS ($p = 0.045$).	[52]
Kasahara et al. (2017)	Japan	27	14 (52%)	Advanced bladder cancer	Systemic chemotherapy	PMI < 2.49 cm^2/m^2 for males and <2.07 cm^2/m^2 for females	The OS of the non-sarcopenic group was significantly better than that of the sarcopenic group (561 vs. 223 days; $p = 0.0150$).	[53]
Abe et al. (2018)	Japan	87	Not reported	Metastatic urothelial carcinoma	Systemic chemotherapy	SMI < 55 cm^2/m^2 for males and <39 cm^2/m^2 for females	Sarcopenia was not significantly associated with OS ($p = 0.11$). SMI stratified by BMI was an independent predictor for shorter OS ($p = 0.026$).	[54]

Abbreviations: BMI = body mass index; CSS = cancer-specific survival; HR = hazard ratio; OS = overall survival; PMI = psoas muscle index; SMI = skeletal muscle index; TPA = total psoas area. [†] TPA was calculated by measuring the cross-sectional area of the right and left psoas muscles on CT using 3-dimensional computerized image analysis.

As shown in Table 1, six studies reported the prognostic role of sarcopenia in bladder cancer patients undergoing a radical cystectomy [45–50]. Five of them revealed that sarcopenia is a significant predictor of cancer-specific survival (CSS) and OS [46–50]. Psutka et al., for the first time demonstrated that sarcopenia is an independent predictor for both poorer CSS and OS [46]. The 5-year CSS and OS rates were lower for sarcopenic patients than for non-sarcopenic counterparts (49% vs. 72% for CSS and 39% vs. 70% for OS, respectively). Three studies from Japan reported similar results to those of Psutka et al. [47–49]. Recently, a multi-center retrospective study from Germany demonstrated that sarcopenia is an independent predictor for both poorer CSS and OS in 500 bladder cancer patients undergoing a radical cystectomy [50]. Only one study, reported by Smith et al., showed no association between sarcopenia and OS [45]. This discrepant result may be due to the different methods for estimating skeletal muscle volume. Four studies calculated SMI, and three of them used the definition of sarcopenia proposed by Martin et al. However, Smith et al. calculated cross-sectional psoas muscle area using 3-dimensional computerized image analysis and defined sarcopenia using their own criteria.

Taken together, most previous studies demonstrated that sarcopenia is a significant poor prognostic factor in bladder cancer patients undergoing a radical cystectomy.

6.2. Survival in Inoperable Advanced Disease

Four studies evaluated the prognostic role of sarcopenia in patients with inoperable advanced bladder cancer (Table 1) [51–54]. Because upper tract urothelial carcinoma is histologically and biologically similar to bladder cancer, three of them included advanced upper tract urothelial carcinoma in their cohorts [51,52,54]. Fukushima et al. showed for the first time that sarcopenia is an independent predictor for shorter OS in patients with advanced urothelial carcinoma (inoperable locoregionally advanced disease and/or metastatic diseases to lymph nodes or distant organs) [51]. The median OS of sarcopenic patients was significantly shorter than that of non-sarcopenic counterparts (11 vs. 31 months). Taguchi et al. reported that sarcopenia is an independent predictor for shorter CSS in metastatic urothelial carcinoma patients receiving systemic chemotherapy as the first-line therapy [52]. Kasahara et al. showed the prognostic significance of sarcopenia in advanced bladder cancer patients receiving gemcitabine and nedaplatin therapy [53]. In addition, Abe et al. could not confirm the significance of sarcopenia in predicting OS, but they showed that SMI stratified by BMI was an independent predictor for shorter OS [54].

Thus, previous studies indicated that sarcopenia is a significant poor prognostic factor in inoperable advanced bladder cancer patients.

7. Prognostic Role of Changes in Skeletal Muscle Mass in Bladder Cancer

Because disease status and patient conditions can affect skeletal muscle mass in cancer-bearing patients, changes in skeletal muscle mass during and after treatment may represent post-therapeutic prognosis. As shown in Table 2, three studies investigated the prognostic role of changes in skeletal muscle mass during treatment in bladder cancer patients [48,55,56]. Miyake et al. reported that a 10% loss in psoas muscle volume before and after a radical cystectomy was an independent predictor for shorter OS [48]. Fukushima et al. reported that post-therapeutic skeletal muscle mass recovery was an independent predictor for both better recurrence-free survival and OS in advanced urothelial carcinoma treated with platinum-based chemotherapy as the first-line therapy [56]. Meanwhile, Zargar et al. showed that decline in psoas muscle volume during neoadjuvant chemotherapy was not predictive of OS in bladder cancer patients treated with neoadjuvant chemotherapy and a radical cystectomy [55].

Table 2. Reported series of the prognostic role of changes in skeletal muscle mass in bladder cancer cancers.

Study (Year)	Country	No. of Total Patients	Cancer Type	Therapeutic Interventions	Evaluation of Skeletal Muscle Mass	Main Findings	Ref.
Miyake et al. (2017)	Japan	89	Bladder cancer	Radical cystectomy	Postoperative changes in psoas major muscle volume were calculated after a radical cystectomy.	A 10% loss in the volume of the psoas muscle was an independent poor prognostic factor with HR 2.4 for OS ($p = 0.02$).	[48]
Zargar et al. (2017)	United States	60	Bladder cancer	NAC and a radical cystectomy	Changes in PMV were calculated from pre- and post-NAC CT images.	The proportion of PMV decline during NAC was not a predictor of OS after a radical cystectomy ($p = 0.85$).	[55]
Fukushima et al. (2018)	Japan	72	Advanced urothelial carcinoma	Systemic chemotherapy	Changes in SMI were calculated from pretherapeutic and posttherapeutic CT images.	Post-therapeutic skeletal muscle mass recovery was an independent favorable prognostic factor with HR 0.24 for RFS ($p < 0.001$) and 0.21 for OS ($p < 0.001$).	[56]

Abbreviations: CT = computed tomography; HR = hazard ratio; NAC = neoadjuvant chemotherapy; OS = overall survival; PMV = psoas muscle volume; RFS = recurrence-free survival; SMI = skeletal muscle index.

Although limited data suggest the prognostic significance of changes in skeletal muscle mass during treatments among bladder cancer patients, further studies are needed to confirm this finding. Therapeutic interventions for cancer might improve cancer cachexia and sarcopenia by eradicating cancer cells. Because adipose tissue depletion precedes skeletal muscle wasting in animal models with cancer cachexia [26], changes in fat and skeletal muscle mass and their patterns might be associated with survival of cancer-bearing patients. Indeed, patterns of fat and skeletal muscle wasting can be associated with survival of patients with pancreatic cancer [57].

8. Therapeutic Interventions for Sarcopenia

Given the prognostic significance of sarcopenia and changes in skeletal muscle mass in bladder cancer patients, prevention of or recovery from sarcopenia and cancer cachexia may contribute to improving their prognosis. There are several studies to investigate nutritional support, medication, and exercise as therapeutic interventions for cancer cachexia and sarcopenia in cancer-bearing patients. However, these current therapies, such as protein supplementation, are limited due to their inefficient efficacy for improving sarcopenia, suggesting the possibility of irreversible damage to skeletal muscles [32].

8.1. Nutritional Support

Several previous studies show the effect of nutritional support on sarcopenia in non-cancer patients. Because sarcopenia results from a decrease in protein synthesis and increase in protein degradation, protein supplementation can play a key role in nutritional support [58]. The effects of protein supplementation on skeletal muscle mass can be increased by adding anabolic agents such as growth hormones and testosterone [58]. However, accumulating evidence suggested that sarcopenia is not fully reversed by conventional nutrition in patients with cancer cachexia [32].

8.2. Medications

8.2.1. *n*-3 Fatty Acids

n-3 Fatty acids, including eicosapentaenoic acid and docosahexaenoic acid, can recover a cancer-induced hyper-catabolic state and improve sarcopenia and cachexia by its anti-inflammatory effects, involving the attenuation of NF-kB signaling, deceleration of the ubiquitin proteasome pathway, and antagonization of superoxide dismutase [59–61]. *n*-3 Fatty acids also reduce the expression of AZGP1 by interfering glucocorticoid receptor [32]. 4-Hydroxyhexenal (HHE) and 4-hydroxynonenal (HNE), lipid peroxidation products of *n*-3 fatty acids, can prevent the blocking of myosin expression and myotube formation caused by tumor cells [62]. *n*-3 Fatty acids can mediate the induction of apoptosis and the reduced proliferation of tumor cells [63]. Moreover, *n*-3 fatty acids have some effects on improving protein anabolism by activating the PI3K/Akt/mTOR pathway [64]. Recently, a randomized controlled study revealed that eicosapentaenoic acid improved postoperative survival in patients undergoing metastasectomy for liver metastases from colorectal cancer [65].

8.2.2. ActR2B Antagonist

ActR2B, a receptor for myostatin and activin A, mediate skeletal muscle protein degradation [31]. Expression of a dominant negative ActR2B in transgenic mice leads to skeletal muscle hypertrophy, which indicates that the ActR2B pathway mediates skeletal muscle growth [66]. In mice models with cancer cachexia, blockage of the ActR2B pathway suppressed skeletal muscle wasting by abolishing activated ubiquitin-proteasome system and inducing atrophy-specific ubiquitin ligases in skeletal muscles, in which tumor growth and fat loss were not inhibited [67]. Therefore, ActR2B antagonism has therapeutic potential for treating cancer cachexia and sarcopenia.

8.2.3. Medications for Insulin Resistance

Insulin resistance is basically enhanced in patients with cancer cachexia, despite the significant loss of adipose tissue [31]. Insulin resistance is related to the reduction of muscle glucose uptake and suppression of protein anabolism. Several medications for diabetes mellitus can be effective for cancer cachexia and sarcopenia. Metformin increases food intake and prolongs survival in cachectic tumor-bearing rat models [68]. Peroxisome proliferator activated receptor γ (PPAR-γ) agonists, including rosiglitazone, troglitazone, and pioglitazone, improve body weight and reduce skeletal muscle protein degradation by enhancing insulin sensitivity [69].

8.2.4. Inhibitors for Lipolysis and Fatty Acid Oxidation

ATGL and HSL regulate lipolysis of triglyceride and their inhibition reduces adipose tissue loss, contributing to maintained skeletal muscle mass [29]. Therefore, inhibitors for ATGL or HSL can be candidates for medications for cancer cachexia and sarcopenia. Moreover, increased oxidative stress caused by excessive fatty acid oxidation leads to skeletal muscle wasting [30]. Therefore, etomoxir, an inhibitor of fatty acid oxidation, can be a new approach for treating cancer cachexia and sarcopenia.

8.2.5. Hormonal Replacement Therapy

Hormonal replacement therapy is used to relieve menopausal symptoms in females. Because estrogen monotherapy can induce endometrial hyperplasia and cancer, progestogens are usually combined with estrogens. Hormonal replacement therapy is also effective for sarcopenia, which is one of the menopausal symptoms [70]. In males, testosterone is usually administered as hormonal replacement therapy. Testosterone improves sarcopenia, especially in combination with protein supplementations [58].

8.3. Exercise

Exercise, including aerobic exercise and resistance training, can contribute to the improvement of sarcopenia in cancer-bearing patients [71,72]. Exercise can overcome sarcopenia by abrogating systemic inflammation and catabolism [73]. Exercise has been reported to contribute to maintaining skeletal muscle mass and function in breast cancer patients treated with systemic chemotherapy [74]. Although the effect of exercise on metabolisms in patients with cancer cachexia is unclear, exercise may have an influence on lipolysis and insulin sensitivity. In addition, several studies demonstrated the anti-tumor effects of exercise. Exercise was shown to induce the secretion of interleukin-6 from muscles and elicit anti-tumor immunity in combination with epinephrine by redistributing natural killer cells to tumor microenvironments [75]. Because exercise enhances anti-tumor immunity, exercise might have a favorable effect on the efficacy of immune-oncology drugs for cancer [76]. Moreover, exercise was shown to inhibit tumor growth by activating the Hippo tumor suppressor pathway via β-adrenergic signaling [77].

9. Future Perspectives

Future studies are expected to clarify how cancer cachexia and sarcopenia progress in bladder cancer patients. Because the loss of adipose tissue precedes skeletal muscle wasting in animal models of cancer cachexia [26], phenotypes of cancer cachexia manifestations can be evaluated using CT images according to the level of fat and skeletal muscle depletion and may be useful in the management of bladder cancer patients [57]. Metabolic and molecular backgrounds of cancer cachexia and sarcopenia should be further elucidated to develop novel therapeutic strategies for sarcopenia. Future clinical trials are expected to assess the efficacy of novel medications and exercise in bladder cancer patients.

10. Conclusions

In this review, we summarized reported series of the prognostic role of sarcopenia in bladder cancer patients. Sarcopenia is significantly associated with unfavorable prognosis in bladder cancer patients undergoing a radical cystectomy. Moreover, sarcopenia is also a significant poor prognostic factor in patients with inoperable advanced bladder cancer. Thus, sarcopenia can be used as a prognostic biomarker in patients with bladder cancer at various stages. We reviewed reported series of the prognostic role of changes in skeletal muscle mass during treatments in bladder cancer patients. Recovery of skeletal muscle mass during treatments can be associated with the improved prognosis of bladder cancer patients, whereas decline of skeletal muscle mass can reflect poor prognosis, indicating its role not only as a prognostic biomarker but also as a surrogate marker for treatment efficacy in bladder cancer patients. In addition, nutritional support, medications, and exercise may improve sarcopenia and cancer cachexia and have a favorable influence on the management of cancer-bearing patients. Future studies may clarify the prognostic value of these interventions in cancer-bearing patients.

Author Contributions: All authors made substantial contributions to this work; acquisition and interpretation of data by online search, H.F. and K.T.; draft and supervision of the work, H.F. and F.K.; revision of the work, H.F., K.T., H.S. and F.K. All authors have approved the final version and agreed to be personally accountable for the author's own contributions.

funding: This work was partly supported by the Clinical Research Fund (H.F., grant number H260301002, URL: http://www.metro.tokyo.jp/) from the Tokyo Metropolitan Government.

Conflicts of Interest: The authors declare no conflicts of interest.

References

1. Antoni, S.; Ferlay, J.; Soerjomataram, I.; Znaor, A.; Jemal, A.; Bray, F. Bladder Cancer Incidence and Mortality: A Global Overview and Recent Trends. *Eur. Urol.* **2017**, *71*, 96–108. [CrossRef] [PubMed]
2. Babjuk, M.; Bohle, A.; Burger, M.; Capoun, O.; Cohen, D.; Comperat, E.M.; Hernandez, V.; Kaasinen, E.; Palou, J.; Roupret, M.; et al. EAU Guidelines on Non-Muscle-invasive Urothelial Carcinoma of the Bladder: Update 2016. *Eur. Urol.* **2017**, *71*, 447–461. [CrossRef] [PubMed]
3. Witjes, J.A.; Lebret, T.; Comperat, E.M.; Cowan, N.C.; De Santis, M.; Bruins, H.M.; Hernandez, V.; Espinos, E.L.; Dunn, J.; Rouanne, M.; et al. Updated 2016 EAU Guidelines on Muscle-invasive and Metastatic Bladder Cancer. *Eur. Urol.* **2017**, *71*, 462–475. [CrossRef] [PubMed]
4. Dalbagni, G.; Genega, E.; Hashibe, M.; Zhang, Z.F.; Russo, P.; Herr, H.; Reuter, V. Cystectomy for bladder cancer: A contemporary series. *J. Urol.* **2001**, *165*, 1111–1116. [CrossRef]
5. Bellmunt, J.; von der Maase, H.; Mead, G.M.; Skoneczna, I.; De Santis, M.; Daugaard, G.; Boehle, A.; Chevreau, C.; Paz-Ares, L.; Laufman, L.R.; et al. Randomized phase III study comparing paclitaxel/cisplatin/gemcitabine and gemcitabine/cisplatin in patients with locally advanced or metastatic urothelial cancer without prior systemic therapy: EORTC Intergroup Study 30987. *J. Clin. Oncol.* **2012**, *30*, 1107–1113. [CrossRef] [PubMed]
6. Sundahl, N.; Rottey, S.; De Maeseneer, D.; Ost, P. Pembrolizumab for the treatment of bladder cancer. *Expert Rev. Anticancer Ther.* **2018**, *18*, 107–114. [CrossRef] [PubMed]
7. Cruz-Jentoft, A.J.; Baeyens, J.P.; Bauer, J.M.; Boirie, Y.; Cederholm, T.; Landi, F.; Martin, F.C.; Michel, J.P.; Rolland, Y.; Schneider, S.M.; et al. Sarcopenia: European consensus on definition and diagnosis: Report of the European Working Group on Sarcopenia in Older People. *Age Ageing* **2010**, *39*, 412–423. [CrossRef] [PubMed]
8. Kim, T.N.; Choi, K.M. Sarcopenia: Definition, epidemiology, and pathophysiology. *J. Bone Metab.* **2013**, *20*, 1–10. [CrossRef] [PubMed]
9. Garatachea, N.; Lucia, A. Genes and the ageing muscle: A review on genetic association studies. *Age* **2013**, *35*, 207–233. [CrossRef] [PubMed]
10. Brown, J.C.; Harhay, M.O.; Harhay, M.N. Sarcopenia and mortality among a population-based sample of community-dwelling older adults. *J. Cachexia Sarcopenia Muscle* **2016**, *7*, 290–298. [CrossRef] [PubMed]
11. Landi, F.; Cruz-Jentoft, A.J.; Liperoti, R.; Russo, A.; Giovannini, S.; Tosato, M.; Capoluongo, E.; Bernabei, R.; Onder, G. Sarcopenia and mortality risk in frail older persons aged 80 years and older: Results from ilSIRENTE study. *Age Ageing* **2013**, *42*, 203–209. [CrossRef] [PubMed]

12. Cosqueric, G.; Sebag, A.; Ducolombier, C.; Thomas, C.; Piette, F.; Weill-Engerer, S. Sarcopenia is predictive of nosocomial infection in care of the elderly. *Br. J. Nutr.* **2006**, *96*, 895–901. [CrossRef] [PubMed]
13. Lee, J.; Hong, Y.P.; Shin, H.J.; Lee, W. Associations of Sarcopenia and Sarcopenic Obesity With Metabolic Syndrome Considering Both Muscle Mass and Muscle Strength. *J. Prev. Med. Public Health* **2016**, *49*, 35–44. [CrossRef] [PubMed]
14. Kim, J.E.; Lee, Y.H.; Huh, J.H.; Kang, D.R.; Rhee, Y.; Lim, S.K. Early-stage chronic kidney disease, insulin resistance, and osteoporosis as risk factors of sarcopenia in aged population: The fourth Korea National Health and Nutrition Examination Survey (KNHANES IV), 2008–2009. *Osteoporos. Int.* **2014**, *25*, 2189–2198. [CrossRef] [PubMed]
15. Kim, J.H.; Cho, J.J.; Park, Y.S. Relationship between sarcopenic obesity and cardiovascular disease risk as estimated by the Framingham risk score. *J. Korean Med. Sci.* **2015**, *30*, 264–271. [CrossRef] [PubMed]
16. Fearon, K.; Strasser, F.; Anker, S.D.; Bosaeus, I.; Bruera, E.; Fainsinger, R.L.; Jatoi, A.; Loprinzi, C.; MacDonald, N.; Mantovani, G.; et al. Definition and classification of cancer cachexia: An international consensus. *Lancet Oncol.* **2011**, *12*, 489–495. [CrossRef]
17. Fearon, K.C.; Voss, A.C.; Hustead, D.S. Definition of cancer cachexia: Effect of weight loss, reduced food intake, and systemic inflammation on functional status and prognosis. *Am. J. Clin. Nutr.* **2006**, *83*, 1345–1350. [CrossRef] [PubMed]
18. Martin, L.; Birdsell, L.; Macdonald, N.; Reiman, T.; Clandinin, M.T.; McCargar, L.J.; Murphy, R.; Ghosh, S.; Sawyer, M.B.; Baracos, V.E. Cancer cachexia in the age of obesity: Skeletal muscle depletion is a powerful prognostic factor, independent of body mass index. *J. Clin. Oncol.* **2013**, *31*, 1539–1547. [CrossRef] [PubMed]
19. Prado, C.M.; Lieffers, J.R.; McCargar, L.J.; Reiman, T.; Sawyer, M.B.; Martin, L.; Baracos, V.E. Prevalence and clinical implications of sarcopenic obesity in patients with solid tumours of the respiratory and gastrointestinal tracts: A population-based study. *Lancet Oncol.* **2008**, *9*, 629–635. [CrossRef]
20. Harimoto, N.; Shirabe, K.; Yamashita, Y.I.; Ikegami, T.; Yoshizumi, T.; Soejima, Y.; Ikeda, T.; Maehara, Y.; Nishie, A.; Yamanaka, T. Sarcopenia as a predictor of prognosis in patients following hepatectomy for hepatocellular carcinoma. *Br. J. Surg.* **2013**, *100*, 1523–1530. [CrossRef] [PubMed]
21. Harada, K.; Ida, S.; Baba, Y.; Ishimoto, T.; Kosumi, K.; Tokunaga, R.; Izumi, D.; Ohuchi, M.; Nakamura, K.; Kiyozumi, Y.; et al. Prognostic and clinical impact of sarcopenia in esophageal squamous cell carcinoma. *Dis. Esophagus* **2016**, *29*, 627–633. [CrossRef] [PubMed]
22. Go, S.I.; Park, M.J.; Song, H.N.; Kim, H.G.; Kang, M.H.; Lee, H.R.; Kim, Y.; Kim, R.B.; Lee, S.I.; Lee, G.W. Prognostic impact of sarcopenia in patients with diffuse large B-cell lymphoma treated with rituximab plus cyclophosphamide, doxorubicin, vincristine, and prednisone. *J. Cachexia Sarcopenia Muscle* **2016**, *7*, 567–576. [CrossRef] [PubMed]
23. Sabel, M.S.; Lee, J.; Cai, S.; Englesbe, M.J.; Holcombe, S.; Wang, S. Sarcopenia as a prognostic factor among patients with stage III melanoma. *Ann. Surg. Oncol.* **2011**, *18*, 3579–3585. [CrossRef] [PubMed]
24. Psutka, S.P.; Boorjian, S.A.; Moynagh, M.R.; Schmit, G.D.; Costello, B.A.; Thompson, R.H.; Stewart-Merrill, S.B.; Lohse, C.M.; Cheville, J.C.; Leibovich, B.C.; et al. Decreased Skeletal Muscle Mass is Associated with an Increased Risk of Mortality after Radical Nephrectomy for Localized Renal Cell Cancer. *J. Urol.* **2016**, *195*, 270–276. [CrossRef] [PubMed]
25. Fukushima, H.; Nakanishi, Y.; Kataoka, M.; Tobisu, K.; Koga, F. Prognostic Significance of Sarcopenia in Patients with Metastatic Renal Cell Carcinoma. *J. Urol.* **2016**, *195*, 26–32. [CrossRef] [PubMed]
26. Kliewer, K.L.; Ke, J.Y.; Tian, M.; Cole, R.M.; Andridge, R.R.; Belury, M.A. Adipose tissue lipolysis and energy metabolism in early cancer cachexia in mice. *Cancer Boil. Ther.* **2015**, *16*, 886–897. [CrossRef] [PubMed]
27. Fearon, K.C.; Glass, D.J.; Guttridge, D.C. Cancer cachexia: Mediators, signaling, and metabolic pathways. *Cell Metab.* **2012**, *16*, 153–166. [CrossRef] [PubMed]
28. Petruzzelli, M.; Schweiger, M.; Schreiber, R.; Campos-Olivas, R.; Tsoli, M.; Allen, J.; Swarbrick, M.; Rose-John, S.; Rincon, M.; Robertson, G.; et al. A switch from white to brown fat increases energy expenditure in cancer-associated cachexia. *Cell Metab.* **2014**, *20*, 433–447. [CrossRef] [PubMed]
29. Das, S.K.; Eder, S.; Schauer, S.; Diwoky, C.; Temmel, H.; Guertl, B.; Gorkiewicz, G.; Tamilarasan, K.P.; Kumari, P.; Trauner, M.; et al. Adipose triglyceride lipase contributes to cancer-associated cachexia. *Science* **2011**, *333*, 233–238. [CrossRef] [PubMed]

30. Fukawa, T.; Yan-Jiang, B.C.; Min-Wen, J.C.; Jun-Hao, E.T.; Huang, D.; Qian, C.N.; Ong, P.; Li, Z.; Chen, S.; Mak, S.Y.; et al. Excessive fatty acid oxidation induces muscle atrophy in cancer cachexia. *Nat. Med.* **2016**, *22*, 666–671. [CrossRef] [PubMed]
31. Argiles, J.M.; Busquets, S.; Stemmler, B.; Lopez-Soriano, F.J. Cancer cachexia: Understanding the molecular basis. *Nat. Rev. Cancer* **2014**, *14*, 754–762. [CrossRef] [PubMed]
32. Tisdale, M.J. Mechanisms of cancer cachexia. *Physiol. Rev.* **2009**, *89*, 381–410. [CrossRef] [PubMed]
33. Schmitt, T.L.; Martignoni, M.E.; Bachmann, J.; Fechtner, K.; Friess, H.; Kinscherf, R.; Hildebrandt, W. Activity of the Akt-dependent anabolic and catabolic pathways in muscle and liver samples in cancer-related cachexia. *J. Mol. Med.* **2007**, *85*, 647–654. [CrossRef] [PubMed]
34. Moylan, J.S.; Smith, J.D.; Chambers, M.A.; McLoughlin, T.J.; Reid, M.B. TNF induction of atrogin-1/MAFbx mRNA depends on Foxo4 expression but not AKT-Foxo1/3 signaling. *Am. J. Physiol. Cell Physiol.* **2008**, *295*, C986–C993. [CrossRef] [PubMed]
35. Julienne, C.M.; Dumas, J.F.; Goupille, C.; Pinault, M.; Berri, C.; Collin, A.; Tesseraud, S.; Couet, C.; Servais, S. Cancer cachexia is associated with a decrease in skeletal muscle mitochondrial oxidative capacities without alteration of ATP production efficiency. *J. Cachexia Sarcopenia Muscle* **2012**, *3*, 265–275. [CrossRef] [PubMed]
36. Stephens, N.A.; Skipworth, R.J.; Macdonald, A.J.; Greig, C.A.; Ross, J.A.; Fearon, K.C. Intramyocellular lipid droplets increase with progression of cachexia in cancer patients. *J. Cachexia Sarcopenia Muscle* **2011**, *2*, 111–117. [CrossRef] [PubMed]
37. Fukushima, H.; Koga, F. Impact of sarcopenia in the management of urological cancer patients. *Expert Rev. Anticancer Ther.* **2017**, *17*, 455–466. [CrossRef] [PubMed]
38. Shen, W.; Punyanitya, M.; Wang, Z.; Gallagher, D.; St-Onge, M.P.; Albu, J.; Heymsfield, S.B.; Heshka, S. Total body skeletal muscle and adipose tissue volumes: Estimation from a single abdominal cross-sectional image. *J. Appl. Physiol.* **2004**, *97*, 2333–2338. [CrossRef] [PubMed]
39. Hamaguchi, Y.; Kaido, T.; Okumura, S.; Kobayashi, A.; Hammad, A.; Tamai, Y.; Inagaki, N.; Uemoto, S. Proposal for new diagnostic criteria for low skeletal muscle mass based on computed tomography imaging in Asian adults. *Nutrition* **2016**, *32*, 1200–1205. [CrossRef] [PubMed]
40. Aubrey, J.; Esfandiari, N.; Baracos, V.E.; Buteau, F.A.; Frenette, J.; Putman, C.T.; Mazurak, V.C. Measurement of skeletal muscle radiation attenuation and basis of its biological variation. *Acta Physiol.* **2014**, *210*, 489–497. [CrossRef] [PubMed]
41. Hulver, M.W.; Dohm, G.L. The molecular mechanism linking muscle fat accumulation to insulin resistance. *Proc. Nutr. Soc.* **2004**, *63*, 375–380. [CrossRef] [PubMed]
42. Moher, D.; Liberati, A.; Tetzlaff, J.; Altman, D.G. Preferred reporting items for systematic reviews and meta-analyses: The PRISMA statement. *Int. J. Surg.* **2010**, *8*, 336–341. [CrossRef] [PubMed]
43. Lawrentschuk, N.; Colombo, R.; Hakenberg, O.W.; Lerner, S.P.; Mansson, W.; Sagalowsky, A.; Wirth, M.P. Prevention and management of complications following radical cystectomy for bladder cancer. *Eur. Urol.* **2010**, *57*, 983–1001. [CrossRef] [PubMed]
44. Wan, F.; Zhu, Y.; Gu, C.; Yao, X.; Shen, Y.; Dai, B.; Zhang, S.; Zhang, H.; Cheng, J.; Ye, D. Lower skeletal muscle index and early complications in patients undergoing radical cystectomy for bladder cancer. *World J. Surg. Oncol.* **2014**, *12*, 14. [CrossRef] [PubMed]
45. Smith, A.B.; Deal, A.M.; Yu, H.; Boyd, B.; Matthews, J.; Wallen, E.M.; Pruthi, R.S.; Woods, M.E.; Muss, H.; Nielsen, M.E. Sarcopenia as a predictor of complications and survival following radical cystectomy. *J. Urol.* **2014**, *191*, 1714–1720. [CrossRef] [PubMed]
46. Psutka, S.P.; Carrasco, A.; Schmit, G.D.; Moynagh, M.R.; Boorjian, S.A.; Frank, I.; Stewart, S.B.; Thapa, P.; Tarrell, R.F.; Cheville, J.C.; et al. Sarcopenia in patients with bladder cancer undergoing radical cystectomy: Impact on cancer-specific and all-cause mortality. *Cancer* **2014**, *120*, 2910–2918. [CrossRef] [PubMed]
47. Hirasawa, Y.; Nakashima, J.; Yunaiyama, D.; Sugihara, T.; Gondo, T.; Nakagami, Y.; Horiguchi, Y.; Ohno, Y.; Namiki, K.; Ohori, M.; et al. Sarcopenia as a Novel Preoperative Prognostic Predictor for Survival in Patients with Bladder Cancer Undergoing Radical Cystectomy. *Ann. Surg. Oncol.* **2016**, *23*, 1048–1054. [CrossRef] [PubMed]
48. Miyake, M.; Morizawa, Y.; Hori, S.; Marugami, N.; Shimada, K.; Gotoh, D.; Tatsumi, Y.; Nakai, Y.; Inoue, T.; Anai, S.; et al. Clinical impact of postoperative loss in psoas major muscle and nutrition index after radical cystectomy for patients with urothelial carcinoma of the bladder. *BMC Cancer* **2017**, *17*, 237. [CrossRef] [PubMed]

49. Saitoh-Maeda, Y.; Kawahara, T.; Miyoshi, Y.; Tsutsumi, S.; Takamoto, D.; Shimokihara, K.; Hayashi, Y.; Mochizuki, T.; Ohtaka, M.; Nakamura, M.; et al. A low psoas muscle volume correlates with a longer hospitalization after radical cystectomy. *BMC Urol.* **2017**, *17*, 87. [CrossRef] [PubMed]
50. Mayr, R.; Gierth, M.; Zeman, F.; Reiffen, M.; Seeger, P.; Wezel, F.; Pycha, A.; Comploj, E.; Bonatti, M.; Ritter, M.; et al. Sarcopenia as a comorbidity-independent predictor of survival following radical cystectomy for bladder cancer. *J. Cachexia Sarcopenia Muscle* **2018**, *9*, 505–513. [CrossRef] [PubMed]
51. Fukushima, H.; Yokoyama, M.; Nakanishi, Y.; Tobisu, K.; Koga, F. Sarcopenia as a prognostic biomarker of advanced urothelial carcinoma. *PLoS ONE* **2015**, *10*, e0115895. [CrossRef] [PubMed]
52. Taguchi, S.; Akamatsu, N.; Nakagawa, T.; Gonoi, W.; Kanatani, A.; Miyazaki, H.; Fujimura, T.; Fukuhara, H.; Kume, H.; Homma, Y. Sarcopenia Evaluated Using the Skeletal Muscle Index Is a Significant Prognostic Factor for Metastatic Urothelial Carcinoma. *Clin. Genitourin. Cancer* **2016**, *14*, 237–243. [CrossRef] [PubMed]
53. Kasahara, R.; Kawahara, T.; Ohtake, S.; Saitoh, Y.; Tsutsumi, S.; Teranishi, J.I.; Miyoshi, Y.; Nakaigawa, N.; Yao, M.; Kobayashi, K.; et al. A Low Psoas Muscle Index before Treatment Can Predict a Poorer Prognosis in Advanced Bladder Cancer Patients Who Receive Gemcitabine and Nedaplatin Therapy. *BioMed Res. Int.* **2017**, *2017*, 7981549. [CrossRef] [PubMed]
54. Abe, H.; Takei, K.; Uematsu, T.; Tokura, Y.; Suzuki, I.; Sakamoto, K.; Nishihara, D.; Yamaguchi, Y.; Mizuno, T.; Nukui, A.; et al. Significance of sarcopenia as a prognostic factor for metastatic urothelial carcinoma patients treated with systemic chemotherapy. *Int. J. Clin. Oncol.* **2018**, *23*, 338–346. [CrossRef] [PubMed]
55. Zargar, H.; Almassi, N.; Kovac, E.; Ercole, C.; Remer, E.; Rini, B.; Stephenson, A.; Garcia, J.A.; Grivas, P. Change in Psoas Muscle Volume as a Predictor of Outcomes in Patients Treated with Chemotherapy and Radical Cystectomy for Muscle-Invasive Bladder Cancer. *Bladder Cancer* **2017**, *3*, 57–63. [CrossRef] [PubMed]
56. Fukushima, H.; Kataoka, M.; Nakanishi, Y.; Sakamoto, K.; Takemura, K.; Suzuki, H.; Ito, M.; Tobisu, K.I.; Fujii, Y.; Koga, F. Posttherapeutic skeletal muscle mass recovery predicts favorable prognosis in patients with advanced urothelial carcinoma receiving first-line platinum-based chemotherapy. *Urol. Oncol.* **2018**, *36*, 156.e9–156.e16. [CrossRef] [PubMed]
57. Kays, J.K.; Shahda, S.; Stanley, M.; Bell, T.M.; O'Neill, B.H.; Kohli, M.D.; Couch, M.E.; Koniaris, L.G.; Zimmers, T.A. Three cachexia phenotypes and the impact of fat-only loss on survival in FOLFIRINOX therapy for pancreatic cancer. *J. Cachexia Sarcopenia Muscle* **2018**. [CrossRef] [PubMed]
58. Ahima, R.S.; Park, H.K. Connecting Myokines and Metabolism. *Endocrinol. Metab.* **2015**, *30*, 235–245. [CrossRef] [PubMed]
59. Vaughan, V.C.; Martin, P.; Lewandowski, P.A. Cancer cachexia: Impact, mechanisms and emerging treatments. *J. Cachexia Sarcopenia Muscle* **2013**, *4*, 95–109. [CrossRef] [PubMed]
60. Whitehouse, A.S.; Smith, H.J.; Drake, J.L.; Tisdale, M.J. Mechanism of attenuation of skeletal muscle protein catabolism in cancer cachexia by eicosapentaenoic acid. *Cancer Res.* **2001**, *61*, 3604–3609. [PubMed]
61. Oh, D.Y.; Talukdar, S.; Bae, E.J.; Imamura, T.; Morinaga, H.; Fan, W.; Li, P.; Lu, W.J.; Watkins, S.M.; Olefsky, J.M. GPR120 is an omega-3 fatty acid receptor mediating potent anti-inflammatory and insulin-sensitizing effects. *Cell* **2010**, *142*, 687–698. [CrossRef] [PubMed]
62. Muzio, G.; Ricci, M.; Traverso, N.; Monacelli, F.; Oraldi, M.; Maggiora, M.; Canuto, R.A. 4-Hydroxyhexenal and 4-hydroxynonenal are mediators of the anti-cachectic effect of n-3 and n-6 polyunsaturated fatty acids on human lung cancer cells. *Free. Radic. Boil. Med.* **2016**, *99*, 63–70. [CrossRef] [PubMed]
63. Newell, M.; Baker, K.; Postovit, L.M.; Field, C.J. A Critical Review on the Effect of Docosahexaenoic Acid (DHA) on Cancer Cell Cycle Progression. *Int. J. Mol. Sci.* **2017**, *18*, 1784. [CrossRef] [PubMed]
64. Smith, G.I.; Atherton, P.; Reeds, D.N.; Mohammed, B.S.; Rankin, D.; Rennie, M.J.; Mittendorfer, B. Omega-3 polyunsaturated fatty acids augment the muscle protein anabolic response to hyperinsulinaemia-hyperaminoacidaemia in healthy young and middle-aged men and women. *Clin. Sci.* **2011**, *121*, 267–278. [CrossRef] [PubMed]
65. Cockbain, A.J.; Volpato, M.; Race, A.D.; Munarini, A.; Fazio, C.; Belluzzi, A.; Loadman, P.M.; Toogood, G.J.; Hull, M.A. Anticolorectal cancer activity of the omega-3 polyunsaturated fatty acid eicosapentaenoic acid. *Gut* **2014**, *63*, 1760–1768. [CrossRef] [PubMed]
66. Lee, S.J.; McPherron, A.C. Regulation of myostatin activity and muscle growth. *Proc. Natl. Acad. Sci. USA* **2001**, *98*, 9306–9311. [CrossRef] [PubMed]

67. Zhou, X.; Wang, J.L.; Lu, J.; Song, Y.; Kwak, K.S.; Jiao, Q.; Rosenfeld, R.; Chen, Q.; Boone, T.; Simonet, W.S.; et al. Reversal of cancer cachexia and muscle wasting by ActRIIB antagonism leads to prolonged survival. *Cell* **2010**, *142*, 531–543. [CrossRef] [PubMed]
68. Oliveira, A.G.; Gomes-Marcondes, M.C. Metformin treatment modulates the tumour-induced wasting effects in muscle protein metabolism minimising the cachexia in tumour-bearing rats. *BMC Cancer* **2016**, *16*, 418. [CrossRef] [PubMed]
69. Beluzi, M.; Peres, S.B.; Henriques, F.S.; Sertie, R.A.; Franco, F.O.; Santos, K.B.; Knobl, P.; Andreotti, S.; Shida, C.S.; Neves, R.X.; et al. Pioglitazone treatment increases survival and prevents body weight loss in tumor-bearing animals: Possible anti-cachectic effect. *PLoS ONE* **2015**, *10*, e0122660. [CrossRef] [PubMed]
70. Dionne, I.J.; Kinaman, K.A.; Poehlman, E.T. Sarcopenia and muscle function during menopause and hormone-replacement therapy. *J. Nutr. Health Aging* **2000**, *4*, 156–161. [PubMed]
71. Stene, G.B.; Helbostad, J.L.; Balstad, T.R.; Riphagen, I.I.; Kaasa, S.; Oldervoll, L.M. Effect of physical exercise on muscle mass and strength in cancer patients during treatment—A systematic review. *Crit. Rev. Oncol. Hematol.* **2013**, *88*, 573–593. [CrossRef] [PubMed]
72. Strasser, B.; Steindorf, K.; Wiskemann, J.; Ulrich, C.M. Impact of resistance training in cancer survivors: A meta-analysis. *Med. Sci. Sports Exerc.* **2013**, *45*, 2080–2090. [CrossRef] [PubMed]
73. Gould, D.W.; Lahart, I.; Carmichael, A.R.; Koutedakis, Y.; Metsios, G.S. Cancer cachexia prevention via physical exercise: Molecular mechanisms. *J. Cachexia Sarcopenia Muscle* **2013**, *4*, 111–124. [CrossRef] [PubMed]
74. Mijwel, S.; Cardinale, D.A.; Norrbom, J.; Chapman, M.; Ivarsson, N.; Wengstrom, Y.; Sundberg, C.J.; Rundqvist, H. Exercise training during chemotherapy preserves skeletal muscle fiber area, capillarization, and mitochondrial content in patients with breast cancer. *FASEB J.* **2018**. [CrossRef] [PubMed]
75. Pedersen, L.; Idorn, M.; Olofsson, G.H.; Lauenborg, B.; Nookaew, I.; Hansen, R.H.; Johannesen, H.H.; Becker, J.C.; Pedersen, K.S.; Dethlefsen, C.; et al. Voluntary Running Suppresses Tumor Growth through Epinephrine- and IL-6-Dependent NK Cell Mobilization and Redistribution. *Cell Metab.* **2016**, *23*, 554–562. [CrossRef] [PubMed]
76. Koelwyn, G.J.; Wennerberg, E.; Demaria, S.; Jones, L.W. Exercise in Regulation of Inflammation-Immune Axis Function in Cancer Initiation and Progression. *Oncology* **2015**, *29*, 908–920, 922. [PubMed]
77. Dethlefsen, C.; Hansen, L.S.; Lillelund, C.; Andersen, C.; Gehl, J.; Christensen, J.F.; Pedersen, B.K.; Hojman, P. Exercise-Induced Catecholamines Activate the Hippo Tumor Suppressor Pathway to Reduce Risks of Breast Cancer Development. *Cancer Res.* **2017**, *77*, 4894–4904. [CrossRef] [PubMed]

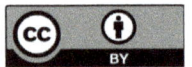

© 2018 by the authors. Licensee MDPI, Basel, Switzerland. This article is an open access article distributed under the terms and conditions of the Creative Commons Attribution (CC BY) license (http://creativecommons.org/licenses/by/4.0/).

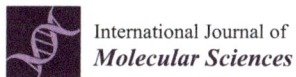

Review

Extracellular Vesicles in Bladder Cancer: Biomarkers and Beyond

Yu-Ru Liu [1], Carlos J. Ortiz-Bonilla [1,2] and Yi-Fen Lee [1,2,*]

1. Department of Urology, University of Rochester Medical Center, Rochester, NY 14642, USA; yu-ru_liu@urmc.rochester.edu (Y.-R.L.); Carlos_ortizbonilla@urmc.rochester.edu (C.J.O.-B.)
2. Department of Pathology and Lab Medicine, University of Rochester Medical Center, Rochester, NY 14642, USA
* Correspondence: yifen_lee@urmc.rochester.edu; Tel.: +1-585-275-9702

Received: 30 July 2018; Accepted: 15 September 2018; Published: 18 September 2018

Abstract: Tumor-derived extracellular vesicles (TEVs) are membrane-bound, nanosized vesicles released by cancer cells and taken up by cells in the tumor microenvironment to modulate the molecular makeup and behavior of recipient cells. In this report, we summarize the pivotal roles of TEVs involved in bladder cancer (BC) development, progression and treatment resistance through transferring their bioactive cargos, including proteins and nucleic acids. We also report on the molecular profiling of TEV cargos derived from urine and blood of BC patients as non-invasive disease biomarkers. The current hurdles in EV research and plausible solutions are discussed.

Keywords: extracellular vesicle; exosome; bladder cancer; biomarkers

1. Introduction

In the past decade, a heterogeneous population of nanograde membrane particles in biological fluids, termed extracellular vesicles (EVs), gained newfound meaning in cancer therapy and diagnosis. EVs is a broad term which generally indicates the heterogeneous vesicles released from cells. In fact, most cells, if not all, shed vesicles constantly. Diverse names have been used to refer to various sorts of EVs, including ectosome, microparticle, exosome and microvesicle. Among them, the biogenesis, specific markers and functions of exosomes and microvesicles have been studied relatively thoroughly. As summarized in Figure 1, the release as well as uptake of EVs occurs simultaneously between cells. Exosomes are 50–100 nm in diameter and their biogenesis starts with the inward budding of a late endosomal membrane which forms a multi-vesicular body (MVB) containing a number of intraluminal vesicles (ILVs) [1]. In contrast, microvesicles (100–1000 nm in diameter) are larger than exosomes and formed by outward budding of the cell membrane. Both exosomes and microvesicles act as "intercellular postal service" [2] since they encapsulate a wide variety of bioactive molecules, including proteins, lipids and nucleic acids (DNA, micro-RNA, mRNA and other noncoding RNA species), and they transport this cargo to recipient cells locally or at a distance, consequently altering their behavior. The uptake of EVs by recipient cells is mediated through fusion, phagocytosis, macropinocytosis and receptor raft-mediated endocytosis. However, the mechanisms by which EV cargo is selected are not yet known.

EVs gained biologists' interest following the groundbreaking finding in 1996 that exosomes transfer Major Histocompatibility Complex (MHC) class II molecules from B cells to T cells, thus mediating activation of the adaptive immune response [3]. Later studies reported on the identification of various functional miRNAs encapsulated in EVs of immune cells. In view of the extensive regulatory capacity of miRNA, Valadi and colleagues in 2007 discovered for the first time that EVs have been exploited by cells as a tool to exchange genetic information [4]. This finding reveals a novel mechanism of gene-based communication between cells via EV cargo transfer. The pivotal roles of EVs are found not only in mediating the immune system but also in regulating various physiological and pathological cellular functions. The urinary bladder is susceptible to diverse EV-containing biological fluids, such as blood, lymphatic fluid and urine, reason why there has been an increased interest in EV roles in bladder cancer (BC) and study of their potential clinical applications. In this review article, we will focus on recent research on EVs derived from BC (BCEVs) and their roles in tumorigenesis and disease progression, as well as emerging applications in therapeutics and diagnostics.

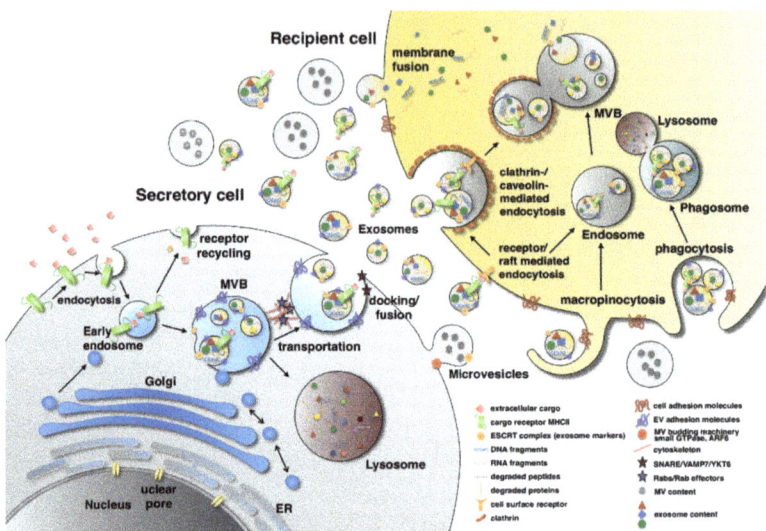

Figure 1. Extracellular vesicles (EV) biogenesis. The EV contents come from three sources: extracellular, intracellular and plasma membrane. Extracellular and plasma membrane molecules enter the early endosome through endocytosis either selectively by cargo receptor (ubiquitinated MHC-II) recognition or non-selectively. In the late endosome, the endosomal sorting complexes required for transport, ESCRT and their associated proteins such as TSG101, Alix, α-arrestin1 and CHMP4 mediate membrane inward invagination and form exosomes within multi-vesicular body (MVB). During the vesicle forming process, certain cytosolic components such as DNA, RNA and proteins are included in the exosome. MVBs can turn into lysosomes and degrade their contents or dock and fuse with the plasma membrane to release their contents to the extracellular space. The transportation and docking of MVBs is mediated by cytoskeleton remodeling which is regulated by Rab GTPase proteins (e.g., Rab27α, Rab27β and Rab7) and their effectors (e.g., SYTL4 and SLAC2B), whereas the fusion of MVBs with the plasma membrane is mediated by SNARE, VAMP7 and YKT6. In contrast, microvesicles are formed by outward budding of the plasma membrane which involves actin-myosin machinery, small GTPase and ARF6. The content sorting in microvesicles also involves TSG101. EV uptake is initiated by adhesion of EVs to the surface adhesion molecules on recipient cells, such as integrins, ICAM-1/LFA-1, CD11a, CD49d, CD44, CD169, heparin sulfate proteoglycans and by CD9, CD81 on EVs. EVs are then internalized through fusion, phagocytosis, macropinocytosis and endocytosis. ESCRT: Endosomal sorting complexes required for transport; TSG101: Tumor susceptibility gene 101; Alix: ALG-2-interacting protein X; CHMP4: Chromatin-modifying protein/charged multivesicular body protein; SYTL4: Synaptotagmin like 4; SLAC2B: Slp homolog lacking C2 domain B; SNARE: SNAP receptor; VAMP7: Vesicle associated membrane protein 7; YKT6: v-SNARE homolog (*S. cerevisiae*); ARF6: ADP-ribosylation factor 6; ICAM1: Intercellulare adhesion molecule 1; LFA1: Lymphocyte function-associated antigen 1.

2. Oncogenic Properties of BCEVs

Cancer cells are known to secrete more EVs than normal cells. The blood plasma of a cancer patient contains approximately 4000 trillion EVs, roughly twice the amount contained in a healthy individual [5]. Numerous studies have shown that EV-mediated cargo transfer to recipient cells affects many stages of cancer progression through communication between the cancer and the surrounding microenvironment, consequently promoting neoplastic transformation, BC proliferation, migration, invasion and angiogenesis. The EV cargo contents and their effects on cancer progression are summarized below.

2.1. BCEVs in Neoplastic Transformation

The transformation of healthy cells into malignant cancer cells involves several pathologic processes and many studies indicate that TEVs participate by transferring oncogenic cargo molecules to recipient cells [6]. A study by Urciuoli et al. [7] reported that treating NIH3T3 fibroblasts with osteosarcoma-derived EVs induced tumor-like phenotypes. Cells gained survival capacity by enhanced proliferation, migration, adhesion and 3D sphere formation and acquired the ability to grow in an anchorage dependent manner. Similar findings were reported in a study by Panagopoulos et al. [8], where they showed that EVs isolated from DU145 prostate cancer cells induced the malignant transformation of non-malignant prostate epithelial cells, possibly via up-regulation of pro-survival protein STAT3 [9,10]. Together, these results demonstrate that TEVs promote malignant transformation.

In the BC field, TEV's role in tumorigenesis is less clear. Goulet et al. recently reported that BCEVs can promote "transformation" of healthy fibroblasts into cancer-associated fibroblasts (CAFs) [11]. They isolated EVs from RT4, T24 and SW1710 BC cells and used them to treat healthy fibroblasts isolated from human bladder biopsies. As a result, recipient fibroblasts gained CAF phenotypes with increased proliferation and migration capacity as well as elevated expression of CAF markers—smooth muscle actin (SMA), fibroblast activation protein (FAP) and Galectin. Interestingly, our unpublished data (12,24,60) reveal that chronically exposing non-malignant immortalized urothelial cells to BCEVs leads to malignant transformation in vitro and in vivo. This might be due to the selection of cells with resistance to a BCEV-induced cellular stress response [12].

2.2. BCEVs Promote Cancer Cell Progression by Mediating Communication between Tumor Cells

2.2.1. Proliferation

The proliferation of tumor cells is an indispensable process for cancer progression, mostly relying on tumor-derived soluble growth factors. TEVs have been shown to promote cancer cell proliferation in leukemia, gastric cancer, glioblastoma, melanoma and prostate cancer, among others [13]. In BC, treating human 5637 and T24 BC cells with BCEVs was shown to stimulate their proliferation, possibly through activation of protein kinase B (Akt) and extracellular signal–regulated kinase (ERK) pathways [14]. Recent research delineating BC proliferation under hypoxia conditions found pivotal roles for BCEVs in transferring long non-coding RNA-urothelial cancer-associated 1 (lncRNA-UCA1) [15]. In this study, Xue et al. demonstrated that BCEVs derived from hypoxic 5637 cells contain high levels of lncRNA-UCA1 which stimulated proliferation, mobility and invasion in human UMUC2 BC recipient cells. In a xenograft model, lncRNA-UCA1-containing EVs facilitated bladder tumor growth and metastasis to the lymph nodes. Knockdown of lncRNA-UCA1 in hypoxic BCEVs increased the expression of E-cadherin while reducing vimentin and MMP9 expression, thereby triggering epithelial-mesenchymal transition (EMT) in the recipient BC cells.

2.2.2. Migration and Invasion

The essential step of tumor progression to metastasis is gaining the ability to migrate and invade. Our previous study showed that EVs derived from high grade TCC-SUP BC cells as well as urinary EVs from patients with muscle invasive bladder cancer (MIBC) facilitated migration and invasion in low grade 5637 BC cells. Two TCC-SUP EV-enriched proteins, EGF-like repeats and discoidin I-like domain-3 (EDIL-3) [16] and periostin [17], were identified. They can activate the ERK1/2 MAP kinase signal pathway in recipient low grade BC cells, thereby promoting migration and invasion and knocking down EDIL-3 and periostin by shRNA disrupted this action. Similar results were reported by other group [18], which showed that EVs derived from T24 and UMUC3 BC cells enhanced urothelial cell migration and invasion. Also, blocking the EV uptake of recipient cells by heparin remarkably reduced BCEV's impact.

In addition to carrying and transferring oncogenic cargos, BCEVs have been found to serve as an apparatus to dispose tumor-suppressor miRNAs (miR23b, miR224 and miR921) [19]. In this study, miRNAs previously identified to possess tumor-suppressor functions, such as miR23b, miR224 and miR921, were identified in BCEVs, implying a cancer character-sustaining mechanism. Silencing of Rab27α and Rab27β, two major EV secretion regulators, indeed halted the tumor-suppressing miRNA secretion. However, the miRNA retained in the cell might be inactivated by sequestration in the MVBs. Suppression of EV release resulted in reduced cellular invasion, which provides a possible explanation for the poor prognosis in BC patients with high expression of RAB27β. The levels of highly exocytosed tumor-suppressor miRNAs were found to be reduced in metastatic lymph nodes relative to primary tumors.

2.3. BCEVs Promote Cancer Cell Progression by Mediating Tumor-Stroma Communication

The tumor microenvironment is composed of a complex and heterogeneous network of different cell types and the extracellular matrix (ECM). Tumor-associated stromal cells arise from various cellular origins: fibroblasts, pericytes, bone marrow mesenchymal stem cells, adipocytes and endothelial cells [20]. The communication between tumor cells and the tumor microenvironment is pivotal to both primary tumor growth and metastatic evolution and this is mediated through direct cell-cell contact as well as via tumor-secreted factors including EVs. One of the most characterized pro-cancer properties of TEVs is their ability to facilitate new growth in vascular networks within tumor microenvironments to sustain the rapidly growing tumor mass during metastasis. TEVs have long been known to be exploited to induce angiogenesis; however, the underlying mechanism was only revealed very recently in a breast cancer study [21]. TEVs derived from breast cancer MDAMB231 cells were reported to contain a unique vascular endothelial growth factor isoform, $VEGF_{90K}$, that was crosslinked with Hsp90 and catalyzed by acyl transferase tissue transglutaminase (tTG). This EV-borne $VEGF_{90K}$-Hsp90 complex stimulates tubulogenesis in HUVEC endothelial cells and this effect was diminished by the use of the HSP90 inhibitor 17AAG to force the release of $VEGF_{90K}$ from the complex. Our group found that EVs from high grade BC cells contain EDIL-3 [16], which is known to promote tumor vascularization through an Arg-Gly-Asp (RGD) motif that interacts with integrin $\alpha v \beta 3$ [22]. We demonstrated that the pro-angiogenic property of these BCEVs was abolished when EDIL-3 was suppressed by shRNA, confirming that EV-borne EDIL-3 mediates recipient endothelial angiogenesis.

Another key event mediated by TEVs during cancer progression is the establishment of a pre-metastatic niche (PMN) in favor of future circulating tumor cell (CTC) adhesion and colonization, which eventually leads to metastatic outgrowth. Growing evidence indicates that TEVs play central roles in PMN establishment and maintenance processes such as vascular remodeling, immune modulation, metabolic environment modification, fibroblast differentiation into CAF, ECM re-organization and organotropic homing [23]. However, the difficulty of obtaining pre-metastatic tissues from cancer patients and the lack of metastatic BC animal models have limited clinical investigation into the significance of this phenomenon. Our laboratory has succeeded in isolating metastasis-prone MB49 sub-lines and we have found that pre-conditioning mice with sub-line EVs promotes lung metastases (manuscript in preparation). A broad panel of ECM components is enriched in MB49 sub-line EVs, suggesting that they may participate in PMN formation principally through ECM re-organization [24].

3. Regulation of Immune Responses by BCEVs

Recent global profiling of the genetic and epigenetic landscape of BC has revealed it to be one of the most mutated cancers after lung cancer and melanoma [25,26]. Many new mutations have been identified; interestingly, many of them coincide with mutations that have been discovered previously in BC. This demonstrates that progressive tumors are heterogeneous, making it difficult to predict their outcome and the signatures of some of these molecular alteration patterns seem to have a prognostic impact [27]. With such a high mutation rate, BC can produce many tumor-associated antigens (TAAs) that are either mutated cellular proteins or molecules with different post-translational modifications [28]. The formation of TAAs leads to the generation of TAA-derived peptides, which are then presented through MHC on the surface of cancer cells to activate immunological surveillance. Since EVs have been known to modulate immune responses by directly or indirectly presenting MHC-antigen peptide complex on their surface, it is likely that these TAA-derived peptides can also be loaded into BCEVs to mediate immune response. In this section, we will discuss BCEVs functional roles in regulating the immune system.

3.1. Immune System Activation by BCEVs

While the activation of the immune system by cancer cell-derived EVs is not a well-studied phenomenon, there are a few reports that support this claim. For example, Rao et al. reported that TEVs elicited an antitumor immune response in a murine hepatocellular carcinoma (HCC) model in vivo [29]. They isolated TEVs from the murine HCC cell line hepa1-6 and used them to activate DC2.4, a murine dendritic cell (DC) line. These TEV-pulsed DCs were orthotopically injected into HCC tumor-bearing C57BL/6 mice, which resulted in increasing infiltration of T lymphocytes and elevated levels of interferon-γ (IFN-γ), consequently suppressing tumor growth. A similar finding was reported by Bu et al., who found that TEV-pulsed DCs elicited a tumor-specific CD8$^+$ cytotoxic T cell response in glioma patients [30]. In this study, they applied patient-derived T cells and CD14$^+$ DC precursor cells and found that EVs from the tumors of the same patients can activate T cell-mediated cytotoxicity. In the context of BC, Zhang et al. found that BCEV-educated DCs elicit T cell cytotoxic activity in vitro [31]. This evidence supports the possibility that BCEVs can promote immune system activation to facilitate the anti-tumor immune response.

3.2. Immune System Suppression by BCEVs

TEVs are known to be able to suppress the immune surveillance system, allowing tumor cells to escape the immune barriers and grow. This role of TEVs has been extensively studied using various cell types involved in the immune surveillance of tumors. In one immune escape strategy, cancer cells downregulate their MHC class I surface expression. However, natural killer (NK) cells are known to recognize and eliminate those non- or low-expressing MHC class I cells [32], so as a defense mechanism cancer cells can secrete EVs bearing transforming growth factor β1 (TGFβ1) to deactivate NK cells and decrease their cytotoxic activity, resulting in the suppression of the anti-tumor immune response [33].

Shinohara et al. reported that the presence of miR145 in colorectal cancer TEVs can polarize classic (M1) type macrophages into M2 type macrophages, thereby supporting cancer cell growth in vitro and in vivo [34]. Further mechanistic dissection revealed that miR145 directly binds to the 3'untrasnlated region (UTR) of *HDAC*II, a histone deacetylase, silencing its expression and promoting interleukin 10 (IL-10) production.

TEV suppression of DC function was demonstrated by Salimu et al. [35]. They treated DC cells with TEVs isolated from DU145 prostate cancer cells and co-cultured them with CD8$^+$ T cells. TEV-educated DCs triggered significantly stronger tumor-antigen-specific T cell responses as determined by IL-2 and IFN-γ production.

TEVs also allow immune escape by inactivating T lymphocytes directly. Rong et al. discovered that breast cancer cells secrete TEVs capable of suppressing T lymphocytes [36]. A similar phenomenon was found in head and neck cancer patients, where TEVs suppressed T lymphocytes, allowing tumor progression [37].

In BC, an important question that remains unanswered is whether EVs have an immunosuppressive character as seen in other cancer types. Last year, Lee et al. found that EVs derived from BC patient urine present an altered protein composition [38]. They found significant upregulation of mucin-1 (MUC1), carcinoembryonic antigen (CEA) and moesin. MUC1 has been reported to contribute to NK cell evasion by cancer cells [39] and its expression level has been associated with BC prognosis [40]. CEA has been correlated with tumor angiogenesis [41] and can inhibit NK cell targeting of cancer cells [42]. Moesin has been associated with metastasis and poor prognosis in a number of different cancers, including pancreatic, colon and laryngeal carcinomas [43–46]. These findings suggest that BCEVs might have immunosuppressive roles and open a new avenue for future research.

3.3. BCEVs in Promoting Inflammation

BCEVs may also have a role in controlling inflammation. We reported that MIBC patient urinary EVs are enriched in transaldolase (TALDO1) [47], an enzyme linked to oxidative stress, inflammation and carcinogenesis [46]. ApoB is another BCEV protein with a functional link to the inflammation process [48]. ApoB is another BCEV protein with a functional link to the inflammation process [49]. Andreu et al. compared the urinary EV protein profiles of BC patients versus healthy non-smokers and found that ApoB expression was significantly increased in BC patient-derived EVs. ApoB is involved in a wide range of biological processes including secretion associated with exosomes [50] and EVs [51]. ApoB has also been reported to play important roles in angiogenesis [52] and inflammation [53].

In summary, our understanding of BCEVs' functional roles in regulation of immune response is still in its initial stage. With recent progress made in cancer immunotherapy and the emerging evidence of BCEVs mediating communication between tumor and immune cells, we anticipate that further research will reveal pathological roles of BCEVs and their cargos in the regulation of immune responses, especially in response to checkpoint inhibitors.

4. Therapeutic Application of BCEVs

4.1. EV-Mediated Delivery of Therapeutic Agents in BC

Nanomedicine was introduced in cancer therapy during the 1990s [54]. With the benefit of small size (usually less than 200 nm), nanoparticles are able to escape from being engulfed by macrophages and neutrophils (which eliminate particles about 250–1000 nm) and then diffuse into the blood circulation and be transported to their target sites. With EVs' small size, various cell origins and low cytotoxicity, EVs have become an ideal nanoparticle drug carrier [55].

EVs were first used as a drug delivery vehicle to transport curcumin, an anti-inflammatory drug, to treat brain inflammatory disease [56]. Administration of exosomes encapsulating curcumin resulted in 5–10 fold higher plasma concentrations than curcumin alone and more effective inhibition of LPS-induced brain inflammation. BC cells are known to take-up EVs in a dose-dependent manner [57]. A recent study also found robust EV internalization in BC cells [58] where human BC cell lines (SW780 and UMUC3) showed 20–50 fold higher EV internalization rates than normal urothelial cells. Such high uptake rates make EV-nanoparticles an attractive method of drug delivery to BC cells. Moreover, the membrane structure of EVs encapsulates and protects vulnerable molecular contents, in particular various RNA species, such as siRNA, miRNA and lncRNA. In a recent study, EVs were exploited as a vector to deliver the designed siRNA to BC cells [58]. EVs were loaded with artificially synthesized siRNAs targeting polo-like kinase-1 (PLK1) by electroporation and then used to treat UMUC3 cells. As a result, the UMUC3 expression of PLK1 was significantly decreased, consequently inducing apoptosis and necrosis.

Chemotherapy following removal of the primary tumor is the standard treatment in many cancers. While chemotherapy is often capable of inducing cell death in tumors, many patients develop more advanced tumor growth due to the appearance of chemo-resistance, which remains one of most challenging problems in cancer research today. A recent study reported an innovative approach of using TEVs to sensitize BC cells to chemotherapeutic agents [59]. In a mouse model, intravesical instillation of TEVs prior to instillation of drugs including doxorubicin, mitomycin C, hydroxycamptothecin and gemcitabine, significantly reduced hematuria and tumor incidence. These TEVs were initially collected from UV-treated tumor cells and ranged in size from 100–1000 nm (microparticles). The recipient BC cells internalized the EVs into lysosomes, increasing lysosomal pH from 4.6 to 5.6, thereby promoting transportation of the lysosome to the nucleus over exocytosis and subsequently retaining drug bioactivity in the BC cells.

In the context of immunotherapy for BC, our group found that Bacillus Calmette–Guérin (BCG) infection stimulated BC cells to release EVs that could activate T lymphocytes, bone marrow-derived DCs and macrophages in vitro. This unpublished data suggests that TEVs are capable of mediating the anti-tumor immune response, possibly from transferring immune-active cargos [60].

4.2. Prognosis and Diagnosis of BC Using EVs

There is a growing trend towards exploring the use of minimally invasive liquid biopsy for early cancer detection and TEVs are attractive sources of cancer diagnostic and prognostic biomarkers for the following reasons: (1) EVs contain a specific cargo of proteins and RNAs that might reflect the status of the originating cells, (2) EVs are membranous structures that can protect the cargo contents from degradation, [61] EVs are relatively accessible as they are found in clinical specimens that can be obtained through non-invasive methods. Apart from plasma/serum, urine is considered the most relevant body fluid in terms of its physical contact with bladder tumor mass. Although EVs compose only 3% of excreted urinary protein [62], with proper isolation methodology and proteomic analysis, many urinary exosomal proteins have been identified to have pathophysiologic significance [61,63–69]. Nawaz et al. in 2014 published a comprehensive review of EVs as biomarkers for urogenital cancers which addressed the great potential of utilizing EVs in prognosis and diagnosis [70].

To define appropriate baselines, proteomic investigation of EVs derived from healthy donors is needed. The first comprehensive study of urinary EV protein contents was performed by Pisitkun et al. in 2004 using liquid chromatography-tandem MS (LC-MS/MS) [71]. Soon after, more detailed proteomic analyses were reported which determined protein profiles for urinary EVs of bladder and prostate gland origin [68,72–76].

Cell-free urine has been used to predict treatment response, recurrence, prognosis and diagnosis by detecting DNA level, methylation, mutation and integrity [77,78]. In BC, DNA level and integrity in cell-free urine were found to be significantly elevated relative to controls [79–81]. Urinary EV profiling of quantity as well as miRNA and protein content has been reported to serve as a prognostic and diagnostic biomarker. Recently, Liang et al. developed an integrated double-filtration microfluidic device to measure EV concentration at the point-of-care. They found higher amounts of EVs in the urine of BC patients compared to healthy controls and this result further suggests that urinary EVs have great potential to be used as a disease biomarker for BC [82]. Profiling miRNAs in cell-free urine was demonstrated to have >80% sensitivity and specificity in detecting different stages of BC [83]. Proteomic analysis of urinary EV cargo provides another prospect for disease prediction. Lin et al. collected urine EVs and analyzed the proteomic data from 129 BC patients versus 62 healthy participants and found SERPINA1 and H2B1K as promising BC biomarkers for prognosis Proteomic analysis of urinary EV cargo provides another prospect for disease prediction. Lin et al. collected urine EVs and analyzed the proteomic data from 129 BC patients versus 62 healthy participants and found alpha-1 antitrypsin (SERPINA1) and Histone H2B type 1-K (H2B1K) as promising BC biomarkers for prognosis [84]. We have searched the cargo contents of EVs derived from BC cells and urine of BC patients from the past 10-year publication and summarized the list of miRNAs and proteins encapsulated in EV cargos in Tables 1 and 2, respectively. The BC patient urinary EVs are a mixture of the whole body EVs and BCEVs, which reflects the clinical reality and relevance. Note that most of the reported cargo molecules are based on global screening that identified differentially displayed miRNAs and proteins between BC samples and controls but their functional roles in BC have not been verified.

Table 1. List of miRNAs identified in BC urinary EVs and/or BC cells EVs.

miRNA	Regulation	Sample Sources	Reference
miR-21	up	urine & BC cells lines	[85–89]
miR-200c	up	urine	[85,86,88]
miR-23b	up	urine	[19,90]
miR-513b-5p	up	urine	[90,91]
miR-183	up	urine	[88,92]
miR-205	up	urine from NMIBC patients	[86,88]
miR-16-1-3p, miR-28-5p, miR-92a-2-5p, miR-142-3p, miR-195-3p, miR-196b-5p, miR-299-3p, miR-492, miR-601, miR-619-5p, miR-3155a, miR-3162-5p, miR-3678-3p, miR-4283, miR-4295, miR-4311, miR-4531, miR-5096, miR-5187-5p	up	urine	[90]
miR-155-5p, miR-132-3p, miR-31-5p, miR-15a-5p	up	urine	[87]
miR-93, miR-940	up	urine	[85]
miR-16, miR-96	up	urine	[92]
miR-486-5p, miR-205-5p, let-7i-5p	up	urine from NMIBC/(G1 + G2)	[88]
miR-106b-3p, let-7c-5p, miR-486-5p, miR-151a-3p, miR-200c-3p, miR-183-5p, miR-185-5p, miR-224-5p	up	urine from NMIBC/G3	
miR-4454, miR-720/3007a, miR-29-3p	up	urine from NMIBC	[86]
miR-214	up	urine from NMIBC	[93]
miR-503-5p, miR-145-5p, miR-3158-3p, miR-30a-3p	up	urine from MIBC	[91]
miR-106b-3p, miR-486-5p, miR-205-5p, miR-451a, miR-25-3p, miR-7-1-5p, miR-146a-3p	up	urine from MIBC	[88]
miR-1, miR-99a, miR-125b, miR-133b, miR-143, miR-1207-5p	down	urine	[92]
let-7f-2-3p, miR-520c-3p, miR-4783-5p	down	urine	[90]
miR-30c-2-5p, miR-30a-5p	down	urine from NMIBC/(G1 + G2)	[88]
miR-30a-5p, miR-30c-2-5p, miR-10b-5p	down	urine from NMIBC/G3	
miR-30a-5p, let-7c-5p	down	urine from MIBC	
miR-27b-3p	down	BC cells	[91]
miR-let-7i-3p	down	BC cells	[89]
miR-29c-5p, miR-146b-5p, miR-200a-3p, miR-200b-3p, miR-141-3p	down	BC cells	[91]

Table 2. List of proteins identified in BC urinary EVs and/or BC cells EVs.

Protein ID	Sample Sources	Validated	Proteomic Detection
EHD4	urine and BC cells		[16,38,94]
HEXB	urine and BC cells		[16,38]
ANXA; SND1	urine and BC cells	[47]	[16,95]
S100A4	urine and BC cells		[16]
TALDO1	urine and BC cells		[16]
MUC1	urine and BC cells	[38,96]	[95]
EPS8	urine	[38]	[94]
CEAM5	urine		
CD44; BSG	BC cells		
ITGB1; ITGA6; CD36; CD73; CD10; CD147; 5T4	BC cells	[96]	

Table 2. *Cont.*

Protein ID	Sample Sources	Validated	Proteomic Detection
NRAS; MUC4	urine	[94]	
SERPINA1 H2B1K	urine	[84]	
TACSTD2	urine	[74]	
EDIL3	urine and BC cells	[16]	
POSTN	urine and BC cells	[17]	
CTNNB1; CDC42	urine and BC cells		[95,97]
14-3-3; ALIX; B2M; EGFR; EZR; FSCN1; LGALS; GST; MSN; PRDX1; PTGFRN; RDX; TAGLN2	BC cells		[95]

5. Current Challenges and Future Prospects

5.1. Current Challenges

Researchers have used dozens of names for various secreted vesicles (including exosomes, microvesicles and EVs), which have been broadly used and are sometimes interchangeable. However, exosomes and microvesicles are functionally and structurally distinct; there are differences in charge, size and molecular composition [98]. Importantly, the size distributions of exosomes and microvesicles overlap significantly and the identity of EVs between 100–150 nm in diameter is ambiguous [12]. Therefore, size alone cannot always be used to distinguish these EV subpopulations from one another. While "extracellular vesicle" is a widely accepted generic term for all secreted vesicles, there is a need for consensus about how to apply the other terms appropriately to different EV subpopulations in terms of vesicle size.

The conflicting names for different EV subpopulations are largely due to the different procedures used in individual laboratories to obtain and sort biological fluids to isolate EVs. Currently, with the rapid increase in the understanding of EV biology, including their function in numerous aspects of human disease and their potential significance in clinical applications, there is a growing demand for simple, efficient and reliable techniques to isolate EVs. Until now, the most standard EV isolation procedure combines filtration and ultracentrifugation, which purify particles based on their size and density [99]. To further purify exosomes from EVs, a common technique uses a continuous sucrose gradient during ultracentrifugation, which distributes particles according to density (exosomes float at densities ranging from 1.15–1.19 g/mL) [100]. In addition, microfluidic techniques combining immune-affinity, sieving and trapping have been applied to concentrate exosomes [101–103]. However, the unavoidable damage to the exosome structure and the low recovery narrows the application of this technique. Another common EV isolation method that has also been widely used for exosome purification is immune-affinity precipitation. This technique captures exosomes using antibodies against exosome surface markers. However, this method is limited by the exclusion of some EV subpopulations that do not carry the well-known markers. Therefore, the identification of general markers for EVs, such as lipid composition, pH value and electrical properties might be useful for capturing whole EV populations [104]. With the rapidly growth of the field, more and more isolation methods are proposed, the most updated EV isolation technic were comprehensively covered by recent reviews [1,12]. The recent launched EV-TRACK database encourages researchers to report their EV isolation details for developing a standardized protocol. (http://evtrack.org).

One of the hurdles to urinary EV isolation is the aggregation of highly abundant non-exosomal proteins, such as Tamm-Horsfall protein (THP), which tends to form fibrillary aggregates at low temperature. This aggregation during the EV isolation process was proposed to be reduced by a disulfide bond reducer, such as dithiothreitol (DTT), or a mild solubilizing detergent, such as CHAPS (3-[(3-cholamidopropyl) dimethylammonio]-1-propanesulfonic), which can separate THP from EVs during differential centrifugation [99,105–107]. However, DTT treatment can cause changes in the extracellular domains of EV proteins that would affect their stability and function. CHAPS treatment is better at preserving EV features but requires longer preparation [99].

The major challenge of EV-based biomarker discovery is the lack of a validated and standardized approach to normalize body-fluid concentrations among patients, especially in urine samples due to variation of water excretion in each individual. Urinary creatinine (UCr) excretion in the renal system is considered to be constant across and within individuals and is commonly used to normalize urinary biomarker concentrations against variations in urine flow rate in the evaluation of chronic kidney disease and prediction of acute kidney injury [108,109]. However, creatinine excretion rates vary widely among individuals with different age, sex, race, diet, physical activity, muscle mass, emotional stress and disease state [110,111], thus potentially masking the true value of EV proteins. Alternatively, specific exosome markers such as TSG101 and Alix can be used for normalization of urinary EV proteins [112]. More studies are needed to evaluate these normalization techniques and/or identify new ones.

Urinary EVs originate from cells throughout the urinary system; therefore, it is important to distinguish BC-specific EVs from the heterogeneous population of urinary EVs shed from other sources such as kidney and prostate. A recent study was able to increase the purity of podocyte-derived exosome isolation using immune-absorption with antibodies against the podocyte-specific complement receptor type 1 (CR1). Proteomic analysis of the podocyte EVs identified 14 new podocyte EV-enriched proteins that can potentially be used as kidney-specific EV markers to distinguish them from the broader urinary EV population [113]. This finding encourages similar efforts to identify BC-specific EV markers that are greatly needed to improve the diagnostic utility of urinary EVs.

5.2. Future Prospects

With accumulating evidence of TEVs' functional roles in cancer progression, depletion of the TEVs in circulation while retaining normal and healthy EVs becomes an ideal therapeutic approach. In 1989, Lentz conducted a primary experiment to remove low molecular weight (<120 kDa) proteins from cancer patients' blood by ultrapheresis, which resulted in tumor size reduction in 6 out of 16 patients [114]. At that time, serum cytokine receptors were proposed to be the key factors in blocking the antineoplastic immune response. However, this therapeutic effect might be because the process also results in the elimination of EVs. Previously, plasmapheresis combined with an affinity matrix containing *Galanthus nivalis* agglutinin to capture hepatitis C viruses has been applied clinically [115]. A similar plasmapheresis system was adapted to capture TEVs using a specific antibody-conjugated cartridge [116]. Therefore, identifying TEV-specific surface markers is the crucial step to take this approach to the next stage.

Another TEV targeting strategy is the inhibition of EV biogenesis and uptake. Amiloride, an endocytic vesicle recycling inhibitor, reduces the EV amount in the circulation and increases chemotherapy effects in mice [117]. Interference with the key proteins in EV biogenesis, such as Rab27β, also results in inhibition of EV release and reduction of tumor progression [118,119]. Theoretically, inhibiting EV uptake can be achieved by blocking surface phosphatidylserine. However, such inhibition can also affect microvesicle uptake by normal cells that might cause off-target side effects. Further dissection of EV machinery might lead to the identification of regulatory pathways in EV biogenesis or internalization that are specifically utilized by cancers.

The mechanisms by which secreted EVs are targeted to recipient cells are not yet well understood. It has been suggested that various integrins expressed on the surface of EVs might determine that they will interact with specific recipients through ligand-receptor binding [56,120,121]. A study by Hoshino et al. found that EVs from a variety of cancer cell types were preferentially taken up by specific cells in various organs depending on their integrin expression [122] This finding raises the possibility of utilizing EVs as therapeutic vectors to deliver RNA, protein or drug cargos to specific targeted cells by genetically engineering the EV integrins [123]. As more understating of the physical and pathological role of EV, more applicable areas of BCEV will be proposed.

6. Conclusions

In this review article, we have discussed various functional roles of BCEVs in mediating BC pathogenesis. As summarized in Figure 2, BCEVs can drive normal urothelial cell malignant transformation, promote BC progression via stimulation of proliferation, invasion and migration of recipient neighboring BC cells and modify the tumor stroma to support tumor growth. BCEVs have been further suggested to have roles in mediating cancer-related immunity, either by promoting inflammation favorable to tumors or by participating in the immune surveillance mechanism. Finally, potential clinical applications of BCEVs, mainly in diagnosis or prognosis or as drug-delivery vehicles, are discussed. However, the normal physiological functions of EVs should not be neglected, so that the off-target side effects of EV-based therapy can be reduced. As to EV-based liquid biopsy development, the identification of tissue/disease-specific EV markers is necessary to facilitate sorting of TEVs from the heterogeneous EV populations in patient specimens. Further investigation of EV biogenesis, content packing and uptake is also critical for future applications.

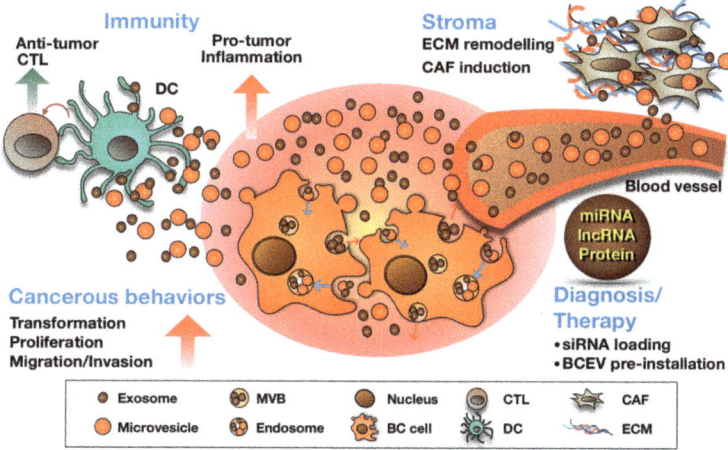

Figure 2. Summary of the roles of BCEVs in cancer, the tumor microenvironment and therapeutic applications. BCEVs are involved in many aspects of cancer development and progression. Like other cancer cells, BC cells release EVs into extracellular spaces and can be received by urothelial cells and immune cells, consequently modifying their behavior to support or suppress tumor growth (red and blue arrows indicate the migrating direction of intracellular vesicles). On the one hand, BCEVs can promote neighboring recipient cells' cancerous behaviors, including malignant transformation, proliferation, migration and invasion, as well as modify the tumor microenvironment in favor of tumor outgrowth, including promoting inflammation, ECM remodeling and fibroblast differentiation to cancer-associated fibroblasts (CAF). In contrast, BCEVs also participate in the immune surveillance system by presenting tumor antigens to provoke dendritic and cytotoxic T cell anti-tumor immunity. With specific cargoes carried by BCEVs such as miRNA, lncRNA and proteins, their clinical application, particularly in disease biomarkers, has rapidly expanded. Moreover, researching the utilization of BCEVs as vesicles to deliver therapeutic materials is also underway.

Funding: This work is supported by NCI R01 CA173986 (Yi-Fen Lee, PI).

Conflicts of Interest: The authors declare no conflicts of interest.

References

1. Ramirez, M.I.; Amorim, M.G.; Gadelha, C.; Milic, I.; Welsh, J.A.; Freitas, V.M.; Nawaz, M.; Akbar, N.; Couch, Y.; Makin, L.; et al. Technical challenges of working with extracellular vesicles. *Nanoscale* **2018**, *10*, 881–906. [CrossRef] [PubMed]
2. Yellon, D.M.; Davidson, S.M. Exosomes: Nanoparticles involved in cardioprotection? *Circ. Res.* **2014**, *114*, 325–332. [CrossRef] [PubMed]
3. Aalberts, M.; Stout, T.A.; Stoorvogel, W. Prostasomes: Extracellular vesicles from the prostate. *Reproduction* **2014**, *147*, R1–R14. [CrossRef] [PubMed]
4. Valadi, H.; Ekstrom, K.; Bossios, A.; Sjostrand, M.; Lee, J.J.; Lotvall, J.O. Exosome-mediated transfer of mRNAs and microRNAs is a novel mechanism of genetic exchange between cells. *Nat. Cell Biol.* **2007**, *9*, 654. [CrossRef] [PubMed]
5. Kalluri, R. The biology and function of exosomes in cancer. *J. Clin. Investig.* **2016**, *126*, 1208–1215. [CrossRef] [PubMed]
6. Choi, D.; Lee, T.H.; Spinelli, C.; Chennakrishnaiah, S.; D'Asti, E.; Rak, J. Extracellular vesicle communication pathways as regulatory targets of oncogenic transformation. *Semin. Cell Dev. Biol.* **2017**, *67*, 11–22. [CrossRef] [PubMed]
7. Urciuoli, E.; Giorda, E.; Scarsella, M.; Petrini, S.; Peruzzi, B. Osteosarcoma-derived extracellular vesicles induce a tumor-like phenotype in normal recipient cells. *J. Cell. Physiol.* **2018**, *233*, 6158–6172. [CrossRef] [PubMed]
8. Panagopoulos, K.; Cross-Knorr, S.; Dillard, C.; Pantazatos, D.; Del Tatto, M.; Mills, D.; Goldstein, L.; Renzulli, J.; Quesenberry, P.; Chatterjee, D. Reversal of chemosensitivity and induction of cell malignancy of a non-malignant prostate cancer cell line upon extracellular vesicle exposure. *Mol. Cancer* **2013**, *12*. [CrossRef] [PubMed]
9. Barton, B.E.; Karras, J.G.; Murphy, T.F.; Barton, A.; Huang, H.F.S. Signal transducer and activator of transcription 3 (STAT3) activation in prostate cancer: Direct STAT3 inhibition induces apoptosis in prostate cancer lines. *Mol. Cancer Ther.* **2004**, *3*, 11–20. [PubMed]
10. Bromberg, J. Stat proteins and oncogenesis. *J. Clin. Investig.* **2002**, *109*, 1139–1142. [CrossRef] [PubMed]
11. Goulet, C.R.; Bernard, G.; Tremblay, S.; Chabaud, S.; Bolduc, S.; Poulit, F. Exosomes induce fibroblast differentiation into cancer-associated fibroblasts through TGFβ signaling. *Mol. Cancer Res.* **2018**. [CrossRef]
12. Mateescu, B.; Kowal, E.J.; van Balkom, B.W.; Bartel, S.; Bhattacharyya, S.N.; Buzas, E.I.; Buck, A.H.; de Candia, P.; Chow, F.W.; Das, S.; et al. Obstacles and opportunities in the functional analysis of extracellular vesicle RNA—An ISEV position paper. *J Extracell. Vesicles* **2017**, *6*, 1286095. [CrossRef] [PubMed]
13. Maia, J.; Caja, S.; Strano Moraes, M.C.; Couto, N.; Costa-Silva, B. Exosome-Based Cell-Cell Communication in the Tumor Microenvironment. *Front. Cell Dev. Biol.* **2018**, *6*, 18. [CrossRef] [PubMed]
14. Yang, L.; Wu, X.H.; Wang, D.; Luo, C.L.; Chen, L.X. Bladder cancer cell-derived exosomes inhibit tumor cell apoptosis and induce cell proliferation in vitro. *Mol. Med. Rep.* **2013**, *8*, 1272–1278. [CrossRef] [PubMed]
15. Xue, M.; Chen, W.; Xiang, A.; Wang, R.Q.; Chen, H.; Pan, J.J.; Pang, H.; An, H.L.; Wang, X.; Hou, H.L.; et al. Hypoxic exosomes facilitate bladder tumor growth and development through transferring long non-coding RNA-UCA1. *Mol. Cancer* **2017**, *16*. [CrossRef] [PubMed]
16. Beckham, C.J.; Olsen, J.; Yin, P.N.; Wu, C.H.; Ting, H.J.; Hagen, F.K.; Scosyrev, E.; Messing, E.M.; Lee, Y.F. Bladder cancer exosomes contain EDIL-3/Del1 and facilitate cancer progression. *J. Urol.* **2014**, *192*, 583–592. [CrossRef] [PubMed]
17. Silvers, C.R.; Liu, Y.R.; Wu, C.H.; Miyamoto, H.; Messing, E.M.; Lee, Y.F. Identification of extracellular vesicle-borne periostin as a feature of muscle-invasive bladder cancer. *Oncotarget* **2016**, *7*, 23335–23345. [CrossRef] [PubMed]
18. Franzen, C.; Greco, K.; Blackwell, R.; Foreman, K.; Gupta, G. Urothelial Cells Undergo Epithelial to Mesenchymal Transition after Exposure to Muscle Invasive Bladder Cancer Exosomes. *J. Urol.* **2015**, *193*, E605–E606. [CrossRef]
19. Ostenfeld, M.S.; Jeppesen, D.K.; Laurberg, J.R.; Boysen, A.T.; Bramsen, J.B.; Primdal-Bengtson, B.; Hendrix, A.; Lamy, P.; Dagnaes-Hansen, F.; Rasmussen, M.H.; et al. Cellular Disposal of miR23b by RAB27-Dependent Exosome Release Is Linked to Acquisition of Metastatic Properties. *Cancer Res.* **2014**, *74*, 5758–5771. [CrossRef] [PubMed]

20. Bussard, K.M.; Mutkus, L.; Stumpf, K.; Gomez-Manzano, C.; Marini, F.C. Tumor-associated stromal cells as key contributors to the tumor microenvironment. *Breast Cancer Res.* **2016**, *18*. [CrossRef] [PubMed]
21. Feng, Q.Y.; Zhang, C.L.; Lum, D.; Druso, J.E.; Blank, B.; Wilson, K.F.; Welm, A.; Antonyak, M.A.; Cerione, R.A. A class of extracellular vesicles from breast cancer cells activates VEGF receptors and tumour angiogenesis. *Nat. Commun.* **2017**, *8*. [CrossRef] [PubMed]
22. Choi, E.Y.; Chavakis, E.; Czabanka, M.A.; Langer, H.F.; Fraemohs, L.; Economopoulou, M.; Kundu, R.K.; Orlandi, A.; Zheng, Y.Y.; Prieto, D.A.; et al. Del-1, an endogenous leukocyte-endothelial adhesion inhibitor, limits inflammatory cell recruitment. *Science* **2008**, *322*, 1101–1104. [CrossRef] [PubMed]
23. Lobb, R.J.; Lima, L.G.; Moller, A. Exosomes: Key mediators of metastasis and pre-metastatic niche formation. *Semin. Cell Dev. Biol.* **2017**, *67*, 3–10. [CrossRef] [PubMed]
24. Liu, Y.R.; Lee, Y.F. Bladder cancer extracellular vesicle facilitate metastasis. Unpublished; manuscript in preparation.
25. Lawrence, M.S.; Stojanov, P.; Polak, P.; Kryukov, G.V.; Cibulskis, K.; Sivachenko, A.; Carter, S.L.; Stewart, C.; Mermel, C.H.; Roberts, S.A.; et al. Mutational heterogeneity in cancer and the search for new cancer-associated genes. *Nature* **2013**, *499*, 214–218. [CrossRef] [PubMed]
26. Weinstein, J.N.; Akbani, R.; Broom, B.M.; Wang, W.Y.; Verhaak, R.G.W.; McConkey, D.; Lerner, S.; Morgan, M.; Creighton, C.J.; Smith, C.; et al. Comprehensive molecular characterization of urothelial bladder carcinoma. *Nature* **2014**, *507*, 315–322. [CrossRef]
27. Sjodahl, G.; Lauss, M.; Lovgren, K.; Chebil, G.; Gudjonsson, S.; Veerla, S.; Patschan, O.; Aine, M.; Ferno, M.; Ringner, M.; et al. A Molecular Taxonomy for Urothelial Carcinoma. *Clin. Cancer Res.* **2012**, *18*, 3377–3386. [CrossRef] [PubMed]
28. Finn, O.J. Immuno-oncology: Understanding the function and dysfunction of the immune system in cancer. *Ann. Oncol.* **2012**, *23*, 6–9. [CrossRef] [PubMed]
29. Rao, Q.; Zuo, B.F.; Lu, Z.; Gao, X.J.; You, A.B.; Wu, C.X.; Du, Z.; Yin, H.F. Tumor-Derived Exosomes Elicit Tumor Suppression in Murine Hepatocellular Carcinoma Models and Humans In Vitro. *Hepatology* **2016**, *64*, 456–472. [CrossRef] [PubMed]
30. Bu, N.; Wu, H.Q.; Sun, B.Z.; Zhang, G.L.; Zhan, S.Q.; Zhang, R.; Zhou, L. Exosome-loaded dendritic cells elicit tumor-specific CD8(+) cytotoxic T cells in patients with glioma. *J. Neurooncol.* **2011**, *104*, 659–667. [CrossRef] [PubMed]
31. Zhang, J.M.; Wu, X.H.; Zhang, Y.; Xia, Y.G.; Luo, C.L. Exosomes derived form bladder transitional cell carcinoma cells induce CTL cytotoxicity in vitro. *Zhonghua Zhong Liu Za Zhi* **2009**, *31*, 738–741. [PubMed]
32. Ljunggren, H.G.; Karre, K. In search of the "missing self": MHC molecules and NK cell recognition. *Immunol. Today* **1990**, *11*, 237–244. [CrossRef]
33. Whiteside, T.L. Immune modulation of T-cell and NK (natural killer) cell activities by TEXs (tumour-derived exosomes). *Biochem. Soc. Trans.* **2013**, *41*, 245–251. [CrossRef] [PubMed]
34. Shinohara, H.; Kuranaga, Y.; Kumazaki, M.; Sugito, N.; Yoshikawa, Y.; Takai, T.; Taniguchi, K.; Ito, Y.; Akao, Y. Regulated Polarization of Tumor-Associated Macrophages by miR-145 via Colorectal Cancer-Derived Extracellular Vesicles. *J. Immunol.* **2017**, *199*, 1505–1515. [CrossRef] [PubMed]
35. Salimu, J.; Webber, J.; Gurney, M.; Al-Taei, S.; Clayton, A.; Tabi, Z. Dominant immunosuppression of dendritic cell function by prostate-cancer-derived exosomes. *J. Extracell. Vesicles* **2017**, *6*, 1368823. [CrossRef] [PubMed]
36. Rong, L.; Li, R.; Li, S.; Luo, R. Immunosuppression of breast cancer cells mediated by transforming growth factor-beta in exosomes from cancer cells. *Oncol. Lett.* **2016**, *11*, 500–504. [CrossRef] [PubMed]
37. Theodoraki, M.N.; Yerneni, S.S.; Hoffmann, T.K.; Gooding, W.E.; Whiteside, T.L. Clinical Significance of PD-L1(+) Exosomes in Plasma of Head and Neck Cancer Patients. *Clin. Cancer Res.* **2018**, *24*, 896–905. [CrossRef] [PubMed]
38. Lee, J.; McKinney, K.Q.; Pavlopoulos, A.J.; Niu, M.; Kang, J.W.; Oh, J.W.; Kim, K.P.; Hwang, S. Altered Proteome of Extracellular Vesicles Derived from Bladder Cancer Patients Urine. *Mol. Cells* **2018**, *41*, 179–187. [CrossRef] [PubMed]
39. Suzuki, Y.; Sutoh, M.; Hatakeyama, S.; Mori, K.; Yamamoto, H.; Koie, T.; Saitoh, H.; Yamaya, K.; Funyu, T.; Habuchi, T.; et al. MUC1 carrying core 2 O-glycans functions as a molecular shield against NK cell attack, promoting bladder tumor metastasis. *Int. J. Oncol.* **2012**, *40*, 1831–1838. [CrossRef] [PubMed]
40. Nielsen, T.O.; Borre, M.; Nexo, E.; Sorensen, B.S. Co-expression of HER3 and MUC1 is associated with a favourable prognosis in patients with bladder cancer. *BJU Int.* **2015**, *115*, 163–165. [CrossRef] [PubMed]

41. Bramswig, K.H.; Poettler, M.; Unseld, M.; Wrba, F.; Uhrin, P.; Zimmermann, W.; Zielinski, C.C.; Prager, G.W. Soluble carcinoembryonic antigen activates endothelial cells and tumor angiogenesis. *Cancer Res.* **2013**, *73*, 6584–6596. [CrossRef] [PubMed]
42. Stern, N.; Markel, G.; Arnon, T.I.; Gruda, R.; Wong, H.; Gray-Owen, S.D.; Mandelboim, O. Carcinoembryonic antigen (CEA) inhibits NK killing via interaction with CEA-related cell adhesion molecule 1. *J. Immunol.* **2005**, *174*, 6692–6701. [CrossRef] [PubMed]
43. Adada, M.M.; Canals, D.; Jeong, N.; Kelkar, A.D.; Hernandez-Corbacho, M.; Pulkoski-Gross, M.J.; Donaldson, J.C.; Hannun, Y.A.; Obeid, L.M. Intracellular sphingosine kinase 2-derived sphingosine-1-phosphate mediates epidermal growth factor-induced ezrin-radixin-moesin phosphorylation and cancer cell invasion. *FASEB J.* **2015**, *29*, 4654–4669. [CrossRef] [PubMed]
44. Jiang, L.; Phang, J.M.; Yu, J.; Harrop, S.J.; Sokolova, A.V.; Duff, A.P.; Wilk, K.E.; Alkhamici, H.; Breit, S.N.; Valenzuela, S.M.; et al. CLIC proteins, ezrin, radixin, moesin and the coupling of membranes to the actin cytoskeleton: A smoking gun? *Biochim. Biophys. Acta* **2014**, *1838*, 643–657. [CrossRef] [PubMed]
45. Piao, J.; Liu, S.; Xu, Y.; Wang, C.; Lin, Z.; Qin, Y.; Liu, S. Ezrin protein overexpression predicts the poor prognosis of pancreatic ductal adenocarcinomas. *Exp. Mol. Pathol.* **2015**, *98*, 1–6. [CrossRef] [PubMed]
46. Wang, Y.; Yago, T.; Zhang, N.; Abdisalaam, S.; Alexandrakis, G.; Rodgers, W.; McEver, R.P. Cytoskeletal regulation of CD44 membrane organization and interactions with E-selectin. *J. Biol. Chem.* **2014**, *289*, 35159–35171. [CrossRef] [PubMed]
47. Silvers, C.R.; Miyamoto, H.; Messing, E.M.; Netto, G.J.; Lee, Y.F. Characterization of urinary extracellular vesicle proteins in muscle-invasive bladder cancer. *Oncotarget* **2017**, *8*, 91199–91208. [CrossRef] [PubMed]
48. Perl, A.; Hanczko, R.; Telarico, T.; Oaks, Z.; Landas, S. Oxidative stress, inflammation and carcinogenesis are controlled through the pentose phosphate pathway by transaldolase. *Trends Mol. Med.* **2011**, *17*, 395–403. [CrossRef] [PubMed]
49. Andreu, Z.; Otta Oshiro, R.; Redruello, A.; Lopez-Martin, S.; Gutierrez-Vazquez, C.; Morato, E.; Marina, A.I.; Olivier Gomez, C.; Yanez-Mo, M. Extracellular vesicles as a source for non-invasive biomarkers in bladder cancer progression. *Eur. J. Pharm. Sci.* **2017**, *98*, 70–79. [CrossRef] [PubMed]
50. Van Niel, G.; Bergam, P.; Di Cicco, A.; Hurbain, I.; Lo Cicero, A.; Dingli, F.; Palmulli, R.; Fort, C.; Potier, M.C.; Schurgers, L.J.; et al. Apolipoprotein E Regulates Amyloid Formation within Endosomes of Pigment Cells. *Cell Rep.* **2015**, *13*, 43–51. [CrossRef] [PubMed]
51. Sodar, B.W.; Kittel, A.; Paloczi, K.; Vukman, K.V.; Osteikoetxea, X.; Szabo-Taylor, K.; Nemeth, A.; Sperlagh, B.; Baranyai, T.; Giricz, Z.; et al. Low-density lipoprotein mimics blood plasma-derived exosomes and microvesicles during isolation and detection. *Sci. Rep.* **2016**, *6*, 24316. [CrossRef] [PubMed]
52. Avraham-Davidi, I.; Ely, Y.; Pham, V.N.; Castranova, D.; Grunspan, M.; Malkinson, G.; Gibbs-Bar, L.; Mayseless, O.; Allmog, G.; Lo, B.; et al. ApoB-containing lipoproteins regulate angiogenesis by modulating expression of VEGF receptor 1. *Nat. Med.* **2012**, *18*, 967–973. [CrossRef] [PubMed]
53. Rao, L.N.; Ponnusamy, T.; Philip, S.; Mukhopadhyay, R.; Kakkar, V.V.; Mundkur, L. Hypercholesterolemia Induced Immune Response and Inflammation on Progression of Atherosclerosis in Apob(tm2Sgy) Ldlr(tm1Her)/J Mice. *Lipids* **2015**, *50*, 785–797. [CrossRef] [PubMed]
54. Bergin, C.; O'Leary, A.; McCreary, C.; Sabra, K.; Mulcahy, F. Treatment of Kaposi's sarcoma with liposomal doxorubicin. *Am. J. Health Syst. Pharm.* **1995**, *52*, 2001–2004. [PubMed]
55. Sun, D.M.; Zhuang, X.Y.; Zhang, S.Q.; Deng, Z.B.; Grizzle, W.; Miller, D.; Zhang, H.G. Exosomes are endogenous nanoparticles that can deliver biological information between cells. *Adv. Drug Deliv. Rev.* **2013**, *65*, 342–347. [CrossRef] [PubMed]
56. Zhuang, X.Y.; Xiang, X.Y.; Grizzle, W.; Sun, D.M.; Zhang, S.Q.; Axtell, R.C.; Ju, S.W.; Mu, J.Y.; Zhang, L.F.; Steinman, L.; et al. Treatment of Brain Inflammatory Diseases by Delivering Exosome Encapsulated Anti-inflammatory Drugs From the Nasal Region to the Brain. *Mol. Ther.* **2011**, *19*, 1769–1779. [CrossRef] [PubMed]
57. Franzen, C.A.; Simms, P.E.; Van Huis, A.F.; Foreman, K.E.; Kuo, P.C.; Gupta, G.N. Characterization of Uptake and Internalization of Exosomes by Bladder Cancer Cells. *Biomed Res. Int.* **2014**. [CrossRef] [PubMed]
58. Greco, K.A.; Franzen, C.A.; Foreman, K.E.; Flanigan, R.C.; Kuo, P.C.; Gupta, G.N. PLK-1 Silencing in Bladder Cancer by siRNA Delivered With Exosomes. *Urology* **2016**, *91*. [CrossRef] [PubMed]

59. Jin, X.; Ma, J.W.; Liang, X.Y.; Tang, K.; Liu, Y.Y.; Yin, X.A.; Zhang, Y.; Zhang, H.F.; Xu, P.W.; Chen, D.G.; et al. Pre-instillation of tumor microparticles enhances intravesical chemotherapy of nonmuscle-invasive bladder cancer through a lysosomal pathway. *Biomaterials* **2017**, *113*, 93–104. [CrossRef] [PubMed]
60. Ortiz-Bonilla, C.J.; Lee, Y.F. BCG internalization releases increased levels of immune-active extracellular vesicles. Unpublished; manuscript in preparation.
61. Zhou, H.; Cheruvanky, A.; Hu, X.; Matsumoto, T.; Hiramatsu, N.; Cho, M.E.; Berger, A.; Leelahavanichkul, A.; Doi, K.; Chawla, L.S.; et al. Urinary exosomal transcription factors, a new class of biomarkers for renal disease. *Kidney Int.* **2008**, *74*, 613–621. [CrossRef] [PubMed]
62. Moon, P.G.; You, S.; Lee, J.E.; Hwang, D.; Baek, M.C. Urinary exosomes and proteomics. *Mass Spectrom. Rev.* **2011**, *30*, 1185–1202. [CrossRef] [PubMed]
63. Adachi, J.; Kumar, C.; Zhang, Y.; Olsen, J.V.; Mann, M. The human urinary proteome contains more than 1500 proteins, including a large proportion of membrane proteins. *Genome Biol.* **2006**, *7*, R80. [CrossRef] [PubMed]
64. Moon, P.G.; Lee, J.E.; You, S.; Kim, T.K.; Cho, J.H.; Kim, I.S.; Kwon, T.H.; Kim, C.D.; Park, S.H.; Hwang, D.; et al. Proteomic analysis of urinary exosomes from patients of early IgA nephropathy and thin basement membrane nephropathy. *Proteomics* **2011**, *11*, 2459–2475. [CrossRef] [PubMed]
65. Knepper, M.A. Common sense approaches to urinary biomarker study design. *J. Am. Soc. Nephrol.* **2009**, *20*, 1175–1178. [CrossRef] [PubMed]
66. Gonzales, P.; Pisitkun, T.; Knepper, M.A. Urinary exosomes: Is there a future? *Nephrol. Dial. Transplant.* **2008**, *23*, 1799–1801. [CrossRef] [PubMed]
67. Keller, S.; Rupp, C.; Stoeck, A.; Runz, S.; Fogel, M.; Lugert, S.; Hager, H.D.; Abdel-Bakky, M.S.; Gutwein, P.; Altevogt, P. CD24 is a marker of exosomes secreted into urine and amniotic fluid. *Kidney Int.* **2007**, *72*, 1095–1102. [CrossRef] [PubMed]
68. Hogan, M.C.; Manganelli, L.; Woollard, J.R.; Masyuk, A.I.; Masyuk, T.V.; Tammachote, R.; Huang, B.Q.; Leontovich, A.A.; Beito, T.G.; Madden, B.J.; et al. Characterization of PKD protein-positive exosome-like vesicles. *J. Am. Soc. Nephrol.* **2009**, *20*, 278–288. [CrossRef] [PubMed]
69. Zhang, Y.; Li, Y.; Qiu, F.; Qiu, Z. Comprehensive analysis of low-abundance proteins in human urinary exosomes using peptide ligand library technology, peptide OFFGEL fractionation and nanoHPLC-chip-MS/MS. *Electrophoresis* **2010**, *31*, 3797–3807. [CrossRef] [PubMed]
70. Nawaz, M.; Camussi, G.; Valadi, H.; Nazarenko, I.; Ekstrom, K.; Wang, X.; Principe, S.; Shah, N.; Ashraf, N.M.; Fatima, F.; et al. The emerging role of extracellular vesicles as biomarkers for urogenital cancers. *Nat. Rev. Urol.* **2014**, *11*, 688–701. [CrossRef] [PubMed]
71. Pisitkun, T.; Shen, R.F.; Knepper, M.A. Identification and proteomic profiling of exosomes in human urine. *Proc. Natl. Acad. Sci. USA* **2004**, *101*, 13368–13373. [CrossRef] [PubMed]
72. Gonzales, P.A.; Pisitkun, T.; Hoffert, J.D.; Tchapyjnikov, D.; Star, R.A.; Kleta, R.; Wang, N.S.; Knepper, M.A. Large-scale proteomics and phosphoproteomics of urinary exosomes. *J. Am. Soc. Nephrol.* **2009**, *20*, 363–379. [CrossRef] [PubMed]
73. Wang, Z.; Hill, S.; Luther, J.M.; Hachey, D.L.; Schey, K.L. Proteomic analysis of urine exosomes by multidimensional protein identification technology (MudPIT). *Proteomics* **2012**, *12*, 329–338. [CrossRef] [PubMed]
74. Chen, C.L.; Lai, Y.F.; Tang, P.; Chien, K.Y.; Yu, J.S.; Tsai, C.H.; Chen, H.W.; Wu, C.C.; Chung, T.; Hsu, C.W.; et al. Comparative and targeted proteomic analyses of urinary microparticles from bladder cancer and hernia patients. *J. Proteome Res.* **2012**, *11*, 5611–5629. [CrossRef] [PubMed]
75. Principe, S.; Jones, E.E.; Kim, Y.; Sinha, A.; Nyalwidhe, J.O.; Brooks, J.; Semmes, O.J.; Troyer, D.A.; Lance, R.S.; Kislinger, T.; et al. In-depth proteomic analyses of exosomes isolated from expressed prostatic secretions in urine. *Proteomics* **2013**, *13*, 1667–1671. [CrossRef] [PubMed]
76. Principe, S.; Kim, Y.; Fontana, S.; Ignatchenko, V.; Nyalwidhe, J.O.; Lance, R.S.; Troyer, D.A.; Alessandro, R.; Semmes, O.J.; Kislinger, T.; et al. Identification of prostate-enriched proteins by in-depth proteomic analyses of expressed prostatic secretions in urine. *J. Proteome Res.* **2012**, *11*, 2386–2396. [CrossRef] [PubMed]
77. Leiblich, A. Recent Developments in the Search for Urinary Biomarkers in Bladder Cancer. *Curr. Urol. Rep.* **2017**, *18*, 100. [CrossRef] [PubMed]

78. Hauser, S.; Kogej, M.; Fechner, G.; Von Ruecker, A.; Bastian, P.J.; Von Pezold, J.; Vorreuther, R.; Lummen, G.; Muller, S.C.; Ellinger, J. Cell-free serum DNA in patients with bladder cancer: Results of a prospective multicenter study. *Anticancer Res.* **2012**, *32*, 3119–3124. [PubMed]
79. Casadio, V.; Calistri, D.; Tebaldi, M.; Bravaccini, S.; Gunelli, R.; Martorana, G.; Bertaccini, A.; Serra, L.; Scarpi, E.; Amadori, D.; et al. Urine cell-free DNA integrity as a marker for early bladder cancer diagnosis: Preliminary data. *Urol. Oncol.* **2013**, *31*, 1744–1750. [CrossRef] [PubMed]
80. Lu, T.; Li, J. Clinical applications of urinary cell-free DNA in cancer: Current insights and promising future. *Am. J. Cancer Res.* **2017**, *7*, 2318–2332. [PubMed]
81. Berrondo, C.; Flax, J.; Kucherov, V.; Siebert, A.; Osinski, T.; Rosenberg, A.; Fucile, C.; Richheimer, S.; Beckham, C.J. Expression of the Long Non-Coding RNA HOTAIR Correlates with Disease Progression in Bladder Cancer and Is Contained in Bladder Cancer Patient Urinary Exosomes. *PLoS ONE* **2016**, *11*, e0147236. [CrossRef] [PubMed]
82. Liang, L.G.; Kong, M.Q.; Zhou, S.; Sheng, Y.F.; Wang, P.; Yu, T.; Inci, F.; Kuo, W.P.; Li, L.J.; Demirci, U.; et al. An integrated double-filtration microfluidic device for isolation, enrichment and quantification of urinary extracellular vesicles for detection of bladder cancer. *Sci. Rep.* **2017**, *7*, 46224. [CrossRef] [PubMed]
83. Juracek, J.; Peltanova, B.; Dolezel, J.; Fedorko, M.; Pacik, D.; Radova, L.; Vesela, P.; Svoboda, M.; Slaby, O.; Stanik, M. Genome-wide identification of urinary cell-free microRNAs for non-invasive detection of bladder cancer. *J. Cell. Mol. Med.* **2018**, *22*, 2033–2038. [CrossRef] [PubMed]
84. Lin, S.Y.; Chang, C.H.; Wu, H.C.; Lin, C.C.; Chang, K.P.; Yang, C.R.; Huang, C.P.; Hsu, W.H.; Chang, C.T.; Chen, C.J. Proteome Profiling of Urinary Exosomes Identifies Alpha 1-Antitrypsin and H2B1K as Diagnostic and Prognostic Biomarkers for Urothelial Carcinoma. *Sci. Rep.* **2016**, *6*, 34446. [CrossRef] [PubMed]
85. Long, J.D.; Sullivan, T.B.; Humphrey, J.; Logvinenko, T.; Summerhayes, K.A.; Kozinn, S.; Harty, N.; Summerhayes, I.C.; Libertino, J.A.; Holway, A.H.; et al. A non-invasive miRNA based assay to detect bladder cancer in cell-free urine. *Am. J. Transl. Res.* **2015**, *7*, 2500–2509. [PubMed]
86. Armstrong, D.A.; Green, B.B.; Seigne, J.D.; Schned, A.R.; Marsit, C.J. MicroRNA molecular profiling from matched tumor and bio-fluids in bladder cancer. *Mol. Cancer* **2015**, *14*, 194. [CrossRef] [PubMed]
87. Matsuzaki, K.; Fujita, K.; Jingushi, K.; Kawashima, A.; Ujike, T.; Nagahara, A.; Ueda, Y.; Tanigawa, G.; Yoshioka, I.; Ueda, K.; et al. MiR-21-5p in urinary extracellular vesicles is a novel biomarker of urothelial carcinoma. *Oncotarget* **2017**, *8*, 24668–24678. [CrossRef] [PubMed]
88. Pardini, B.; Cordero, F.; Naccarati, A.; Viberti, C.; Birolo, G.; Oderda, M.; Di Gaetano, C.; Arigoni, M.; Martina, F.; Calogero, R.A.; et al. microRNA profiles in urine by next-generation sequencing can stratify bladder cancer subtypes. *Oncotarget* **2018**, *9*, 20658–20669. [CrossRef] [PubMed]
89. Heba Fanous, T.S. Kimberly Rieger-Christ. Distinct exosomalL miRNA profiles in chemoresistant bladder carcinoma cell lines. *J. Urol.* **2017**, *197*, 2.
90. Yasui, T.; Yanagida, T.; Ito, S.; Konakade, Y.; Takeshita, D.; Naganawa, T.; Nagashima, K.; Shimada, T.; Kaji, N.; Nakamura, Y.; et al. Unveiling massive numbers of cancer-related urinary-microRNA candidates via nanowires. *Sci. Adv.* **2017**, *3*, e1701133. [CrossRef] [PubMed]
91. Baumgart, S.; Holters, S.; Ohlmann, C.H.; Bohle, R.; Stockle, M.; Ostenfeld, M.S.; Dyrskjot, L.; Junker, K.; Heinzelmann, J. Exosomes of invasive urothelial carcinoma cells are characterized by a specific miRNA expression signature. *Oncotarget* **2017**, *8*, 58278–58291. [CrossRef] [PubMed]
92. Zhang, D.Z.; Lau, K.M.; Chan, E.S.; Wang, G.; Szeto, C.C.; Wong, K.; Choy, R.K.; Ng, C.F. Cell-free urinary microRNA-99a and microRNA-125b are diagnostic markers for the non-invasive screening of bladder cancer. *PLoS ONE* **2014**, *9*, e100793. [CrossRef] [PubMed]
93. Kim, S.M.; Kang, H.W.; Kim, W.T.; Kim, Y.J.; Yun, S.J.; Lee, S.C.; Kim, W.J. Cell-Free microRNA-214 From Urine as a Biomarker for Non-Muscle-Invasive Bladder Cancer. *Korean J. Urol.* **2013**, *54*, 791–796. [CrossRef] [PubMed]
94. Smalley, D.M.; Sheman, N.E.; Nelson, K.; Theodorescu, D. Isolation and identification of potential urinary microparticle biomarkers of bladder cancer. *J. Proteome Res.* **2008**, *7*, 2088–2096. [CrossRef] [PubMed]
95. Fontana, S.; Saieva, L.; Taverna, S.; Alessandro, R. Contribution of proteomics to understanding the role of tumor-derived exosomes in cancer progression: State of the art and new perspectives. *Proteomics* **2013**, *13*, 1581–1594. [CrossRef] [PubMed]
96. Welton, J.L.; Khanna, S.; Giles, P.J.; Brennan, P.; Brewis, I.A.; Staffurth, J.; Mason, M.D.; Clayton, A. Proteomics analysis of bladder cancer exosomes. *Mol. Cell. Proteom.* **2010**, *9*, 1324–1338. [CrossRef] [PubMed]

97. Kumari, N.; Saxena, S.; Agrawal, U. Exosomal protein interactors as emerging therapeutic targets in urothelial bladder cancer. *J. Egypt. Natl. Cancer Inst.* **2015**, *27*, 51–58. [CrossRef] [PubMed]
98. Alvarez, M.L.; Khosroheidari, M.; Ravi, R.K.; DiStefano, J.K. Comparison of protein, microRNA and mRNA yields using different methods of urinary exosome isolation for the discovery of kidney disease biomarkers. *Kidney Int.* **2012**, *82*, 1024–1032. [CrossRef] [PubMed]
99. Musante, L.; Saraswat, M.; Duriez, E.; Byrne, B.; Ravida, A.; Domon, B.; Holthofer, H. Biochemical and physical characterisation of urinary nanovesicles following CHAPS treatment. *PLoS ONE* **2012**, *7*, e37279. [CrossRef] [PubMed]
100. Thery, C.; Amigorena, S.; Raposo, G.; Clayton, A. Isolation and characterization of exosomes from cell culture supernatants and biological fluids. *Curr. Protoc. Cell Biol.* **2006**, *3*, 3–22. [CrossRef] [PubMed]
101. Liga, A.; Vliegenthart, A.D.B.; Oosthuyzen, W.; Dear, J.W.; Kersaudy-Kerhoas, M. Exosome isolation: A microfluidic road-map. *Lab Chip* **2015**, *15*, 2388–2394. [CrossRef] [PubMed]
102. Kanwar, S.S.; Dunlay, C.J.; Simeone, D.M.; Nagrath, S. Microfluidic device (ExoChip) for on-chip isolation, quantification and characterization of circulating exosomes. *Lab Chip* **2014**, *14*, 1891–1900. [CrossRef] [PubMed]
103. Santana, S.M.; Antonyak, M.A.; Cerione, R.A.; Kirby, B.J. Microfluidic isolation of cancer-cell-derived microvesicles from hetergeneous extracellular shed vesicle populations. *Biomed. Microdevices* **2014**, *16*, 869–877. [CrossRef] [PubMed]
104. Momen-Heravi, F.; Balaj, L.; Alian, S.; Mantel, P.Y.; Halleck, A.E.; Trachtenberg, A.J.; Soria, C.E.; Oquin, S.; Bonebreak, C.M.; Saracoglu, E.; et al. Current methods for the isolation of extracellular vesicles. *Biol. Chem.* **2013**, *394*, 1253–1262. [CrossRef] [PubMed]
105. Fernandez-Llama, P.; Khositseth, S.; Gonzales, P.A.; Star, R.A.; Pisitkun, T.; Knepper, M.A. Tamm-Horsfall protein and urinary exosome isolation. *Kidney Int.* **2010**, *77*, 736–742. [CrossRef] [PubMed]
106. Witwer, K.W.; Buzas, E.I.; Bemis, L.T.; Bora, A.; Lasser, C.; Lotvall, J.; Nolte-'t Hoen, E.N.; Piper, M.G.; Sivaraman, S.; Skog, J.; et al. Standardization of sample collection, isolation and analysis methods in extracellular vesicle research. *J. Extracell. Vesicles* **2013**, *2*. [CrossRef] [PubMed]
107. Lotvall, J.; Rajendran, L.; Gho, Y.S.; Thery, C.; Wauben, M.; Raposo, G.; Sjostrand, M.; Taylor, D.; Telemo, E.; Breakefield, X.O. The launch of Journal of Extracellular Vesicles (JEV), the official journal of the International Society for Extracellular Vesicles—About microvesicles, exosomes, ectosomes and other extracellular vesicles. *J. Extracell. Vesicles* **2012**, *1*. [CrossRef] [PubMed]
108. Waikar, S.S.; Sabbisetti, V.S.; Bonventre, J.V. Normalization of urinary biomarkers to creatinine during changes in glomerular filtration rate. *Kidney Int.* **2010**, *78*, 486–494. [CrossRef] [PubMed]
109. Tang, K.W.A.; Toh, Q.C.; Teo, B.W. Normalisation of urinary biomarkers to creatinine for clinical practice and research—When and why. *Singapore Med. J.* **2015**, *56*, 7–10. [CrossRef] [PubMed]
110. Mattix, H.J.; Hsu, C.Y.; Shaykevich, S.; Curhan, G. Use of the albumin/creatinine ratio to detect microalbuminuria: Implications of sex and race. *J. Am. Soc. Nephrol.* **2002**, *13*, 1034–1039. [PubMed]
111. Mitch, W.E.; Collier, V.U.; Walser, M. Creatinine Metabolism in Chronic Renal-Failure. *Clin. Res.* **1978**, *26*, A636. [CrossRef]
112. Zhou, H.; Yuen, P.S.; Pisitkun, T.; Gonzales, P.A.; Yasuda, H.; Dear, J.W.; Gross, P.; Knepper, M.A.; Star, R.A. Collection, storage, preservation and normalization of human urinary exosomes for biomarker discovery. *Kidney Int.* **2006**, *69*, 1471–1476. [CrossRef] [PubMed]
113. Prunotto, M.; Farina, A.; Lane, L.; Pernin, A.; Schifferli, J.; Hochstrasser, D.F.; Lescuyer, P.; Moll, S. Proteomic analysis of podocyte exosome-enriched fraction from normal human urine. *J. Proteom.* **2013**, *82*, 193–229. [CrossRef] [PubMed]
114. Lentz, M.R. Continuous whole blood UltraPheresis procedure in patients with metastatic cancer. *J. Biol. Response Mod.* **1989**, *8*, 511–527. [PubMed]
115. Tullis, R.H.; Duffin, R.P.; Handley, H.H.; Sodhi, P.; Menon, J.; Joyce, J.A.; Kher, V. Reduction of hepatitis C virus using lectin affinity plasmapheresis in dialysis patients. *Blood Purif.* **2009**, *27*, 64–69. [CrossRef] [PubMed]
116. Marleau, A.M.; Chen, C.S.; Joyce, J.A.; Tullis, R.H. Exosome removal as a therapeutic adjuvant in cancer. *J. Transl. Med.* **2012**, *10*, 134. [CrossRef] [PubMed]

117. Chalmin, F.; Ladoire, S.; Mignot, G.; Vincent, J.; Bruchard, M.; Remy-Martin, J.P.; Boireau, W.; Rouleau, A.; Simon, B.; Lanneau, D.; et al. Membrane-associated Hsp72 from tumor-derived exosomes mediates STAT3-dependent immunosuppressive function of mouse and human myeloid-derived suppressor cells. *J. Clin. Investig.* **2010**, *120*, 457–471. [CrossRef] [PubMed]
118. Jiang, Y.; Wang, X.; Zhang, J.; Lai, R. MicroRNA-599 suppresses glioma progression by targeting RAB27B. *Oncol. Lett.* **2018**, *16*, 1243–1252. [CrossRef] [PubMed]
119. Ostrowski, M.; Carmo, N.B.; Krumeich, S.; Fanget, I.; Raposo, G.; Savina, A.; Moita, C.F.; Schauer, K.; Hume, A.N.; Freitas, R.P.; et al. Rab27a and Rab27b control different steps of the exosome secretion pathway. *Nat. Cell Biol.* **2010**, *12*, 19–30. [CrossRef] [PubMed]
120. Sun, D.; Zhuang, X.; Xiang, X.; Liu, Y.; Zhang, S.; Liu, C.; Barnes, S.; Grizzle, W.; Miller, D.; Zhang, H.G. A novel nanoparticle drug delivery system: The anti-inflammatory activity of curcumin is enhanced when encapsulated in exosomes. *Mol. Ther.* **2010**, *18*, 1606–1614. [CrossRef] [PubMed]
121. Tian, Y.; Li, S.; Song, J.; Ji, T.; Zhu, M.; Anderson, G.J.; Wei, J.; Nie, G. A doxorubicin delivery platform using engineered natural membrane vesicle exosomes for targeted tumor therapy. *Biomaterials* **2014**, *35*, 2383–2390. [CrossRef] [PubMed]
122. Hoshino, A.; Costa-Silva, B.; Shen, T.L.; Rodrigues, G.; Hashimoto, A.; Tesic Mark, M.; Molina, H.; Kohsaka, S.; Di Giannatale, A.; Ceder, S.; et al. Tumour exosome integrins determine organotropic metastasis. *Nature* **2015**, *527*, 329–335. [CrossRef] [PubMed]
123. Xitong, D.; Xiaorong, Z. Targeted therapeutic delivery using engineered exosomes and its applications in cardiovascular diseases. *Gene* **2016**, *575*, 377–384. [CrossRef] [PubMed]

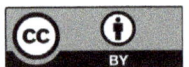

© 2018 by the authors. Licensee MDPI, Basel, Switzerland. This article is an open access article distributed under the terms and conditions of the Creative Commons Attribution (CC BY) license (http://creativecommons.org/licenses/by/4.0/).

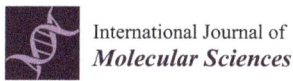

Review

Biomarkers for Predicting Clinical Outcomes of Chemoradiation-Based Bladder Preservation Therapy for Muscle-Invasive Bladder Cancer

Fumitaka Koga *, Kosuke Takemura and Hiroshi Fukushima

Department of Urology, Tokyo Metropolitan Cancer and Infectious diseases Center Komagome Hospital, 3-18-22 Honkomagome, Bunkyo-ku, Tokyo 113-8677, Japan; takemura-uro@cick.jp (K.T.); fukuuro@tmd.ac.jp (H.F.)
* Correspondence: f-koga@cick.jp; Tel.: +81-3-3823-2101; Fax: +81-3-3823-5433

Received: 27 August 2018; Accepted: 14 September 2018; Published: 15 September 2018

Abstract: Chemoradiation-based bladder preservation therapy (BPT) is currently a curative option for non-metastatic muscle-invasive bladder cancer (MIBC) patients at favorable risk or an alternative to radical cystectomy (RC) for those who are unfit for RC. In BPT, only patients who achieve complete response (CR) after chemoradiation have a favorable prognosis and quality of life with a preserved functional bladder. Thus, predicting CR and favorable prognosis is important for optimal patient selection for BPT. We reviewed biomarkers for predicting the clinical outcomes of chemoradiation-based BPT. The biomarkers studied were categorized into those related to apoptosis, cell proliferation, receptor tyrosine kinases, DNA damage response genes, hypoxia, molecular subtype, and others. Among these biomarkers, the Ki-67 labeling index (Ki-67 LI) and meiotic recombination 11 may be used for selecting BPT or RC. Ki-67 LI and erythroblastic leukemia viral oncogene homolog 2 (erbB2) may be used for predicting both the chemoradiation response and the prognosis of patients on BPT. Concurrent use of trastuzumab and a combination of carbogen and nicotinamide can overcome chemoradiation resistance conferred by erbB2 overexpression and tumor hypoxia. Further studies are needed to confirm the practical utility of these biomarkers for progress on biomarker-directed personalized management of MIBC patients.

Keywords: biomarker; chemoradiation; prognosis; bladder preservation; bladder neoplasm; urothelial carcinoma

1. Introduction

Bladder cancer is the second most common malignancy of the genitourinary tract after prostate cancer in the United States, with approximately 81,000 new cases and 17,000 deaths each year as of 2018 [1]. Approximately 75% of bladder cancer patients present with non-muscle-invasive bladder cancer confined to the mucosa and submucosa (Tis, Ta, and T1), while the rest present with muscle-invasive bladder cancer (MIBC) [2]. The reference standard of care for MIBC patients has long been radical cystectomy (RC) with urinary diversion and lymph node dissection. However, this surgical procedure is complex and invasive and could have long-term adverse effects on urinary, gastrointestinal, and sexual functions. A recent systematic review on the surgical outcomes of robot-assisted laparoscopic RC demonstrated a 90-day overall complication rate of 59%, a 90-day major complication rate of 15%, and a 90-day mortality rate of 3% [3]. The long-term adverse effects on urinary, gastrointestinal, and sexual functions significantly compromised quality of life (QOL) in patients undergoing RC and urinary diversion when compared with those retaining their native bladders [4].

Bladder preservation therapy (BPT), consisting of transurethral resection, chemotherapy, and radiation, has yielded oncological outcomes and QOL comparable to or more favorable than RC when select MIBC patients undergo BPT [5]. Because of the lack of randomized control trials, BPT used to be an alternative to RC for MIBC patients medically unfit for RC. However, accumulated clinical evidence reported from centers of excellence has demonstrated favorable oncological and QOL outcomes [6–8]. Consequently, guidelines of the American Urological Association, American Society of Clinical Oncology, American Society for Radiation Oncology, and Society of Urologic Oncology mention that chemoradiation-based BPT should be offered as an option of standard therapies for non-metastatic MIBC patients who desire to retain their bladders and for whom RC is not a treatment option [2].

MIBC patients with favorable oncological and QOL outcomes after BPT are those achieving complete response (CR) to chemoradiation; such patients account for 50–90% of MIBC patients treated with chemoradiation-based BPT [5]. Although those who do not achieve CR are advised to undergo salvage RC, MIBC patients who do not achieve CR to chemoradiation show unfavorable cancer-specific survival (CSS) regardless of salvage RC with curative intent due to metastatic recurrences [5,9]; such patients may benefit from neoadjuvant chemotherapy plus RC in terms of CSS. Thus, prediction of chemoradiation response enables selection of optimal candidates for BPT and may ultimately improve prognosis and QOL of MIBC patients.

In this study, we conducted a non-systematic review to identify studies investigating biomarkers associated with chemoradiation response and prognosis on chemoradiation-based BPT among MIBC patients. Some biomarkers can be used as targets for therapeutic intervention to improve clinical outcomes by modifying the functions of biomarkers (e.g., concurrent use of trastuzumab for erythroblastic leukemia viral oncogene homolog 2 (erbB2)-overexpressing tumors to improve chemoradiation response).

2. Current Practice on Bladder Preservation Therapy in Muscle-Invasive Bladder Cancer Patients

BPT in the form most widely utilized and recommended by guidelines comprises transurethral resection and chemoradiation. Randomized controlled phase III trials demonstrated oncological advantages of concurrent administration of chemotherapeutic agents over radiotherapy alone in non-metastatic MIBC patients. In a Canadian trial reported in 1996, adding cisplatin as a radiosensitizer significantly improved local control [10]. However, this study did not have adequate power to show the survival advantages of chemoradiation over radiotherapy alone. A randomized trial in the United Kingdom investigated fluorouracil and mitomycin-C as radiosensitizers in MIBC patients [11]. The concurrent use of these agents significantly improved the 2-year locoregional disease-free survival from 54% to 67%. In this trial, the 5-year overall survival (OS) improved from 35% to 48% but there was no statistical significance. Case series and phase I/II studies demonstrated possible activity of gemcitabine [12] and paclitaxel [13] as radiosensitizers for MIBC.

2.1. Indications

Indications of BPT in MIBC patients are quite different according to whether they are fit for RC or not. BPT for those who are fit for RC and who desire their native bladders is regarded as selective BPT. On the other hand, those who are unfit for RC due to severe comorbidity or poor performance status receive BPT as an alternative to RC.

Selective BPT is generally given to patients with low-risk MIBC in whom favorable oncological outcomes are expected to be comparable to those of RC. Favorable clinical features of MIBC include small, solitary and non-metastatic low stage (clinical T2N0) diseases, the absence of hydronephrosis, and the absence of extensive carcinoma in situ [5]. Such tumors are amenable to complete transurethral resection prior to chemoradiation; indeed, the visibly complete transurethral resection of primary tumors is associated with favorable prognosis in patients treated with BPT [5,8].

In contrast to the RC-fit patients, those unfit for RC would receive BPT with chemoradiation as a curative option alternative to RC. These patients would have diseases of higher risks than those who are subjected to selective BPT. Therefore, RC-unfit patients treated with BPT generally have a worse prognosis than those treated with selective BPT.

2.2. Therapeutic Protocols

Two typical templates for chemoradiation were reported: Split- or single-course protocol [5]. A split-course protocol consists of induction chemoradiation of 40–45 Gy, followed by evaluation of any residual tumor with imaging studies and transurethral biopsy, and then consolidative chemoradiation of 20–25 Gy if CR is achieved. Patients who do not achieve CR undergo salvage RC. In contrast, a single-course protocol includes full-dose chemoradiation of 55–65 Gy followed by response evaluation and surveillance if CR is achieved. Although salvage RC is planned for patients who do not achieve CR, high-dose (>60 Gy) pelvic irradiation increases both the morbidity and mortality of RC; in patients undergoing salvage RC after high-dose radiotherapy, mortality rates range from 6% to 33%, higher than the rates reported in published contemporary RC series for non-irradiated subjects, which range up to 4% [5]. The split-course protocol places priority on cancer control by carrying out salvage RC with minimal delay for non-CR patients in selective BPT. A lower dose of preoperative irradiation also reduces the risk of RC-associated complications for non-CR patients after induction chemoradiation [14]. However, splitting of radiotherapy could reduce antitumor effects of the split-course protocol compared with those of the single-course protocol. In this respect, the single-course protocol is more suitable than the split-course protocol for BPT in patients unfit for RC.

Other protocols involve consolidative partial cystectomy with pelvic lymph node dissection following induction chemoradiation [15,16] and intraarterial chemotherapy [17] to increase therapeutic intensity.

2.3. Prognosis

A published series of chemoradiation-based BPT reported OS comparable to that of RC (50–70% at 5 years) while preserving the native bladder in 40–60% of MIBC patients [5]. There is no randomized controlled trial comparing outcomes between BPT and RC in MIBC patients. Recently, 3 studies retrospectively compared prognosis of MIBC patients between BPT and RC using a propensity score matching analysis: 2 studies derived from the National Cancer Database (NCD) [18,19] and one study from a Canadian multidisciplinary bladder cancer clinic [20]. The 2 NCD studies demonstrated more favorable OS for RC than that for BPT. Because of the lack of adjustment for performance status, an established prognostic factor in MIBC patients, in these NCD studies, the results would be biased by patients who were unfit for RC due to poor performance status and thus received BPT [18,19]. In the Canadian study, subjects were matched for more prognostic factors including performance status than those of the NCD studies, and BPT yielded OS and CSS similar to RC after propensity score matching [20].

2.4. Clinicopathologic Factors Associated with Outcomes of Bladder Preservation Therapy

Clinicopathologic parameters associated with outcomes of chemoradiation-based BPT are classified into tumor and therapeutic factors. The clinical tumor parameters associated with favorable chemoradiation response include small tumor size (<5 cm), clinical T2 stage, unifocal disease, and the absence of hydronephrosis [8,16]. The most important therapeutic parameter is completeness of transurethral resection [8]. Thus, it is mandatory to attempt transurethral resection of tumors as thoroughly as is safely possible for candidates of BPT. Prognostic factors after BPT include completeness of transurethral resection, clinical T stage, and lymphovascular invasion [8].

Coen et al. developed comprehensive nomograms predicting outcomes of BPT including therapeutic response to chemoradiation, CSS, and bladder-intact disease-free survival in a cohort of 325 MIBC patients who were treated with selective BPT of split-course chemoradiation [21]. The most important clinical parameters for CR after chemoradiation are the absence of hydronephrosis and complete transurethral resection followed by younger age (<65 years) and female gender. For

CSS, the most favorable parameters include clinical T2 disease (versus T3–4) and the absence of hydronephrosis followed by histological grade 2 disease (versus grade 3). For favorable bladder-intact disease-free survival, the most relevant parameter is the absence of hydronephrosis followed by complete transurethral resection, clinical T2 disease, and younger age (<65 years). Such nomograms may assist patients and clinicians making treatment decisions.

3. Biomarkers Associated with Chemoradiation Response and Prognosis

Summaries of studies that reported emerging biomarkers associated with chemoradiation response and prognosis on BPT for MIBC are listed in Tables 1 and 2, respectively. These biomarkers are categorized as follows: (1) apoptosis-related biomarkers, (2) cell proliferation-related biomarkers, (3) receptor tyrosine kinases (RTK), (4) DNA damage response (DDR)-related biomarkers, (5) hypoxia-related biomarkers, (6) molecular subtypes, and (7) others.

Table 1. Biomarkers associated with chemoradiation response.

Biomarkers	Samples Used (No. Patients)	Chemoradiation Regimen	Associations with Response	Study Type	Reference
Apoptosis-related					
Apoptotic index	Tumor tissues (n = 70)	RT 59.4 Gy + cisplatin	Higher apoptotic index was associated with a higher CR rate (86% vs. 57%, p = 0.02)	Retrospective	[22]
bax/bcl-2 ratio	Tumor tissues (n = 62)	RT 40.5 Gy (median) + cisplatin	Higher Bax/Bcl-2 ratio was associated with a higher CR rate (p = 0.029)	Retrospective	[23]
Cell proliferation-related					
Ki-67 LI	Tumor tissues (n = 70)	RT 59.4 Gy + cisplatin	Higher Ki-67 LI was associated with a higher CR rate (86% vs. 57%, p = 0.02)	Retrospective	[22]
Ki-67 LI	Tumor tissues (n = 94)	RT 40 Gy + cisplatin, 69 (73%) underwent partial or salvage radical cystectomy	Higher Ki-67 LI (continuous variable) was associated with a higher CR rate (p = 0.0004)	Retrospective	[24]
ADC value	MRI (n = 23)	RT 40 Gy + cisplatin	Sensitivity/specificity/accuracy = 92/90/91% when ADC < 0.74×10^{-3} mm^2/s	Retrospective	[25]
RTKs					
erbB2	Tumor tissues (n = 55)	RT 40 Gy + cisplatin + other agents	CR rates, 50% vs. 81% for positive vs. negative (p = 0.026)	Retrospective	[26]
erbB2	Tumor tissues (n = 119)	RT 40 Gy + cisplatin	CR rates, 29% vs. 53% for positive vs. negative (p = 0.01)	Retrospective	[27]
erbB2	Tumor tissues (n = 66)	RT 64.8 Gy + paclitaxel with (group 1: erbB2+) or without trastuzumab (group 2: erbB2-)	CR rates, 72% for group 1 and 68% for group 2	Prospective	[28]
DDR-related					
ERCC1	Tumor tissues (n = 22)	RT 40-66 Gy + cisplatin or nedaplatin	CR rates, 25% vs. 86% for positive vs. negative (p = 0.008)	Retrospective	[29]
Molecular subtype					
Molecular subtype	Tumor tissues (n = 118)	RT 40 Gy + cisplatin	CR rates, 52%/45%/15% for GU/SCC-like/Uro (p < 0.001)	Retrospective	[30]
Others					
Hsp60	Tumor tissues (n = 54)	RT 40 Gy + cisplatin	Positive Hsp60 was associated with better response (p = 0.05)	Retrospective	[31]

RT, radiotherapy; CR, complete response; LI, labeling index; ADC, apparent diffusion coefficient; MRI, magnetic resonance imaging; RTK, receptor tyrosine kinases; erbB2, erythroblastic leukemia viral oncogene homolog 2; DDR, DNA damage response; ERCC1, excision repair cross-complementing group 1; GU, genomically unstable subtype; SCC-like, squamous cell cancer-like subtype; Uro, urobasal subtype; Hsp60, heat shock protein 60.

Table 2. Biomarkers associated with prognosis of muscle invasive bladder cancer patients on chemoradiation-based bladder preservation therapy.

Biomarkers	Samples Used (No. Patients)	Chemoradiation Regimen	Associations with Prognosis	Study Type	Reference
Cell proliferation-related					
Ki-67 LI	Tumor tissues ($n = 70$)	RT 59.4 Gy + cisplatin	Better CSS with preserved bladder for higher Ki-67 LI (50% vs. 36% at 5-year, $p = 0.04$)	Retrospective	[22]
Ki-67 LI	Tumor tissues ($n = 62$)	RT 40.5 Gy (median) + cisplatin	Worse CSS for high Ki-67 LI of > 20% ($p = 0.014$)	Retrospective	[23]
Ki-67 LI	Tumor tissues ($n = 94$)	RT 40 Gy + cisplatin, 69 (73%) underwent partial or salvage radical cystectomy	Better CSS for high Ki-67 LI of > 20% (HR 0.3, $p = 0.01$)	Retrospective	[24]
RTKs					
EGFR	Tumor tissues ($n = 73$)	RT 40 Gy + cisplatin + other agents	Better CSS for positive EGFR ($p = 0.042$)	Retrospective	[26]
erbB2	Tumor tissues ($n = 119$)	RT 40 Gy + cisplatin	Worse CSS for erbB2 overexpression (56% vs. 87%, $p = 0.001$)	Retrospective	[27]
VEGF-B/C and VEGFR2	Tumor tissues ($n = 43$)	RT 64.8 Gy + cisplatin + other agents	Worse OS for high VEGF-B/C/R2 expression ($p = 0.01$-0.02), higher distant failure rate for high VEGF-R2 expression ($p = 0.01$)	Retrospective	[32]
VEGF-C/NRP2	Tumor tissues ($n = 247$)	RT 56.3 Gy + cisplatin	Worse OS for high NRP2 or VEGFC expression (HR 4.25, $p = 0.023$)	Retrospective	[33]
DDR-related					
MRE11	Tumor tissues ($n = 179$)	RT 55 Gy	Better CSS for high MRE11 expression (HR 0.36, $p = 0.01$)	Retrospective	[34]
ERCC1/XRCC1	Tumor tissues ($n = 157$)	RT 48.6 Gy (median) + cisplatin	Better CSS for positive ERCC1 or XRCC1 (HR 0.64, $p = 0.024$)	Retrospective	[35]
DDR alterations	Tumor tissues ($n = 48$)	RT or chemoradiation (details unavailable)	Trend for better RFS for the presence of DDR alterations (HR 0.37, $p = 0.07$)	Retrospective	[36]
Hypoxia-related					
Necrosis	Tumor tissues ($n = 220$)	RT vs. RT + CON	The presence of necrosis predicted better OS for RT + CON than RT alone (HR 0.43, $p = 0.004$)	Retrospective	[37]
HIF-1α	Tumor tissues ($n = 137$)	RT vs. RT + CON	Positive HIF-1α predicted better DFS for RT + CON than RT alone (HR 0.48, $p = 0.02$)	Retrospective	[38]
Others					
CRP	Serum ($n = 88$)	RT 40 Gy + cisplatin	Worse CSS for high CRP of > 0.5 mg/dL (HR 1.8, $p = 0.046$)	Retrospective	[39]
Lymphocytopenia	Blood ($n = 74$)	RT 52.5 Gy + gemcitabine	Worse RFS for lymphocytopenia of < 1.5×10^9/L (HR 3.9, $p = 0.003$)	Retrospective	[40]

LI, labeling index; RT, radiotherapy; CSS, cancer-specific survival; HR, hazard ratio; RTK, receptor tyrosine kinases; EGFR, epidermal growth factor receptor; erbB2, erythroblastic leukemia viral oncogene homolog 2; VEGF(R), vascular endothelial growth factor (receptor); OS, overall survival; NRP2, neutropilin 2; DDR, DNA damage response; MRE11, meiotic recombination 11; ERCC1, excision repair cross-complementing group 1; XRCC1, X-ray repair cross-complementing group 1; RFS, recurrence-free survival; CON, carbogen and nicotinamide; HIF-1α, hypoxia-inducible factor-1α; DFS, disease-free survival; CRP, C-reactive protein.

3.1. Apoptosis-Related Biomarkers

Apoptosis is a key mechanism by which DNA-damaging stimuli, including chemotherapeutic agents and ionizing radiation, exhibit therapeutic effects. Apoptosis-related biomarkers, including apoptotic index (AI), p53, bcl-2, and bax, were investigated in relation to chemoradiation response and prognosis following BPT. Bax and bcl-2 regulate apoptosis downstream of p53 in response to DNA damage, and bax and bcl-2 have a pro-apoptotic and anti-apoptotic effect, respectively [41].

Rodel et al. reported that a higher AI was associated with a higher CR rate (86% vs. 57%, $p = 0.02$) among 70 invasive bladder cancer (cT1-4) patients treated with chemoradiation (59.4 Gy + cisplatin) [22]. However, no significant association with chemoradiation response was observed for immunohistochemical expression p53 or bcl-2. Neither AI, nor p53, nor bcl-2 was associated with CSS in this study. Matsumoto et al. investigated associations of p53, bcl-2, bax, and apoptotic index with clinical response among 62 invasive bladder cancer patients (cT1G3-T4N0) receiving chemoradiation (median dose 40.5 Gy + cisplatin) [23]. They found no significant association between immunohistochemical expression of each biomarker and chemoradiation response. However, higher bax/bcl-2 ratios were significantly associated with higher CR rates ($p = 0.029$). No association with prognosis was observed for any of these biomarkers.

Thus, some apoptosis-related biomarkers (AI and bax/bcl-2 ratios) are predictive of chemoradiation response but not of prognosis of patients treated with BPT.

3.2. Cell Proliferation-Related Biomarkers

Ki-67 is an established marker of cell proliferation and a biomarker reflecting the biological aggressiveness of malignancies. In fact, a high Ki-67 labeling index (LI) was an independent risk factor for recurrence and cancer death in bladder cancer patients undergoing RC [42]. In contrast, Ki-67 LI could be a biomarker predicting favorable clinical outcomes for MIBC patients when they are treated with chemoradiation.

Rodel et al. [22] and Tanabe et al. [24] reported that a higher Ki-67 LI was significantly associated with a higher CR rate among bladder cancer patients receiving chemoradiation. These two studies also demonstrated significantly better CSS for patients with tumors of higher Ki-67 LI. However, Matsumoto et al. reported conflicting results; Ki-67 LI was not associated with chemoradiation response and higher Ki-67 LI was significantly associated with worse CSS [23]. In the latter study [10], the total radiation dose of chemoradiation (median 40.5 Gy) and CR rate (34%) were lower than those of a study by Rodel et al. (59.4 Gy and 71%, respectively) [9]. In a study by Tanabe et al., patients received chemoradiation at 40 Gy, and 73% eventually underwent partial cystectomy of the original MIBC site or salvage RC to completely eradicate possible residual cancer cells [12]. The above conflicting results may be attributed to the difference in therapeutic intensity and the probability of the presence of residual disease; residual cancer cells of high Ki-67 LI, which survive chemoradiation at a relatively low dose, may progress and be associated with worse prognosis in a study by Matsumoto et al. [10].

Magnetic resonance imaging (MRI) is routinely used for staging of bladder cancer. Diffusion-weighted MRI is constructed by quantifying the diffusion of water molecules and malignant lesions exhibit high signal intensity in this modality as a result of higher cellularity, tissue disorganization, and decreased extracellular space, all of which restrict water diffusion [43]. The extent of the water diffusion is quantitatively expressed as apparent diffusion coefficient (ADC) values. Yoshida et al. demonstrated that ADC values were inversely correlated with Ki-67 LI in MIBC tissues and that tumors with lower ADC values were more sensitive to chemoradiation [25]. However, the prognostic significance of ADC values has not yet been assessed among MIBC patients treated with BPT.

Taken together, cell proliferation-related biomarkers (Ki-67 LI and ADC values) are likely to be predictive of the chemoradiation response and prognosis of MIBC patients treated with BPT. However, validation studies are needed to confirm the prognostic significance of Ki-67 LI.

3.3. Receptor Tyrosine Kinases

Signaling via receptor tyrosine kinases (RTKs) promotes cell proliferation, tumor invasion, and therapeutic resistance [44]. Among RTKs, erbB2, epidermal growth factor receptor (EGFR), and vascular endothelial growth factor (VEGF)-family proteins are associated with clinical outcomes of chemoradiation in MIBC patients. Notably, a biomarker-driven clinical trial was conducted to overcome chemoradiation resistance of erbB2-overexpressing bladder cancer [28].

Chakravarti, et al. investigated the associations of erbB2 and EGFR with chemoradiation response and prognosis following BPT. They reported that positive erbB2 was significantly associated with lower CR rates (50% vs. 81% for negative erbB2, $p = 0.026$) and that positive EGFR was significantly associated with better CSS ($p = 0.042$) [26]. However, the reasons for the association between positive EGFR and better CSS remain to be elucidated. Inoue et al. confirmed the association between erbB2 overexpression and lower CR rates, and demonstrated, for the first time, adverse CSS for erbB2 overexpression among 119 MIBC patients receiving chemoradiation [27]. These data suggest that erbB2 inhibitors improve clinical outcomes of chemoradiation in patients with MIBC overexpressing erbB2. A recent study by Michaelson et al. showed possible improvement of chemoradiation response with erbB2 targeted therapy [28]; 66 evaluable bladder cancer patients were treated with radiation (64.8 Gy) and either paclitaxel + anti-erbB2 monoclonal antibody, trastuzumab (group 1, $n = 20$) or paclitaxel alone (group 2, $n = 46$) according to the presence (group 1) or absence of erbB2 overexpression (group 2) in tumor tissues. The CR rate at 1 year for group 1 was equivalent to that for group 2 (72% vs. 68%, respectively) with comparable toxicity profiles between the 2 groups. In this phase I/II clinical trial, mid- to long-term prognostic outcomes were not reported.

VEGFs have important functions in tumor angiogenesis and lymphangiogenesis, promoting cancer progression [45]. Two studies demonstrated prognostic significance of expression of VEGF family proteins among bladder cancer patients treated with chemoradiation. Lautenschlaeger et al. reported that overexpression of VEGF-B and C and their receptor VEGFR2 were significantly associated with worse OS [32]. However, no association was observed between these biomarkers and the chemoradiation response. Keck et al. demonstrated that overexpression of VEGF-C or its receptor neutropilin-2 was independently associated with worse OS [33]. In this study, the associations of VEGF-C/neutropilin-2 expression with chemoradiation response were not assessed.

3.4. DNA Damage Response-Related Biomarkers

Ionizing radiation induces cell death primarily via DNA double-strand breaks. Upon exposure to ionizing radiation, the damage is detected by the meiotic recombination 11 (MRE11)-RAD50-NBS1 complex, resulting in activation of the DDR pathway [46]. DNA cross-links induced by cisplatin are repaired by the nucleotide excision repair pathway, including excision repair cross-complementing group 1 (ERCC1) [47]. Failure to repair such DNA damage results in tumor cell death.

No DDR-related biomarkers except ERCC1 were associated with chemoradiation response. Kawashima et al. demonstrated that loss of ERCC1 expression was significantly associated with better chemoradiation response (CR rate, 86% vs. 25% for positive ERCC1) in a cohort of 22 MIBC patients [29]. These investigators also showed that loss of ERCC1 expression canceled resistance to ionizing radiation in bladder cancer cells in vitro.

Choudhury et al. reported that higher MRE11 expression was significantly associated with better CSS in 179 invasive bladder cancer patients treated with definitive radiotherapy at 55 Gy (hazard ratio (HR) 0.36, $p = 0.01$) [34]. A trend for an inverse prognostic effect of higher MRE11 expression was observed among patients undergoing RC, and CSS was significantly better for those treated with radiotherapy than RC among patients with tumors of higher MRE11 expression (HR 0.60, $p = 0.02$). This study suggests that MRE11 expression status may allow patient selection for radiotherapy or RC. Sakano et al. reported that positive expression of ERCC1 or X-ray repair cross-complementing group 1 (XRCC1) was significantly associated with better CSS (HR 0.64, $p = 0.024$) among 157 invasive bladder cancer patients undergoing cisplatin-based chemoradiation [35]. Given that chemoradiation sensitivity is a critical surrogate for prognosis among MIBC patients treated with BPT [5,9], findings of this study and the abovementioned ERCC1 study [29] appear to be conflicting. Desai et al. investigated the prognostic impact of DDR gene alterations, which were analyzed using a next-generation sequencing assay, in 48 invasive bladder cancer patients undergoing chemoradiation or radiotherapy [36]. The presence of DDR gene alterations, most commonly identified in *ERCC2*, showed a trend for better bladder or metastatic recurrence-free survival (HR 0.47, $p = 0.070$); this finding is in line with studies on neoadjuvant chemotherapy for MIBC [48,49] and systemic chemotherapy for advanced urothelial carcinoma [50], showing significantly better clinical outcomes for tumors with DDR gene alterations.

Thus, the roles of DNA damage response-related genes or proteins as practical biomarkers for predicting outcomes of chemoradiation seem to be largely unknown. The presence of DDR gene alterations may be a biomarker to predict favorable clinical outcomes of MIBC patients undergoing chemoradiation. MRE11 expression status may be used for selecting BPT or RC. However, further validation studies are needed to confirm the practical utility of DDR-related biomarkers in predicting clinical outcomes of BPT for MIBC patients.

3.5. Hypoxia-Related Biomarkers

Tumor hypoxia contributes to tumor progression, invasion, metastasis, and resistance to chemotherapy and radiotherapy [45]. A phase III clinical trial showed that hypoxia modification with carbogen and nicotinamide (CON) significantly improved prognosis of invasive bladder cancer patients treated with radiotherapy [51]. Ad hoc analyses of this clinical trial identified hypoxia-related biomarkers for predicting patients who benefit from concurrent CON [37,38]. Tumor hypoxia induces hypoxia-inducible factor-1α (HIF-1α) expression and necrosis in bladder cancer tissues. The presence of histological necrosis in tumor tissues was predictive of benefit from CON; radiotherapy + CON showed significantly better OS than radiotherapy alone in the presence of necrosis (HR 0.43, $p = 0.02$) but not in the absence of necrosis (HR 1.64, $p = 0.08$) [37]. Similarly, the addition of CON provided survival benefit for patients with higher HIF-1α-expressing tumors (HR 0.48, $p = 0.02$) but not for those with lower HIF-1α-expressing ones (HR 0.81, $p = 0.5$) [38].

3.6. Molecular Subtypes

Molecular subtypes of bladder cancer can characterize their clinical behaviors and can help predict therapeutic responses to neoadjuvant chemotherapy prior to RC [52,53]. Tanaka et al. demonstrated that molecular subtypes may be used to predict chemoradiation response in 118 MIBC patients [30]. The subtyping model used was the Lund University model, which characterizes three subtypes based on immunohistochemical expression patterns of cyclin B1 and keratin 5: Urobasal (Uro), genomically unstable (GU), and squamous cell cancer-like (SCC-like) [54]. CR rates after chemoradiation (40 Gy + cisplatin) were 52%, 45%, and 15% for GU, SCC-like, and Uro, respectively ($p < 0.001$). Molecular subtypes were not associated with CSS probably because most non-CR patients underwent salvage cystectomy [30].

3.7. Others

Urushibara et al. investigated the associations of heat shock proteins (Hsp), which play key roles in cellular stress responses and can be involved in therapeutic resistance and tumor aggressiveness, with clinical outcomes of 54 invasive bladder cancer patients treated with chemoradiation (40 Gy + cisplatin) [31]. Among Hsp27, Hsp60, Hsp70, and Hsp90, positive Hsp60 expression was independently associated with favorable responses ($p = 0.05$). However, no survival advantage was observed for Hsp60-positive tumors.

Two studies demonstrated the possible utility of serum and blood biomarkers, C-reactive protein (CRP) and lymphocytopenia, in predicting prognosis of MIBC patients treated with BPT [39,40]. Yoshida et al. reported that elevated serum CRP (>0.5 mg/dL) was independently associated with worse CSS (HR 1.8, $p = 0.046$) among 88 MIBC patients undergoing chemoradiation-based BPT [39]. CRP was not associated with chemoradiation response. Joseph et al. reported that lymphocytopenia (<1.5 × 10^9 /L) was significantly associated with worse disease-free survival (HR 3.9, $p = 0.003$) among 74 MIBC patients receiving chemoradiation (52.5 Gy + gemcitabine) [40].

4. Conclusions

Possible roles of the abovementioned biomarkers in predicting chemoradiation response and prognosis on chemoradiation-based BPT in MIBC patients are summarized in Figures 1 and 2, respectively. Higher Ki-67 LI, negative erbB2, higher expression of MRE11, higher AI, higher Bax/Bcl-2 ratio, lower ADC values, negative ERCC1, Uro subtype in the Lund University subtyping model, positive Hsp60, positive EGFR, lower expression of VEGF-related proteins, presence of DDR gene alterations, lower serum CRP, and absence of lymphocytopenia are possible biomarkers to predict favorable clinical outcomes in these patients. Of these biomarkers, Ki-67 LI and MRE11 may be used for selecting BPT or RC because a higher Ki-67 LI and higher MRE11 expression appear to favor BPT rather than RC in terms of post-therapeutic survival. Ki-67 LI and erbB2 may be used for predicting both chemoradiation response and prognosis of patients on BPT. Concurrent use of trastuzumab and CON can overcome chemoradiation resistance conferred by erbB2 overexpression and tumor hypoxia.

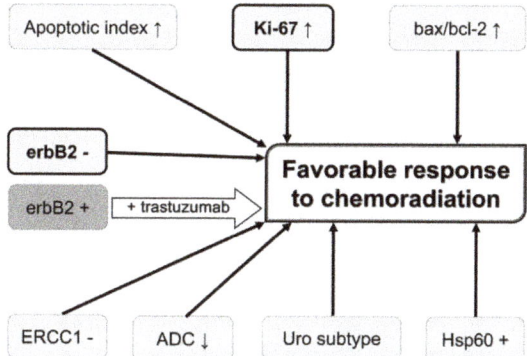

Figure 1. Biomarkers that may be used for predicting and improving the chemoradiation response. Biomarkers in bold letter are also associated with favorable prognosis on bladder preservation therapy. Overexpression of erbB2 is associated with unfavorable chemoradiation response, which can be overcome by trastuzumab. ADC, apparent diffusion coefficient value on diffusion-weighted magnetic resonance imaging; erbB2, erythroblastic leukemia viral oncogene homolog 2; ERCC1, excision repair cross-complementing group 1; Hsp60, heat shock protein 60; Uro subtype, urobasal subtype in the Lund University subtyping model;↑, high value;↓, low value.

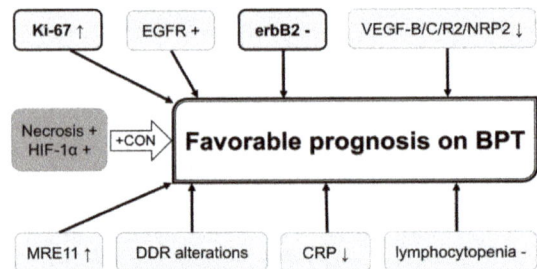

Figure 2. Biomarkers that may be used for predicting and improving prognosis on bladder preservation therapy. Biomarkers in bold letter are also associated with favorable chemoradiation response. Biomarkers in dark shadow are associated with unfavorable clinical outcomes, which can be overcome by CON. BPT, bladder preservation therapy; CON, carbogen and nicotinamide; CRP, C-reactive protein; DDR, DNA damage response; EGFR, epidermal growth factor receptor; erbB2, erythroblastic leukemia viral oncogene homolog 2; HIF-1α, hypoxia-inducible factor-1α; MRE11, meiotic recombination 11; NRP2, neutropilin 2; VEGF, vascular endothelial growth factor;↑, increased expression;↓, decreased expression or low value.

The introduction of immune-oncology drugs (IODs) to daily clinical practices may create a paradigm shift in the management of bladder cancer patients. IODs have the potential to provide long-term survival to a subset of metastatic bladder cancer patients who are considered incurable in the pre-IOD era [55]. Currently, chemoradiation-based BPT is proposed for non-metastatic MIBC patients who desire to retain their bladders and for whom RC is not a treatment option [2]. Hereafter, indications of intensive therapy to the primary site, including chemoradiation and RC, may expand to metastatic MIBC patients for whom long-term survival is expected on IODs. In this respect, identification of biomarkers and development of biomarker panels for comprehensively predicting clinical courses of bladder cancer patients are in increasing demand. In the near future, progress on biomarker research could allow for personalized management of MIBC patients, including those with metastatic disease, eventually providing better prognosis and QOL with BPT and IODs for optimally select patients.

Author Contributions: All authors made substantial contributions to this work; acquisition and interpretation of data by online search, F.K., K.T., and H.F.; draft and supervision of the work, F.K.; revision of the work, F.K., K.T., and H.F. All authors have approved the final version and agree to be personally accountable for the author's own contributions.

funding: This research was funded by JSPS KAKENHI grant number JP 17K11167 (F.K.).

Acknowledgments: This work was partly supported by JSPS KAKENHI Grant Number JP 17K11167 (F.K.).

Conflicts of Interest: The authors declare no conflict of interest.

References

1. Siegel, R.L.; Miller, K.D.; Jemal, A. Cancer statistics, 2018. *CA Cancer J. Clin.* **2018**, *68*, 7–30. [CrossRef] [PubMed]
2. Chang, S.S.; Bochner, B.H.; Chou, R.; Dreicer, R.; Kamat, A.M.; Lerner, S.P.; Lotan, Y.; Meeks, J.J.; Michalski, J.M.; Morgan, T.M.; et al. Treatment of Non-Metastatic Muscle-Invasive Bladder Cancer: AUA/ASCO/ASTRO/SUO Guideline. *J. Urol.* **2017**, *198*, 552–559. [CrossRef] [PubMed]
3. Novara, G.; Catto, J.W.; Wilson, T.; Annerstedt, M.; Chan, K.; Murphy, D.G.; Motttrie, A.; Peabody, J.O.; Skinner, E.C.; Wiklund, P.N.; et al. Systematic review and cumulative analysis of perioperative outcomes and complications after robot-assisted radical cystectomy. *Eur. Urol.* **2015**, *67*, 376–401. [CrossRef] [PubMed]
4. Gilbert, S.M.; Wood, D.P.; Dunn, R.L.; Weizer, A.Z.; Lee, C.T.; Montie, J.E.; Wei, J.T. Measuring health-related quality of life outcomes in bladder cancer patients using the Bladder Cancer Index (BCI). *Cancer* **2007**, *109*, 1756–1762. [CrossRef] [PubMed]

5. Koga, F.; Kihara, K. Selective bladder preservation with curative intent for muscle-invasive bladder cancer: A contemporary review. *Int. J. Urol.* **2012**, *19*, 388–401. [CrossRef] [PubMed]
6. Giacalone, N.J.; Shipley, W.U.; Clayman, R.H.; Niemierko, A.; Drumm, M.; Heney, N.M.; Michaelson, M.D.; Lee, R.J.; Saylor, P.J.; Wszolek, M.F.; et al. Long-term Outcomes After Bladder-preserving Tri-modality Therapy for Patients with Muscle-invasive Bladder Cancer: An Updated Analysis of the Massachusetts General Hospital Experience. *Eur. Urol.* **2017**, *71*, 952–960. [CrossRef] [PubMed]
7. Ploussard, G.; Daneshmand, S.; Efstathiou, J.A.; Herr, H.W.; James, N.D.; Rodel, C.M.; Shariat, S.F.; Shipley, W.U.; Sternberg, C.N.; Thalmann, G.N.; et al. Critical analysis of bladder sparing with trimodal therapy in muscle-invasive bladder cancer: A systematic review. *Eur. Urol.* **2014**, *66*, 120–137. [CrossRef] [PubMed]
8. Rodel, C.; Grabenbauer, G.G.; Kuhn, R.; Papadopoulos, T.; Dunst, J.; Meyer, M.; Schrott, K.M.; Sauer, R. Combined-modality treatment and selective organ preservation in invasive bladder cancer: Long-term results. *J. Clin. Oncol.* **2002**, *20*, 3061–3071. [CrossRef] [PubMed]
9. Koga, F.; Numao, N.; Saito, K.; Masuda, H.; Fujii, Y.; Kawakami, S.; Kihara, K. Sensitivity to chemoradiation predicts development of metastasis in muscle-invasive bladder cancer patients. *Urol. Oncol.* **2013**, *31*, 1270–1275. [CrossRef] [PubMed]
10. Coppin, C.M.; Gospodarowicz, M.K.; James, K.; Tannock, I.F.; Zee, B.; Carson, J.; Pater, J.; Sullivan, L.D. Improved local control of invasive bladder cancer by concurrent cisplatin and preoperative or definitive radiation. The National Cancer Institute of Canada Clinical Trials Group. *J. Clin. Oncol.* **1996**, *14*, 2901–2907. [CrossRef] [PubMed]
11. James, N.D.; Hussain, S.A.; Hall, E.; Jenkins, P.; Tremlett, J.; Rawlings, C.; Crundwell, M.; Sizer, B.; Sreenivasan, T.; Hendron, C.; et al. Radiotherapy with or without chemotherapy in muscle-invasive bladder cancer. *N. Engl. J. Med.* **2012**, *366*, 1477–1488. [CrossRef] [PubMed]
12. Choudhury, A.; Swindell, R.; Logue, J.P.; Elliott, P.A.; Livsey, J.E.; Wise, M.; Symonds, P.; Wylie, J.P.; Ramani, V.; Sangar, V.; et al. Phase II study of conformal hypofractionated radiotherapy with concurrent gemcitabine in muscle-invasive bladder cancer. *J. Clin. Oncol.* **2011**, *29*, 733–738. [CrossRef] [PubMed]
13. Muller, A.C.; Diestelhorst, A.; Kuhnt, T.; Kuhn, R.; Fornara, P.; Scholz, H.J.; Dunst, J.; Zietman, A.L. Organ-sparing treatment of advanced bladder cancer: Paclitaxel as a radiosensitizer. *Strahlenther. Onkol.* **2007**, *183*, 177–183. [CrossRef] [PubMed]
14. Iwai, A.; Koga, F.; Fujii, Y.; Masuda, H.; Saito, K.; Numao, N.; Sakura, M.; Kawakami, S.; Kihara, K. Perioperative complications of radical cystectomy after induction chemoradiotherapy in bladder-sparing protocol against muscle-invasive bladder cancer: A single institutional retrospective comparative study with primary radical cystectomy. *Jpn. J. Clin. Oncol.* **2011**, *41*, 1373–1379. [CrossRef] [PubMed]
15. Koga, F.; Kihara, K.; Yoshida, S.; Yokoyama, M.; Saito, K.; Masuda, H.; Fujii, Y.; Kawakami, S. Selective bladder-sparing protocol consisting of induction low-dose chemoradiotherapy plus partial cystectomy with pelvic lymph node dissection against muscle-invasive bladder cancer: Oncological outcomes of the initial 46 patients. *BJU Int.* **2012**, *109*, 860–866. [CrossRef] [PubMed]
16. Koga, F.; Yoshida, S.; Kawakami, S.; Kageyama, Y.; Yokoyama, M.; Saito, K.; Fujii, Y.; Kobayashi, T.; Kihara, K. Low-dose chemoradiotherapy followed by partial or radical cystectomy against muscle-invasive bladder cancer: An intent-to-treat survival analysis. *Urology* **2008**, *72*, 384–388. [CrossRef] [PubMed]
17. Azuma, H.; Inamoto, T.; Takahara, K.; Nomi, H.; Hirano, H.; Ibuki, N.; Uehara, H.; Komura, K.; Minami, K.; Uchimoto, T.; et al. Novel bladder preservation therapy with Osaka Medical College regimen. *J. Urol.* **2015**, *193*, 443–450. [CrossRef] [PubMed]
18. Cahn, D.B.; Handorf, E.A.; Ghiraldi, E.M.; Ristau, B.T.; Geynisman, D.M.; Churilla, T.M.; Horwitz, E.M.; Sobczak, M.L.; Chen, D.Y.T.; Viterbo, R.; et al. Contemporary use trends and survival outcomes in patients undergoing radical cystectomy or bladder-preservation therapy for muscle-invasive bladder cancer. *Cancer* **2017**, *123*, 4337–4345. [CrossRef] [PubMed]
19. Ritch, C.R.; Balise, R.; Prakash, N.S.; Alonzo, D.; Almengo, K.; Alameddine, M.; Venkatramani, V.; Punnen, S.; Parekh, D.J.; Gonzalgo, M.L. Propensity matched comparative analysis of survival following chemoradiation or radical cystectomy for muscle-invasive bladder cancer. *BJU Int.* **2018**, *121*, 745–751. [CrossRef] [PubMed]
20. Kulkarni, G.S.; Hermanns, T.; Wei, Y.; Bhindi, B.; Satkunasivam, R.; Athanasopoulos, P.; Bostrom, P.J.; Kuk, C.; Li, K.; Templeton, A.J.; et al. Propensity Score Analysis of Radical Cystectomy Versus Bladder-Sparing

Trimodal Therapy in the Setting of a Multidisciplinary Bladder Cancer Clinic. *J. Clin. Oncol.* **2017**, *35*, 2299–2305. [CrossRef] [PubMed]
21. Coen, J.J.; Paly, J.J.; Niemierko, A.; Kaufman, D.S.; Heney, N.M.; Spiegel, D.Y.; Efstathiou, J.A.; Zietman, A.L.; Shipley, W.U. Nomograms predicting response to therapy and outcomes after bladder-preserving trimodality therapy for muscle-invasive bladder cancer. *Int. J. Radiat. Oncol. Biol. Phys.* **2013**, *86*, 311–316. [CrossRef] [PubMed]
22. Rodel, C.; Grabenbauer, G.G.; Rodel, F.; Birkenhake, S.; Kuhn, R.; Martus, P.; Zorcher, T.; Fursich, D.; Papadopoulos, T.; Dunst, J.; et al. Apoptosis, p53, bcl-2, and Ki-67 in invasive bladder carcinoma: Possible predictors for response to radiochemotherapy and successful bladder preservation. *Int. J. Radiat. Oncol. Biol. Phys.* **2000**, *46*, 1213–1221. [CrossRef]
23. Matsumoto, H.; Wada, T.; Fukunaga, K.; Yoshihiro, S.; Matsuyama, H.; Naito, K. Bax to Bcl-2 ratio and Ki-67 index are useful predictors of neoadjuvant chemoradiation therapy in bladder cancer. *Jpn. J. Clin. Oncol.* **2004**, *34*, 124–130. [CrossRef] [PubMed]
24. Tanabe, K.; Yoshida, S.; Koga, F.; Inoue, M.; Kobayashi, S.; Ishioka, J.; Tamura, T.; Sugawara, E.; Saito, K.; Akashi, T.; et al. High Ki-67 Expression Predicts Favorable Survival in Muscle-Invasive Bladder Cancer Patients Treated with Chemoradiation-Based Bladder-Sparing Protocol. *Clin. Genitourin. Cancer* **2015**, *13*, e243-51. [CrossRef] [PubMed]
25. Yoshida, S.; Koga, F.; Kobayashi, S.; Ishii, C.; Tanaka, H.; Tanaka, H.; Komai, Y.; Saito, K.; Masuda, H.; Fujii, Y.; et al. Role of diffusion-weighted magnetic resonance imaging in predicting sensitivity to chemoradiotherapy in muscle-invasive bladder cancer. *Int. J. Radiat. Oncol. Biol. Phys.* **2012**, *83*, e21-7. [CrossRef] [PubMed]
26. Chakravarti, A.; Winter, K.; Wu, C.L.; Kaufman, D.; Hammond, E.; Parliament, M.; Tester, W.; Hagan, M.; Grignon, D.; Heney, N.; et al. Expression of the epidermal growth factor receptor and Her-2 are predictors of favorable outcome and reduced complete response rates, respectively, in patients with muscle-invading bladder cancers treated by concurrent radiation and cisplatin-based chemotherapy: A report from the Radiation Therapy Oncology Group. *Int. J. Radiat. Oncol. Biol. Phys.* **2005**, *62*, 309–317. [PubMed]
27. Inoue, M.; Koga, F.; Yoshida, S.; Tamura, T.; Fujii, Y.; Ito, E.; Kihara, K. Significance of ERBB2 overexpression in therapeutic resistance and cancer-specific survival in muscle-invasive bladder cancer patients treated with chemoradiation-based selective bladder-sparing approach. *Int. J. Radiat. Oncol. Biol. Phys.* **2014**, *90*, 303–311. [CrossRef] [PubMed]
28. Michaelson, M.D.; Hu, C.; Pham, H.T.; Dahl, D.M.; Lee-Wu, C.; Swanson, G.P.; Vuky, J.; Lee, R.J.; Souhami, L.; Chang, B.; et al. A Phase 1/2 Trial of a Combination of Paclitaxel and Trastuzumab With Daily Irradiation or Paclitaxel Alone with Daily Irradiation After Transurethral Surgery for Noncystectomy Candidates With Muscle-Invasive Bladder Cancer (Trial NRG Oncology RTOG 0524). *Int. J. Radiat. Oncol. Biol. Phys.* **2017**, *97*, 995–1001. [CrossRef] [PubMed]
29. Kawashima, A.; Nakayama, M.; Kakuta, Y.; Abe, T.; Hatano, K.; Mukai, M.; Nagahara, A.; Nakai, Y.; Oka, D.; Takayama, H.; et al. Excision repair cross-complementing group 1 may predict the efficacy of chemoradiation therapy for muscle-invasive bladder cancer. *Clin. Cancer Res.* **2011**, *17*, 2561–2569. [CrossRef] [PubMed]
30. Tanaka, H.; Yoshida, S.; Koga, F.; Toda, K.; Yoshimura, R.; Nakajima, Y.; Sugawara, E.; Akashi, T.; Waseda, Y.; Inoue, M.; et al. Impact of Immunohistochemistry-Based Subtypes in Muscle-Invasive Bladder Cancer on Response to Chemoradiotherapy. *Int. J. Radiat. Oncol. Biol. Phys.* **2018**. [CrossRef] [PubMed]
31. Urushibara, M.; Kageyama, Y.; Akashi, T.; Otsuka, Y.; Takizawa, T.; Koike, M.; Kihara, K. HSP60 may predict good pathological response to neoadjuvant chemoradiotherapy in bladder cancer. *Jpn. J. Clin. Oncol.* **2007**, *37*, 56–61. [CrossRef] [PubMed]
32. Lautenschlaeger, T.; George, A.; Klimowicz, A.C.; Efstathiou, J.A.; Wu, C.L.; Sandler, H.; Shipley, W.U.; Tester, W.J.; Hagan, M.P.; Magliocco, A.M.; et al. Bladder preservation therapy for muscle-invading bladder cancers on Radiation Therapy Oncology Group trials 8802, 8903, 9506, and 9706: Vascular endothelial growth factor B overexpression predicts for increased distant metastasis and shorter survival. *Oncologist* **2013**, *18*, 685–686. [CrossRef] [PubMed]
33. Keck, B.; Wach, S.; Taubert, H.; Zeiler, S.; Ott, O.J.; Kunath, F.; Hartmann, A.; Bertz, S.; Weiss, C.; Honscheid, P.; et al. Neuropilin-2 and its ligand VEGF-C predict treatment response after transurethral resection and radiochemotherapy in bladder cancer patients. *Int. J. Cancer* **2015**, *136*, 443–451. [CrossRef] [PubMed]

34. Choudhury, A.; Nelson, L.D.; Teo, M.T.; Chilka, S.; Bhattarai, S.; Johnston, C.F.; Elliott, F.; Lowery, J.; Taylor, C.F.; Churchman, M.; et al. MRE11 expression is predictive of cause-specific survival following radical radiotherapy for muscle-invasive bladder cancer. *Cancer Res.* **2010**, *70*, 7017–7026. [CrossRef] [PubMed]
35. Sakano, S.; Ogawa, S.; Yamamoto, Y.; Nishijima, J.; Miyachika, Y.; Matsumoto, H.; Hara, T.; Matsuyama, H. ERCC1 and XRCC1 expression predicts survival in bladder cancer patients receiving combined trimodality therapy. *Mol. Clin. Oncol.* **2013**, *1*, 403–410. [CrossRef] [PubMed]
36. Desai, N.B.; Scott, S.N.; Zabor, E.C.; Cha, E.K.; Hreiki, J.; Sfakianos, J.P.; Ramirez, R.; Bagrodia, A.; Rosenberg, J.E.; Bajorin, D.F.; et al. Genomic characterization of response to chemoradiation in urothelial bladder cancer. *Cancer* **2016**, *122*, 3715–3723. [CrossRef] [PubMed]
37. Eustace, A.; Irlam, J.J.; Taylor, J.; Denley, H.; Agrawal, S.; Choudhury, A.; Ryder, D.; Ord, J.J.; Harris, A.L.; Rojas, A.M.; et al. Necrosis predicts benefit from hypoxia-modifying therapy in patients with high risk bladder cancer enrolled in a phase III randomised trial. *Radiother. Oncol.* **2013**, *108*, 40–47. [CrossRef] [PubMed]
38. Hunter, B.A.; Eustace, A.; Irlam, J.J.; Valentine, H.R.; Denley, H.; Oguejiofor, K.K.; Swindell, R.; Hoskin, P.J.; Choudhury, A.; West, C.M. Expression of hypoxia-inducible factor-1alpha predicts benefit from hypoxia modification in invasive bladder cancer. *Br. J. Cancer* **2014**, *111*, 437–443. [CrossRef] [PubMed]
39. Yoshida, S.; Saito, K.; Koga, F.; Yokoyama, M.; Kageyama, Y.; Masuda, H.; Kobayashi, T.; Kawakami, S.; Kihara, K. C-reactive protein level predicts prognosis in patients with muscle-invasive bladder cancer treated with chemoradiotherapy. *BJU Int.* **2008**, *101*, 978–981. [CrossRef] [PubMed]
40. Joseph, N.; Dovedi, S.J.; Thompson, C.; Lyons, J.; Kennedy, J.; Elliott, T.; West, C.M.; Choudhury, A. Pre-treatment lymphocytopaenia is an adverse prognostic biomarker in muscle-invasive and advanced bladder cancer. *Ann. Oncol.* **2016**, *27*, 294–299. [CrossRef] [PubMed]
41. Zinkel, S.; Gross, A.; Yang, E. BCL2 family in DNA damage and cell cycle control. *Cell Death Differ.* **2006**, *13*, 1351–1359. [CrossRef] [PubMed]
42. Margulis, V.; Lotan, Y.; Karakiewicz, P.I.; Fradet, Y.; Ashfaq, R.; Capitanio, U.; Montorsi, F.; Bastian, P.J.; Nielsen, M.E.; Muller, S.C.; et al. Multi-institutional validation of the predictive value of Ki-67 labeling index in patients with urinary bladder cancer. *J. Natl. Cancer Inst.* **2009**, *101*, 114–119. [CrossRef] [PubMed]
43. Koh, D.M.; Collins, D.J. Diffusion-weighted MRI in the body: Applications and challenges in oncology. *AJR Am. J. Roentgenol.* **2007**, *188*, 1622–1635. [CrossRef] [PubMed]
44. Mitsudomi, T.; Yatabe, Y. Epidermal growth factor receptor in relation to tumor development: EGFR gene and cancer. *FEBS J.* **2010**, *277*, 301–308. [CrossRef] [PubMed]
45. Harris, A.L. Hypoxia—A key regulatory factor in tumour growth. *Nat. Rev. Cancer* **2002**, *2*, 38–47. [CrossRef] [PubMed]
46. Thompson, L.H. Recognition, signaling, and repair of DNA double-strand breaks produced by ionizing radiation in mammalian cells: The molecular choreography. *Mutat. Res.* **2012**, *751*, 158–246. [CrossRef] [PubMed]
47. Hanawalt, P.C.; Spivak, G. Transcription-coupled DNA repair: Two decades of progress and surprises. *Nat. Rev. Mol. Cell Biol.* **2008**, *9*, 958–970. [CrossRef] [PubMed]
48. Iyer, G.; Balar, A.V.; Milowsky, M.I.; Bochner, B.H.; Dalbagni, G.; Donat, S.M.; Herr, H.W.; Huang, W.C.; Taneja, S.S.; Woods, M.; et al. Multicenter Prospective Phase II Trial of Neoadjuvant Dose-Dense Gemcitabine Plus Cisplatin in Patients with Muscle-Invasive Bladder Cancer. *J. Clin. Oncol.* **2018**, *36*, 1949–1956. [CrossRef] [PubMed]
49. Plimack, E.R.; Dunbrack, R.L.; Brennan, T.A.; Andrake, M.D.; Zhou, Y.; Serebriiskii, I.G.; Slifker, M.; Alpaugh, K.; Dulaimi, E.; Palma, N.; et al. Defects in DNA Repair Genes Predict Response to Neoadjuvant Cisplatin-based Chemotherapy in Muscle-invasive Bladder Cancer. *Eur. Urol.* **2015**, *68*, 959–967. [CrossRef] [PubMed]
50. Teo, M.Y.; Bambury, R.M.; Zabor, E.C.; Jordan, E.; Al-Ahmadie, H.; Boyd, M.E.; Bouvier, N.; Mullane, S.A.; Cha, E.K.; Roper, N.; et al. DNA Damage Response and Repair Gene Alterations Are Associated with Improved Survival in Patients with Platinum-Treated Advanced Urothelial Carcinoma. *Clin. Cancer Res.* **2017**, *23*, 3610–3618. [CrossRef] [PubMed]
51. Hoskin, P.J.; Rojas, A.M.; Bentzen, S.M.; Saunders, M.I. Radiotherapy with concurrent carbogen and nicotinamide in bladder carcinoma. *J. Clin. Oncol.* **2010**, *28*, 4912–4918. [CrossRef] [PubMed]

52. Cancer Genome Atlas Research Network. Comprehensive molecular characterization of urothelial bladder carcinoma. *Nature* **2014**, *507*, 315–322. [CrossRef] [PubMed]
53. Choi, W.; Porten, S.; Kim, S.; Willis, D.; Plimack, E.R.; Hoffman-Censits, J.; Roth, B.; Cheng, T.; Tran, M.; Lee, I.L.; et al. Identification of distinct basal and luminal subtypes of muscle-invasive bladder cancer with different sensitivities to frontline chemotherapy. *Cancer Cell* **2014**, *25*, 152–165. [CrossRef] [PubMed]
54. Sjodahl, G.; Lovgren, K.; Lauss, M.; Patschan, O.; Gudjonsson, S.; Chebil, G.; Aine, M.; Eriksson, P.; Mansson, W.; Lindgren, D.; et al. Toward a molecular pathologic classification of urothelial carcinoma. *Am. J. Pathol.* **2013**, *183*, 681–691. [CrossRef] [PubMed]
55. Bellmunt, J.; de Wit, R.; Vaughn, D.J.; Fradet, Y.; Lee, J.L.; Fong, L.; Vogelzang, N.J.; Climent, M.A.; Petrylak, D.P.; Choueiri, T.K.; et al. Pembrolizumab as Second-Line Therapy for Advanced Urothelial Carcinoma. *N. Engl. J. Med.* **2017**, *376*, 1015–1026. [CrossRef] [PubMed]

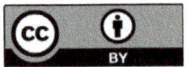

© 2018 by the authors. Licensee MDPI, Basel, Switzerland. This article is an open access article distributed under the terms and conditions of the Creative Commons Attribution (CC BY) license (http://creativecommons.org/licenses/by/4.0/).

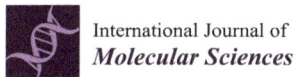

Review

Circulating Tumour DNA in Muscle-Invasive Bladder Cancer

Melissa P. Tan [1,2], Gerhardt Attard [3] and Robert A. Huddart [1,2,*]

1. Division of Radiotherapy & Imaging, Institute of Cancer Research, 15 Cotswold Road, Sutton, Surrey SM2 5NG, UK; melissa.tan@icr.ac.uk
2. Academic Urology Unit, The Royal Marsden NHS Foundation Trust, Downs Road, Sutton, Surrey SM2 5PT, UK
3. Research Department of Oncology, UCL Cancer Institute, University College London, 72 Huntley Street, London WC1E 6DD, UK; g.attard@ucl.ac.uk
* Correspondence: robert.huddart@icr.ac.uk; Tel.: +44-20-8661-3271

Received: 31 July 2018; Accepted: 27 August 2018; Published: 29 August 2018

Abstract: Circulating tumour DNA (ctDNA) is an attractive tool in cancer research, offering many advantages over tissue samples obtained using traditional biopsy methods. There has been increasing interest in its application to muscle-invasive bladder cancer (MIBC), which is recognised to be a heterogeneous disease with overall poor prognosis. Using a range of platforms, studies have shown that ctDNA is detectable in MIBC and may be a useful biomarker in monitoring disease status and guiding treatment decisions in MIBC patients. Currently, with no such predictive or prognostic biomarkers in clinical practice to guide treatment strategy, there is a real unmet need for a personalised medicine approach in MIBC, and ctDNA offers an exciting avenue through which to pursue this goal. In this article, we present an overview of work to date on ctDNA in MIBC, and discuss the inherent challenges present as well as the potential future clinical applications.

Keywords: circulating tumour DNA (ctDNA); muscle-invasive bladder cancer (MIBC); biomarker

1. Introduction

In the drive towards personalised medicine, circulating tumour DNA (ctDNA) is an invaluable tool in cancer research, offering unique advantages over tissue samples collected using traditional biopsy methods. Its collection via a simple blood draw allows serial samples to be conveniently and safely taken over a course of treatment, thus facilitating the study of tumour dynamics, treatment resistance, and disease progression. Furthermore, it has been suggested that ctDNA samples are likely to provide a more representative snapshot of an individual's cancer compared with biopsy samples as tumour clones from the primary, micro-, and macro-metastatic deposits are present in a single sample [1,2].

These advantages have been exploited in numerous studies across various cancers including colorectal, breast, prostate, and lung malignancies [3–6]. ctDNA levels have been shown to be associated with disease burden [7,8] and in an analysis of serial samples, increasing levels have been shown to pre-date radiological progression [4,9,10]. Analysis of sequential samples taken over a course of treatment have also demonstrated tumour evolution with the emergence of subclones documented at disease progression [11–13]. In addition to plasma, tumour DNA fragments have also been detected in other body fluids such as urine and cerebrospinal fluid [14].

There has been a surge of interest in recent years focusing on ctDNA in muscle-invasive bladder cancer (MIBC); a heterogeneous disease with an aggressive natural history and poor prognosis. With no predictive or prognostic biomarkers in current clinical practice to guide treatment strategy, there is a real need to develop a personalised medicine approach to optimise patient outcomes, and ctDNA offers an innovative approach to address this challenge.

In this review article, we provide a brief background on ctDNA before summarising research to date on ctDNA in MIBC, discussing the challenges present and future clinical applications.

2. Circulating Tumour DNA: Background

2.1. Biology of Circulating DNA

It has long been known that plasma contains nucleic acid fragments including those of DNA (genomic, mitochondrial, and viral), RNA, and micro-RNA; these have been collectively termed circulating nucleic acids. The mechanism by which nucleic acid fragments are released into the circulation remains under debate, but is thought to involve apoptosis, necrosis, and secretion [15]. Circulating DNA (cDNA) fragments are typically less than 200 bp in length. They are thought to undergo hepatic and renal excretion, and the reported half-life of cDNA fragments ranges between 16 min and 2.5 h [9,15,16]. While increased levels of cDNA are seen in malignancy and have been reported to be associated with tumour burden and prognosis in some cancer sites [17–19], raised levels are also seen in benign conditions such as pregnancy, trauma, or inflammation, meaning that cDNA levels alone are not necessarily a specific biomarker in the diagnosis or management of cancer [15].

In the majority of patients with malignancies, cDNA is mainly composed of wildtype, i.e., normal DNA, but may also contain fragments derived from the primary tumor, distant metastases, and micrometastases. The proportion of circulating tumour DNA (ctDNA) fragments (tumour fraction) has been shown to increase with disease burden [3,4,7], and also to vary between tumour types [7]. Although some patients with very advanced disease have demonstrated high tumour fractions above 50% [11], these are the minority and in numerous studies of metastatic disease, tumour fractions as low as 0.04% [4,20] have been reported. Indeed, a recent abstract reported an estimated median tumour fraction of 1.9% in metastatic urothelial cancer [21]. One of the challenges of working with ctDNA, therefore, is in detecting and quantifying the tumour fraction, particularly in the setting of early disease where levels may be in region of 0.01% [3].

2.2. Circulating DNA vs. Circulating Tumour DNA

In order to distinguish ctDNA from wildtype DNA, it is necessary to identify and detect somatic aberrations harboured by the tumour fragments. Quantification of fragments containing aberrations, which may include single nucleotide variants (SNVs), copy number alterations (CNAs), or structural variants, is used as a surrogate of tumour fraction.

There are various approaches to achieve this. One strategy is to first identify aberrations present in a patient's tumour tissue using either a broad de novo sequencing approach (e.g., whole exome or whole genome sequencing) or using a pre-determined set of assays or targeted sequencing panels encompassing known relevant aberrations in the cancer of interest. Aberrations identified in tumour tissue can then be detected in cDNA using polymerase chain reaction (PCR)-based specific assays or a focused next generation sequencing (NGS) approach. An alternative is to sequence the cDNA upfront using either of the approaches described above. However, in order to perform whole genome or whole exome sequencing on cDNA, a minimum tumour fraction is required, in the order of at least 10–20% [22,23], and so this approach is precluded in a significant proportion of cases where tumour fraction does not meet this threshold.

While employing a broad sequencing approach allows an overview of aberrations present, allows assessment of copy number alterations, and supports the design of patient-specific plasma assays, cost may often be a prohibitive factor, particularly if high levels of coverage are sought to identify low frequency aberrations with confidence.

A targeted panel or pre-determined set of assays is more cost-effective, but there is the risk that tumour fraction may be underestimated or ctDNA may not be detected if the individual's relevant mutations are not included in the panel. Furthermore, using specific assays means that mutations arising over time or under selective pressure from treatment will not be identified unless included on the panel. There is thus a balance to be achieved in selecting an approach with sufficient breadth and depth that allows the question being asked to be answered. In the context of MIBC, we shall see that both approaches have been employed, and we discuss this further in the next section of this review.

In trying to improve detection rates of ctDNA, it has been suggested that as tumour fragments are shorter than wildtype DNA fragments [24–26], fragment size selection will be enriched for ctDNA and thus allow very low frequency aberrations to be more readily detected [27]. This approach may be useful for increasing detection of ctDNA in patients with early disease or rare variants.

Whichever approach is employed, ultra-sensitive techniques are required to detect the low levels of ctDNA present. Digital PCR techniques such as BEAMing or droplet digital PCR (ddPCR) have allowed research in this area to progress with sensitivity thresholds of 0.01% [3,28]. However, these approaches only allow a few aberrations to be interrogated at a time, and thus require a priori knowledge regarding aberrations to be detected.

3. Muscle-Invasive Bladder Cancer

3.1. Overview

Muscle-invasive bladder cancer is a heterogeneous disease with an overall poor prognosis [29]. Several molecular profiling studies have identified a number of molecular subtypes that are suggested to have different spectrums of mutations and clinical behaviour [30–32]. Sequencing studies have demonstrated that it has a high mutational burden, third only to melanoma and lung [30], but yet, in contrast to other tumour types, there are currently no approved biomarkers to guide its management. Radical treatment options in MIBC include neoadjuvant platinum-based combination chemotherapy followed by surgery, or in patients where surgery is deemed unsuitable or a bladder preservation strategy is being pursued, chemoradiation may be offered as part of a trimodality approach. In the palliative setting, platinum-based chemotherapy remains the mainstay of treatment, with the recently approved immune checkpoint inhibitors offering a further line of treatment. There is a real unmet clinical need for predictive and prognostic biomarkers in MIBC in order to develop a personalised approach if outcomes are to be improved. ctDNA in MIBC thus promises to be an exciting avenue to enable researchers to better understand the molecular biology, study treatment resistance and disease progression, and identify potential therapeutic targets.

3.2. Potential Clinical Applications of ctDNA in MIBC

ctDNA has the potential to be clinically useful at every step of the treatment pathway in MIBC, from early diagnosis, monitoring or predicting response to treatment in both the radical and palliative settings, assessing the need for adjuvant treatment, and in monitoring for recurrence or progression. Currently, one area of particular interest is in predicting and monitoring response to neoadjuvant chemotherapy. International guidelines [33,34] currently recommend all patients with localised disease are offered neoadjuvant cisplatin-based chemotherapy. However, up to 60% of patients do not respond [35,36] and these patients have thus not only been subjected to unnecessary toxicity, but have also experienced a delay to their definitive treatment, with a potential detrimental effect on outcome [37]. A minimally invasive biomarker to predict response or more sensitively monitor response would thus be of huge clinical benefit, and ctDNA offers the potential to achieve this.

4. CtDNA in MIBC

4.1. Overview

Some of the first work on ctDNA in MIBC dates back to 1991 when Sidransky et al. demonstrated the presence of *p53* mutations in the urinary sediment of three patients with MIBC [38]. Over a decade later, cDNA and ctDNA levels in plasma were shown to be higher in bladder cancer patients than in healthy controls [39,40]. Then, there followed a hiatus in publications on ctDNA in MIBC until Bettegowda et al.'s landmark paper [7], where next generation sequencing was performed on tumour tissue from three patients with metastatic MIBC as part of a broader pan-cancer cohort. A *p53* mutation was identified in each of the patients and was successfully detected in plasma in all three cases. In this small subset of patients, clinical outcomes were not reported, although the paper overall reported increased ctDNA levels with advanced disease. In the last two years, there has been a surge of publications looking at ctDNA in MIBC. Table 1 summarises representative publications including select poster abstracts as of June 2018. Some of the earlier studies have included superficial, i.e., <T2 disease; non-muscle-invasive bladder cancer (NMIBC), and MIBC in a cohort. However, more recently, MIBC has been considered separately and this is in keeping with fact that NMIBC and MIBC have been shown to have different molecular profiles [41].

4.2. ctDNA Is Detectable Using Commercially Available Panels

In 2016, Sonpavde et al. [42] presented work showing that aberrations in cDNA could be detected in 25/29 (86.2%) patients with metastatic urothelial cancer using a commercially available panel composed of 68 cancer-related genes. Using the updated, now 73-gene panel (Guardant360), the group further went on to demonstrate aberrations in plasma from 265/294 (90%) patients with metastatic lower tract urothelial cancer [43]. *TP53* (48%), *ARID1A* (17%), and *PIK3CA* (14%) were the most commonly reported aberrations. They also compared these results from plasma with publically available data from previous NGS studies reporting aberrations in tumour tissue, and reported similar results in terms of the frequency of reported aberrations included on the panel.

Using an alternative 62-gene panel (FoundationACT), McGregor et al. [21] found at least one aberration in plasma of 48/66 (73%) patients with metastatic urothelial cancer. A proportion of their cohort also had sequencing data on baseline tumour tissue available, and the authors reported an example where plasma taken at the time of cisplatin resistance showed persistence of *ERBB2* and *TP53* mutations identified in baseline tumour tissue alongside a new *NF1* aberration. This demonstrates a potential application of ctDNA in furthering our understanding of disease progression and treatment resistance in MIBC, with the potential ability to monitor patients during treatment for evidence of response or the emergence of new potential targets.

Of note, both of these ctDNA panels that were used contained at most only 9 of the most frequent 23 gene mutations documented in the TCGA report [30], and omitted many of the chromatin-modifying gene alterations frequently seen in MIBC, for example, *KMT2D* and *KDM6A* (observed in 28% and 26% of TCGA MIBC cases, respectively). *ERCC2*, which has been put forward as a potential biomarker of sensitivity to cisplatin chemotherapy [44], is also absent. However, as the primary aim of these panels is to identify potential targeted therapy options in the clinical setting, it could be argued that these omissions do not have any clinical impact for MIBC patients, given that there are currently no associated therapies for these targets. However, in the research setting, the omission of these frequently mutated genes is a limitation of these panels in the exploration of potential targets and the study of disease biology.

Table 1. Representative publications including select poster abstracts as of June 2018.

Reference	Year	n	Cohort	Method	Key Findings
Bettegowda et al. [7]	2014	3	Metastatic MIBC	One-hundred-gene panel on tumour tissue; SafeSeq on plasma for patient-specific aberrations	TP53 mutations detected in tumour tissue of 3/3 patients, and detectable in plasma of all three patients
Sonpavde et al. $ [42]	2016	29	Advanced urothelial cancer (MIBC = 27/29)	Sixty-eight-gene commercially available panel to sequence a single plasma sample from each patient (Guardant360)	Aberrations detected in 86.2% patients
Birkenkamp-Demtröder et al. [45]	2016	12	NMIBC: six with recurrence and six with progression to MIBC	WES/WGS/mate-pair sequencing on tumour tissue; personalised ddPCR on sequential plasma samples	ctDNA detectable in 10/12; ctDNA detected several months before clinical diagnosis of progression to MIBC in 4/6 patients
Christensen et al. [46]	2017	1: 363; 2: 468	1: NMIBC 2: Cx (MIBC ≥ 363/468)	ddPCR assays to screen for PIK3CA and FGFR3 hotspots in tissue, urinary supernatant, and plasma	Eleven percent of Cx cohort had ≥1 mutation detected in tumour tissue. Analysis of 23 paired urine and plasma showed higher levels of ctDNA in urine. In 27 Cx plasma samples analysed, high levels of ctDNA in plasma associated with disease recurrence
Vandekerkhove et al. [47]	2017	51	MIBC: 14/51 N0M0 disease; 27/51 N+ve/M1 disease	Bladder cancer-specific targeted panel (50 genes) on plasma from 44 patients including sequential samples; WES on plasma from eight patients to assess mutational burden	ctDNA detected in 25/44 (56.8%) patients with tumour fractions ranging from 3.9–72.6%; All with tumour fraction >30% had distant metastatic disease. Mutational burden derived from targeted sequencing panel consistent with that from WES
Patel et al. [48]	2017	17	MIBC (starting NAC)	Eight-gene TAm-Seq panel (for SNVs) and shallow WGS for copy number assessment on tumour tissue, plasma, urinary cell pellet, and urinary supernatant	Aberration detected in plasma or urine of 10/17 patients pre-NAC. Greater levels of ctDNA detection in urine. Detection of plasma or urine ctDNA pre-cycle two NAC associated with disease recurrence
Birkenkamp-Demtröder et al. [49]	2017	60	MIBC: 50 NAC; 10 palliative chemotherapy	Three ddPCR assays to screen for PIK3CA and FGFR3 mutation in tumour tissue; WES on tumour tissue and germline in 24. Personalised ddPCR assays in plasma for 26 patients	PIK3CA/FGFR3 assays positive in 19/60; ctDNA detectable in patients prior to clinically detected recurrence with median lead time 101 days
McGregor et al. $ [21]	2018	66	Metastatic urothelial cancer	Commercially available 62-gene panel to sequence plasma (FoundationACT)	ctDNA aberrations detected in 48/66 (73%); Estimated median tumour fraction 1.9%
Barata et al. [50]	2017	22	Metastatic urothelial cancer	Compared sequencing results from tumour tissue and plasma sequenced using two different commercially available panels	Concordance between the two tests was 16.4%
Soave et al. [51]	2017	72	Radical Cx (>46/72 MIBC)	Tested 43 regions covering 37 genes for copy number variations (multiplex ligation dependent probe amplification)	cDNA had CNV in 48.6% samples; Overall CNV status not associated with clinical outcome; gain in KLF5, ZFHX3, and CDH1 associated with reduced cancer-specific survival

Table 1. Cont.

Reference	Year	n	Cohort	Method	Key Findings
Agarwal et al. [43]	2018	369	Metastatic urinary tract cancer (294/369—lower urinary tract cancer)	Commercially available 73-gene panel (Guardant360) used to sequence plasma	Similar aberrations seen when compared with publically available NGS data on tumour tissue
Cheng et al. $ [52]	2017	26	Metastatic urothelial cancer	Used a 341–468-gene NGS assay (MSK-IMPACT) to sequence plasma (n = 26) and archival tumour tissue (n = 15)	ctDNA detected in 69% patients. Interval between plasma sampling and tissue collection was 35 days to >4 years; Identical tissue and plasma profiles in 20% (3/15)

Abbreviations: MIBC: muscle-invasive bladder cancer; NMIBC: non-MIBC; ctDNA: circulating tumour DNA; NAC: neoadjuvant chemotherapy; WES: whole exome sequencing; WGS: whole genome sequencing; Cx: cystectomy; NGS: next generation sequencing; CNV: copy number variation; SNV: single nucleotide variation; ddPCR: droplet digital polymerase chain reaction; N+ve: node positive; M1: distant metastases; TAm-Seq: tagged amplicon sequencing. $: poster abstract.

The high aberration detection rates of up to 90%, however, are not to be ignored as other groups using custom, albeit much smaller panels/assays have reported lower ctDNA detection rates. Of note, the above cohorts were composed exclusively of patients with advanced disease where ctDNA levels would be expected to be higher and thus more readily detectable. As yet in the literature, there are no reports of using such commercially available panels to profile patients with non-metastatic disease.

4.3. Using Patient-Specific Assays to Detect ctDNA

4.3.1. In NMIBC Cohorts

In one of the first papers to apply a personalised approach to bladder cancer, Birkenkamp-Demtröder et al. [45] used whole exome sequencing (WES), whole genome sequencing (WGS) and/or matepair sequencing to identify mutations in fresh frozen tumour tissue before designing personalised ddPCR assays for use on urine and plasma in a cohort comprising of 12 patients with NMIBC with either disease recurrence or progression to MIBC. ctDNA was detectable in 10/12 (83.3%) patients, including those with non-invasive disease only. In 4/6 (66.7%) patients progressing to muscle-invasive disease, detection of ctDNA pre-dated clinical diagnosis of MIBC by several months.

Christensen et al. [46] also detected ctDNA in patients with NMIBC and MIBC, but used a targeted approach with ddPCR assays to detect three hotspot mutations in *PIK3CA* (E545K) and *FGFR3* (S249C, Y373C), first in tumour tissue and then in plasma and urinary supernatant. In 201 urine samples from patients with NMIBC taken during their disease course, they reported overall higher urinary ctDNA levels in those later progressing to MIBC when compared with those with no progression. Kaplan-Meier progression free survival estimates for a subset of 25 showed that those with ctDNA urinary levels above the median at initial visit had increased progression rates to MIBC (7/13; 54%) compared with those with ctDNA levels below the median (1/12; 8%; $p = 0.036$).

However, within their cystectomy cohort of 468 patients, of whom at least 363 had MIBC, only 44/403 (11%; 65 excluded as insufficient material) had at least one mutation detected in tissue using the *PIK3CA* and *FGFR3* assays. Of those, 27 urine and 27 plasma samples were analysed. A third of patients (9/27) had detectable ctDNA in plasma. Increased ctDNA levels in plasma were associated with lower recurrence-free survival and overall survival. ctDNA levels were overall found to be higher in urine than in plasma [46].

Using the TCGA data portal [53], it can be shown that 62/412 (15%) MIBC patients possess at least one of the three hotspot mutations tested by Christensen et al. [46], which is slightly higher than the detection rate of 11% reported. The authors suggest that the procurement of tissue from a tissue microarray contributed to a low yield of DNA at the tumour tissue screening step, which may have resulted in missed cases. The subsequent low detection rate (33%) in plasma, despite the use of ddPCR, likely reflects the fact that as a cystectomy cohort, patients had localised disease with very low ctDNA fractions. This study highlights the importance of selecting aberrations to capture as many patients as possible, especially when utilising techniques where only a few aberrations can be interrogated at one time.

However, despite small numbers and heterogeneous cohorts consisting mainly of NMIBC, these studies demonstrate proof-of-concept in using both broad and targeted approaches in screening tumour tissue for aberrations to subsequently detect in plasma and urine in patients with bladder cancer. The results raise the possibility of using ctDNA to monitor patients with NMIBC for progression to MIBC. However much work is needed before this can be explored in the setting of a prospective clinical trial, and one of the key steps will be in determining the optimal aberration panel with which to identify and quantify ctDNA.

4.3.2. In MIBC Cohorts

Building upon previous work, Birkenkamp-Demtröder et al. [49] used the same three ddPCR assays for *PIK3CA* and *FGFR3* hotspot mutations in combination with WES to screen diagnostic tumour tissue taken at transurethral resection (TUR) in 60 patients with MIBC, comprising of 50 commencing NAC and 10 commencing palliative chemotherapy. Using the three assays, at least one mutation was found in 19/60 patients (31.7%). WES was additionally performed on tissue from 24 patients and aberrations identified in 100%. The authors went on to design 84 personalised assays for 61 genes for a final cohort of 26 patients. Of note, only 2/26 (7.7%) had aberrations identified using only the *PIK3CA/FGFR3* assays. Plasma and urine samples were tested although longitudinal results were available only for plasma. Blood was taken at pre-defined time points during treatment and follow-up.

Of the 24 patients proceeding to radical cystectomy following chemotherapy, 12/24 (50%) relapsed at a median of 275 days. In 6/12 (50%) of relapsing patients, ctDNA was detectable at a median of 137 days resulting in a median positive lead time of 101 days. However, ctDNA was also detected at some time point in 50% of patients who remained disease-free post-surgery, so the presence of ctDNA post-cystectomy is not specific for relapse [49]. However, the authors noted a significant association between high plasma ctDNA levels in samples taken at one week to four months post-cystectomy, and disease relapse, thus suggesting that ctDNA may allow more sensitive detection of disease recurrence post-surgery, and may be useful in the selection of patients for further treatment. Samples taken before, during, and after treatment for disease relapse were also analysed with an overall decrease in levels after 2–5 cycles of treatment correlating with radiological response, and subsequent increase in levels correlating with progression.

While this paper omits some technical details from its methodology, it sets the scene for the potential use of ctDNA in the post-operative setting to assess risk of recurrence and perhaps guide decisions on adjuvant treatment. Once again, the importance of selecting an appropriate panel of aberrations to target is highlighted, given that in 92.3%, personalised assay design was dependent upon data from whole exome sequencing.

The potential for ctDNA to detect recurrence before clinical or radiological confirmation was also demonstrated by Patel et al. [48]. In a cohort of 17 MIBC patients embarking on neoadjuvant platinum-based chemotherapy, the authors performed tagged amplicon sequencing (TAm-Seq) using a bladder cancer-specific panel of eight genes to detect mutant DNA in TUR tumour tissue, plasma, urinary cell pellet (UCP), and urinary supernatant (USN). The eight genes were *BRAF*, *CTNNB1*, *FGFR3*, *HRAS*, *KRAS*, *NFE2L2*, *PIK3CA*, and *TP53*, and were anticipated to encompass 72% of patients based upon TCGA data. A *TERT* promoter assay did not perform well and so was excluded. They also performed shallow whole genome sequencing in order to assess copy number alterations (CNAs). Samples were collected over a median period of 83 days from commencing NAC, with a median of 15 samples per patient. Patients were followed up for a median of 742 days from commencing NAC, and 588 days after completing definitive therapy.

On sequencing the available tumour tissue from 16 patients, single nucleotide variations (SNVs) were detected in 12/16 (75%) patients. The most frequent SNVs were in *TP53*, *KRAS*, and *PIK3CA*. Copy number alterations were identified in all 16 TUR samples, with the most frequent being *CDKN2A* loss, *E2F3/SOX4* gain, and *PPARG* gain.

Subsequent testing in plasma, UCP, and USN in the 12 patients with tumour tissue SNVs showed detection of mutant DNA in 4/12 (33%), 5/12 (42%), and 5/12 (42%), respectively. CNAs were detected in 4/16 (33%), 8/15 (53%), and 8/16 (50%) of plasma, UCP, and USN samples, respectively. Of note, shallow WGS on serial samples from five patients showed evidence of tumour evolution under the selective pressure of NAC. Overall, aberrations were detected in 10/17 (59%) patients in plasma and urine samples taken prior to commencing NAC. Detection of aberrations at this point did not predict the response to treatment. However, upon analysing samples taken prior to cycle two NAC, the authors found that mutant DNA was present in 5/6 (83%) patients that relapsed, but was not detected in relapse-free patients (specificity 100%, sensitivity 83%). The median lead time over radiological diagnosis of progression was 243 days. Of note, of the five patients with mutant DNA present, only one patient had aberrations detected in plasma. Overall, higher levels of detection were noted in urine compared with plasma, although no single sample type captured all the aberrations present [48].

Although this was a relatively small cohort, the comprehensive assessment of plasma and urine shows great promise for ctDNA as a potential biomarker of response to treatment in the radical setting, and suggests that assessment of both plasma and urine is warranted at least in the neoadjuvant setting. In both these studies, it is again demonstrated that the optimal panel of genes and platform to interrogate MIBC remains unclear with *PIK3CA* and *FGFR3* assays allowing ctDNA analysis in only 7.7%, and a combination of eight TAm-Seq assays and shallow WGS detecting ctDNA in 59%. However, with sequencing costs continuing to fall, it may be that broad approaches such as WES, which identified aberrations in 100% of tumour tissue samples, become more accessible. This strategy, however, would depend upon the availability of contemporary tissue samples and would thus likely necessitate repeat biopsies, particularly in those previously treated or with relapsed disease, which may be neither achievable on a practical level nor acceptable to patients.

Another question to consider is whether the identification of aberrations in tumour tissue first is necessary or indeed useful given potential intra-tumour heterogeneity and tumour evolution over time. Cheng et al. [52] used the 341–468 gene MSK IMPACT panel to profile plasma samples from 26 patients with metastatic urothelial cancer. At least one mutation was detected in 18/26 (69%). For 15 patients, archived tumour tissue was also sequenced using the same panel. The interval between tissue and plasma sampling ranged from 35 days to >4 years, and 11/15 patients had received treatment during this period. They reported that the tissue and plasma profiles were identical in only 3/15 (20%) of patients where the interval between samples ranged from 35 days to <1.5 years. Six out of fifteen (40%) had mutations identified in plasma, but not in tissue, and vice versa in 11/15 (73%). They concluded that the differences may reflect tumour evolution or intratumour heterogeneity. It may then be that sequencing archived tissue to detect aberrations of interest may not always identify the most appropriate targets in ctDNA, and may not be the ideal strategy particularly in patients who have received treatment or demonstrated a change in disease status in the intervening period. In these situations, upfront analysis of ctDNA is an attractive option, particularly when repeat up to date tissue biopsies are not possible.

4.4. Using a MIBC-Specific Panel to Sequence Plasma Upfront

Vandekerkhove et al. [47] designed a 50-gene bladder cancer-specific panel based upon published data on recurrent mutations and copy number changes in bladder cancer, including the TCGA report. In designing the panel, the authors noted that 98% of patients from the TCGA MIBC dataset (consisting primarily of subjects with non-metastatic disease) had a non-synonymous mutation in at least one of the 50 genes included on their panel. With target depth of 500–1000×, aberrations would be detected in those with tumour fraction of 5% or more.

Fifty-one patients with MIBC were recruited, including 37 with nodal or distant metastases. Plasma from all those with nodal or distant metastases, and seven with organ-confined disease were sequenced using the targeted panel. Overall, 25/44 (56.8%) patients demonstrated a ctDNA fraction above the 2% detection threshold set. The tumour fraction ranged from 3.9 to 72.6% with all samples demonstrating greater than 30% tumour fraction originating from patients with distant metastatic disease. In those with tumour fractions between 3.9–30%, 52% had distant metastatic disease. Only one of the seven patients with localised disease had detectable ctDNA [47]. This association of higher tumour content with higher disease burden is in keeping with previous work in other tumour types [7]. In three patients with metastatic disease where ctDNA was detected at more than one time-point over the course of chemotherapy, aberrations identified were consistent [47]. Frequently mutated genes included *TP53*, *PIK3CA*, and *ARID1A*; over 50% of patients had chromatin-modifying gene aberrations and this work has demonstrated that like the commercially available panels, upfront NGS analysis of plasma cDNA can identify potentially actionable aberrations. Of note, the only recurrent mutations seen were known hotspot regions in *ERBB2*, *PIK3CA*, and the *TERT* promoter. All other mutations were unique to individual patients and this highlights the incredible (and challenging) heterogeneity seen in MIBC.

Whole exome sequencing was also performed on 11 samples with tumour fraction over 25% from eight patients, with the primary aim of comparing mutation rates derived from the targeted sequencing data with that from WES data. The WES results correlated with targeted sequencing data, although the difference in sequencing depth meant that mutations seen on targeted panel were not always called on exome data [47]. Mutation rates derived from whole exome data and targeted sequencing data were also correlated, which is of interest given that mutational burden has been put forward as a predictor of response to immune checkpoint agents. The potential to assess mutational burden on a plasma sample rather than tissue biopsy is a potential advantage in the clinical trial setting, where patients may not otherwise be able or willing to undergo an invasive procedure as part of trial entry.

5. Conclusions

In the last two years, significant progress has been made in the field of ctDNA in MIBC and the knowledge base has grown rapidly. We have seen that ctDNA can be detected, with varying degrees of sensitivity, in the plasma and urine of patients with localised and metastatic MIBC. The levels detected have been demonstrated to be associated with tumour burden and while samples taken at one time-point are able to allow the identification of potentially actionable aberrations, the real value of ctDNA lies in the ease of obtaining sequential samples. By analysing samples taken over a course of treatment or during follow-up, early results in small trials suggest that the presence of ctDNA may indicate minimal residual disease following surgery, or predict for future disease recurrence with greater sensitivity than that offered by current standard radiological assessment. This is hugely exciting and the implications are potentially practice changing, but there is much work to be done before ctDNA can be applied in the clinical setting.

A key challenge is in refining the detection of ctDNA. MIBC is somewhat unique from other cancer types where ctDNA research is perhaps more established. Whereas a select few assays, for example, *APC* or *KRAS* mutations in colorectal cancer, *BRAF* in melanoma encompass a significant proportion of patients, and are thus reliable aberrations to use a surrogate for tumour fraction, the equivalent targets have yet to be demonstrated in MIBC. While this is in part because of the heterogeneity of the disease, it is also likely attributable to the fact that the molecular landscape of MIBC was only more recently explored when compared with other cancer subtypes. It has since been put forward that 90% MIBC patients have at least one mutation in hotspot regions of *PIK3CA*, *TP53*, or the *TERT* promoter, and so a panel encompassing these should be of relevance to the vast majority [23]. While these genes were included in the 50-gene bladder cancer specific panel by Vandekerkhove et al. [47], the detection threshold set of 2% for tumour fraction likely accounts for their plasma ctDNA detection rate of 56.8% falling short of the theoretical 90% described. It will be of great interest to see whether more sensitive methods, for example, ddPCR assays for this three-gene panel, will indeed encompass the majority of MIBC patients, including those with localised disease where low tumour fractions make detection more technically challenging. Furthermore, the use of so-called molecular barcodes, as recently explored in MIBC samples, offer another method to improve detection thresholds [54].

A unique feature of bladder cancer is the availability of ctDNA in urine. We have seen that ctDNA was more readily detectable in urine in a cohort of patients undergoing neoadjuvant treatment [48], and it seems reasonable to suggest that this is by virtue of the close proximity of the primary tumour to urine, i.e., the shedding of tumour DNA fragments directly into urine. It may well be that urinary ctDNA is most relevant in patients with localised disease, while plasma ctDNA reflects the systemic burden of disease.

While great promise is shown in the use of ctDNA to detect recurrence earlier than current standard approaches, an important consideration is also whether or not detecting recurrence earlier has any impact on clinical outcomes, and this can only be determined through prospective clinical trials.

MIBC is rapidly catching up with other more established tumour sites in the field of ctDNA research, and the clinical implications are huge in this poor prognosis disease where there are currently no biomarkers in everyday clinical use. By fully harnessing the potential of ctDNA, a truly personalised approach bypassing spatial and temporal barriers in cancer research appears possible and is key in furthering our understanding of MIBC and ultimately improving clinical outcomes.

funding: MPT is supported by funding from the National Institute for Health Research (NIHR) Biomedical Research Centre at the Royal Marsden NHS Foundation Trust and the Institute of Cancer Research. The views expressed are those of the authors and not necessarily those of the NHS, the NIHR, or the Department of Health. Funds were received from the Institute of Cancer Research to cover the costs to publish in open access.

Conflicts of Interest: The authors declare no conflict of interest

Abbreviations

bp	Base pairs
cDNA	Circulating DNA
ctDNA	Circulating tumour DNA
CNA	Copy number alteration
MIBC	Muscle-invasive bladder cancer
NAC	Neoadjuvant chemotherapy
NGS	Next generation sequencing
PCR	Polymerase chain reaction
TUR	Transurethral resection
SNV	Single nucleotide variant
WES	Whole exome sequencing
WGS	Whole genome sequencing

References

1. Chan, K.C.; Jiang, P.; Zheng, Y.W.; Liao, G.J.; Sun, H.; Wong, J.; Siu, S.S.; Chan, W.C.; Chan, S.L.; Chan, A.T.; et al. Cancer genome scanning in plasma: Detection of tumor-associated copy number aberrations, single-nucleotide variants, and tumoral heterogeneity by massively parallel sequencing. *Clin. Chem.* **2013**, *59*, 211–224. [CrossRef] [PubMed]
2. Murtaza, M.; Dawson, S.J.; Pogrebniak, K.; Rueda, O.M.; Provenzano, E.; Grant, J.; Chin, S.F.; Tsui, D.W.; Marass, F.; Gale, D.; et al. Multifocal clonal evolution characterized using circulating tumour DNA in a case of metastatic breast cancer. *Nat. Commun.* **2015**, *6*, 8760. [CrossRef] [PubMed]
3. Diehl, F.; Li, M.; Dressman, D.; He, Y.; Shen, D.; Szabo, S.; Diaz, L.A., Jr.; Goodman, S.N.; David, K.A.; Juhl, H.; et al. Detection and quantification of mutations in the plasma of patients with colorectal tumors. *Proc. Natl. Acad. Sci. USA* **2005**, *102*, 16368–16373. [CrossRef] [PubMed]
4. Dawson, S.J.; Tsui, D.W.; Murtaza, M.; Biggs, H.; Rueda, O.M.; Chin, S.F.; Dunning, M.J.; Gale, D.; Forshew, T.; Mahler-Araujo, B.; et al. Analysis of circulating tumor DNA to monitor metastatic breast cancer. *N. Engl. J. Med.* **2013**, *368*, 1199–1209. [CrossRef] [PubMed]
5. Romanel, A.; Tandefelt, D.G.; Conteduca, V.; Jayaram, A.; Casiraghi, N.; Wetterskog, D.; Salvi, S.; Amadori, D.; Zafeiriou, Z.; Rescigno, P.; et al. Plasma AR abiraterone-resistant prostate cancer. *Sci. Transl. Med.* **2015**, *7*, 312. [CrossRef] [PubMed]
6. Jamal-Hanjani, M.; Wilson, G.A.; Horswell, S.; Mitter, R.; Sakarya, O.; Constantin, T.; Salari, R.; Kirkizlar, E.; Sigurjonsson, S.; Pelham, R.; et al. Detection of ubiquitous and heterogeneous mutations in cell-free DNA from patients with early-stage non-small-cell lung cancer. *Ann. Oncol.* **2016**, *27*, 862–867. [CrossRef] [PubMed]
7. Bettegowda, C.; Sausen, M.; Leary, R.J.; Kinde, I.; Wang, Y.; Agrawal, N.; Bartlett, B.R.; Wang, H.; Luber, B.; Alani, R.M.; et al. Detection of circulating tumor DNA in early- and late-stage human malignancies. *Sci. Transl. Med.* **2014**, *6*, 224. [CrossRef] [PubMed]
8. Parkinson, C.A.; Gale, D.; Piskorz, A.M.; Biggs, H.; Hodgkin, C.; Addley, H.; Freeman, S.; Moyle, P.; Sala, E.; Sayal, K.; et al. Exploratory analysis of tp53 mutations in circulating tumour DNA as biomarkers of treatment

9. Diehl, F.; Schmidt, K.; Choti, M.A.; Romans, K.; Goodman, S.; Li, M.; Thornton, K.; Agrawal, N.; Sokoll, L.; Szabo, S.A.; et al. Circulating mutant DNA to assess tumor dynamics. *Nat. Med.* **2008**, *14*, 985–990. [CrossRef] [PubMed]
10. Garcia-Murillas, I.; Schiavon, G.; Weigelt, B.; Ng, C.; Hrebien, S.; Cutts, R.J.; Cheang, M.; Osin, P.; Nerurkar, A.; Kozarewa, I.; et al. Mutation tracking in circulating tumor DNA predicts relapse in early breast cancer. *Sci. Transl. Med.* **2015**, *7*, 302. [CrossRef] [PubMed]
11. Murtaza, M.; Dawson, S.J.; Tsui, D.W.; Gale, D.; Forshew, T.; Piskorz, A.M.; Parkinson, C.; Chin, S.F.; Kingsbury, Z.; Wong, A.S.; et al. Non-invasive analysis of acquired resistance to cancer therapy by sequencing of plasma DNA. *Nature* **2013**, *497*, 108–112. [CrossRef] [PubMed]
12. Carreira, S.; Romanel, A.; Goodall, J.; Grist, E.; Ferraldeschi, R.; Miranda, S.; Prandi, D.; Lorente, D.; Frenel, J.S.; Pezaro, C.; et al. Tumor clone dynamics in lethal prostate cancer. *Sci. Transl. Med.* **2014**, *6*, 254. [CrossRef] [PubMed]
13. Abbosh, C.; Birkbak, N.J.; Wilson, G.A.; Jamal-Hanjani, M.; Constantin, T.; Salari, R.; Quesne, J.L.; Moore, D.A.; Veeriah, S.; Rosenthal, R.; et al. Phylogenetic ctdna analysis depicts early stage lung cancer evolution. *Nature* **2017**, *545*, 446. [CrossRef] [PubMed]
14. Peng, M.; Chen, C.; Hulbert, A.; Brock, M.V.; Yu, F. Non-blood circulating tumor DNA detection in cancer. *Oncotarget* **2017**, *8*, 69162–69173. [CrossRef] [PubMed]
15. Schwarzenbach, H.; Hoon, D.S.; Pantel, K. Cell-free nucleic acids as biomarkers in cancer patients. *Nat. Rev. Cancer* **2011**, *11*, 426–437. [CrossRef] [PubMed]
16. Wan, J.C.M.; Massie, C.; Garcia-Corbacho, J.; Mouliere, F.; Brenton, J.D.; Caldas, C.; Pacey, S.; Baird, R.; Rosenfeld, N. Liquid biopsies come of age: Towards implementation of circulating tumour DNA. *Nat. Rev. Cancer* **2017**, *17*, 223–238. [CrossRef] [PubMed]
17. Ellinger, J.; Muller, S.C.; Stadler, T.C.; Jung, A.; von Ruecker, A.; Bastian, P.J. The role of cell-free circulating DNA in the diagnosis and prognosis of prostate cancer. *Urol. Oncol.* **2011**, *29*, 124–129. [CrossRef] [PubMed]
18. Cargnin, S.; Canonico, P.L.; Genazzani, A.A.; Terrazzino, S. Quantitative analysis of circulating cell-free DNA for correlation with lung cancer survival: A systematic review and meta-analysis. *J. Thorac. Oncol.* **2017**, *12*, 43–53. [CrossRef] [PubMed]
19. Valpione, S.; Gremel, G.; Mundra, P.; Middlehurst, P.; Galvani, E.; Girotti, M.R.; Lee, R.J.; Garner, G.; Dhomen, N.; Lorigan, P.C.; et al. Plasma total cell-free DNA (cfDNA) is a surrogate biomarker for tumour burden and a prognostic biomarker for survival in metastatic melanoma patients. *Eur. J. Cancer* **2018**, *88*, 1–9. [CrossRef] [PubMed]
20. Newman, A.M.; Bratman, S.V.; To, J.; Wynne, J.F.; Eclov, N.C.; Modlin, L.A.; Liu, C.L.; Neal, J.W.; Wakelee, H.A.; Merritt, R.E.; et al. An ultrasensitive method for quantitating circulating tumor DNA with broad patient coverage. *Nat. Med.* **2014**, *20*, 548–554. [CrossRef] [PubMed]
21. McGregor, B.A.; Chung, J.; Bergerot, P.G.; Forcier, B.; Grivas, P.; Choueiri, T.K.; Ross, J.S.; Ali, S.M.; Stephens, P.J.; Miller, V.A.; et al. Correlation of circulating tumor DNA (ctDNA) ssessment with tissue-based comprehensive genomic profiling (CGP) in metastatic urothelial cancer (MUC). *J. Clin. Oncol.* **2018**, *36*, 453. [CrossRef]
22. Adalsteinsson, V.A.; Ha, G.; Freeman, S.S.; Choudhury, A.D.; Stover, D.G.; Parsons, H.A.; Gydush, G.; Reed, S.C.; Rotem, D.; Rhoades, J.; et al. Scalable whole-exome sequencing of cell-free DNA reveals high concordance with metastatic tumors. *Nat. Commun.* **2017**, *8*, 1324. [CrossRef] [PubMed]
23. Todenhofer, T.; Struss, W.J.; Seiler, R.; Wyatt, A.W.; Black, P.C. Liquid biopsy-analysis of circulating tumor DNA (ctDNA) in bladder cancer. *Bladder Cancer* **2018**, *4*, 19–29. [CrossRef] [PubMed]
24. Mouliere, F.; Robert, B.; Arnau Peyrotte, E.; Del Rio, M.; Ychou, M.; Molina, F.; Gongora, C.; Thierry, A.R. High fragmentation characterizes tumour-derived circulating DNA. *PLoS ONE* **2011**, *6*, e23418. [CrossRef] [PubMed]
25. Volik, S.; Alcaide, M.; Morin, R.D.; Collins, C. Cell-free DNA (cfDNA): Clinical significance and utility in cancer shaped by emerging technologies. *Mol. Cancer Res.* **2016**, *14*, 898–908. [CrossRef] [PubMed]
26. Thierry, A.R.; El Messaoudi, S.; Gahan, P.B.; Anker, P.; Stroun, M. Origins, structures, and functions of circulating DNA in oncology. *Cancer Metastasis Rev.* **2016**, *35*, 347–376. [CrossRef] [PubMed]

27. Underhill, H.R.; Kitzman, J.O.; Hellwig, S.; Welker, N.C.; Daza, R.; Baker, D.N.; Gligorich, K.M.; Rostomily, R.C.; Bronner, M.P.; Shendure, J. Fragment length of circulating tumor DNA. *PLoS Genet.* **2016**, *12*, e1006162. [CrossRef] [PubMed]
28. Conteduca, V.; Wetterskog, D.; Sharabiani, M.T.A.; Grande, E.; Fernandez-Perez, M.P.; Jayaram, A.; Salvi, S.; Castellano, D.; Romanel, A.; Lolli, C.; et al. Androgen receptor gene status in plasma DNA associates with worse outcome on enzalutamide or abiraterone for castration-resistant prostate cancer: A multi-institution correlative biomarker study. *Ann. Oncol.* **2017**, *28*, 1508–1516. [CrossRef] [PubMed]
29. Stein, J.P.; Lieskovsky, G.; Cote, R.; Groshen, S.; Feng, A.C.; Boyd, S.; Skinner, E.; Bochner, B.; Thangathurai, D.; Mikhail, M.; et al. Radical cystectomy in the treatment of invasive bladder cancer: Long-term results in 1054 patients. *J. Clin. Oncol.* **2001**, *19*, 666–675. [CrossRef] [PubMed]
30. Robertson, A.G.; Kim, J.; Al-Ahmadie, H.; Bellmunt, J.; Guo, G.; Cherniack, A.D.; Hinoue, T.; Laird, P.W.; Hoadley, K.A.; Akbani, R.; et al. Comprehensive molecular characterization of muscle-invasive bladder cancer. *Cell* **2017**, *171*, 540–556. [CrossRef] [PubMed]
31. Choi, W.; Porten, S.; Kim, S.; Willis, D.; Plimack, E.R.; Hoffman-Censits, J.; Roth, B.; Cheng, T.; Tran, M.; Lee, I.L.; et al. Identification of distinct basal and luminal subtypes of muscle-invasive bladder cancer with different sensitivities to frontline chemotherapy. *Cancer Cell* **2014**, *25*, 152–165. [CrossRef] [PubMed]
32. Seiler, R.; Ashab, H.A.; Erho, N.; van Rhijn, B.W.; Winters, B.; Douglas, J.; Van Kessel, K.E.; Fransen van de Putte, E.E.; Sommerlad, M.; Wang, N.Q.; et al. Impact of molecular subtypes in muscle-invasive bladder cancer on predicting response and survival after neoadjuvant chemotherapy. *Eur. Urol.* **2017**, *72*, 544–554. [CrossRef] [PubMed]
33. Alfred Witjes, J.; Lebret, T.; Comperat, E.M.; Cowan, N.C.; De Santis, M.; Bruins, H.M.; Hernandez, V.; Espinos, E.L.; Dunn, J.; Rouanne, M.; et al. Updated 2016 eau guidelines on muscle-invasive and metastatic bladder cancer. *Eur. Urol.* **2017**, *71*, 462–475. [CrossRef] [PubMed]
34. Chang, S.S.; Bochner, B.H.; Chou, R.; Dreicer, R.; Kamat, A.M.; Lerner, S.P.; Lotan, Y.; Meeks, J.J.; Michalski, J.M.; Morgan, T.M.; et al. Treatment of non-metastatic muscle-invasive bladder cancer: Aua/asco/astro/suo guideline. *J. Urol.* **2017**, *198*, 552–559. [CrossRef] [PubMed]
35. Zargar, H.; Espiritu, P.N.; Fairey, A.S.; Mertens, L.S.; Dinney, C.P.; Mir, M.C.; Krabbe, L.M.; Cookson, M.S.; Jacobsen, N.E.; Gandhi, N.M.; et al. Multicenter assessment of neoadjuvant chemotherapy for muscle-invasive bladder cancer. *Eur. Urol.* **2015**, *67*, 241–249. [CrossRef] [PubMed]
36. Zargar, H.; Shah, J.B.; van Rhijn, B.W.; Daneshmand, S.; Bivalacqua, T.J.; Spiess, P.E.; Black, P.C.; Kassouf, W. Neoadjuvant dose dense mvac versus gemcitabine and cisplatin in patients with cT3-4aN0M0 bladder cancer treated with radical cystectomy. *J. Urol.* **2018**, *199*, 1452–1458. [CrossRef] [PubMed]
37. Lee, C.T.; Madii, R.; Daignault, S.; Dunn, R.L.; Zhang, Y.; Montie, J.E.; Wood, D.P. Cystectomy delay more than 3 months from initial bladder cancer diagnosis results in decreased disease specific and overall survival. *J. Urol.* **2006**, *175*, 1262–1267. [CrossRef]
38. Sidransky, D.; Voneschenbach, A.; Tsai, Y.C.; Jones, P.; Summerhayes, I.; Marshall, F.; Paul, M.; Green, P.; Hamilton, S.R.; Frost, P.; et al. Identification of p53 gene-mutations in bladder cancers and urine samples. *Science* **1991**, *252*, 706–709. [CrossRef] [PubMed]
39. Utting, M.; Werner, W.; Dahse, R.; Schubert, J.; Junker, K. Microsatellite analysis of free tumor DNA in urine, serum and plasma of patients: A minimally invasive method for the detection fo bladder cancer. *Clin. Cancer Res.* **2002**, *8*, 35–40. [PubMed]
40. Ellinger, J.; Bastian, P.J.; Ellinger, N.; Kahl, P.; Perabo, F.G.; Buttner, R.; Muller, S.C.; Ruecker, A. Apoptotic DNA fragments in serum of patients with muscle invasive bladder cancer: A prognostic entity. *Cancer Lett.* **2008**, *264*, 274–280. [CrossRef] [PubMed]
41. Knowles, M.A.; Hurst, C.D. Molecular biology of bladder cancer: New insights into pathogenesis and clinical diversity. *Nat. Rev. Cancer* **2015**, *15*, 25–41. [CrossRef] [PubMed]
42. Sonpavde, G.; Nagy, R.; Apolo, N.; Pal, S.; Grivas, P.; Vaishampayan, U.; Lanman, R.; Talasaz, A. Circulating cell-free DNA profiling of patients with advanced urothelial carcinoma. *J. Clin. Oncol.* **2016**, *34*, 358. [CrossRef]
43. Agarwal, N.; Pal, S.K.; Hahn, A.W.; Nussenzveig, R.H.; Pond, G.R.; Gupta, S.V.; Wang, J.; Bilen, M.A.; Naik, G.; Ghatalia, P.; et al. Characterization of metastatic urothelial carcinoma via comprehensive genomic profiling of circulating tumor DNA. *Cancer* **2018**, *124*, 2115–2124. [CrossRef] [PubMed]

44. Van Allen, E.M.; Mouw, K.W.; Kim, P.; Iyer, G.; Wagle, N.; Al-Ahmadie, H.; Zhu, C.; Ostrovnaya, I.; Kryukov, G.V.; O'Connor, K.W.; et al. Somatic *ERCC2* mutations correlate with cisplatin sensitivity in muscle-invasive urothelial carcinoma. *Cancer Discov.* **2014**, *4*, 1140–1153. [CrossRef] [PubMed]
45. Birkenkamp-Demtröder, K.; Nordentoft, I.; Christensen, E.; Hoyer, S.; Reinert, T.; Vang, S.; Borre, M.; Agerbaek, M.; Jensen, J.B.; Orntoft, T.F.; et al. Genomic alterations in liquid biopsies from patients with bladder cancer. *Eur. Urol.* **2016**, *70*, 75–82. [CrossRef] [PubMed]
46. Christensen, E.; Birkenkamp-Demtröder, K.; Nordentoft, I.; Hoyer, S.; van der Keur, K.; van Kessel, K.; Zwarthoff, E.; Agerbaek, M.; Orntoft, T.F.; Jensen, J.B.; et al. Liquid biopsy analysis of *FGFR3* and *PIK3CA* hotspot mutations for disease surveillance in bladder cancer. *Eur. Urol.* **2017**, *71*, 961–969. [CrossRef] [PubMed]
47. Vandekerkhove, G.; Todenhofer, T.; Annala, M.; Struss, W.J.; Wong, A.; Beja, K.; Ritch, E.; Brahmbhatt, S.; Volik, S.V.; Hennenlotter, J.; et al. Circulating tumor DNA reveals clinically actionable somatic genome of metastatic bladder cancer. *Clin. Cancer Res.* **2017**, *23*, 6487–6497. [CrossRef] [PubMed]
48. Patel, K.M.; van der Vos, K.E.; Smith, C.G.; Mouliere, F.; Tsui, D.; Morris, J.; Chandrananda, D.; Marass, F.; van den Broek, D.; Neal, D.E.; et al. Association of plasma and urinary mutant DNA with clinical outcomes in muscle invasive bladder cancer. *Sci. Rep.* **2017**, *7*, 5554. [CrossRef] [PubMed]
49. Birkenkamp-Demtröder, K.; Christensen, E.; Nordentoft, I.; Knudsen, M.; Taber, A.; Hoyer, S.; Lamy, P.; Agerbaek, M.; Jensen, J.B.; Dyrskjot, L. Monitoring treatment response and metastatic relapse in advanced bladder cancer by liquid biopsy analysis. *Eur. Urol.* **2017**, *73*, 535–540. [CrossRef] [PubMed]
50. Barata, P.C.; Koshkin, V.S.; Funchain, P.; Sohal, D.; Pritchard, A.; Klek, S.; Adamowicz, T.; Gopalakrishnan, D.; Garcia, J.; Rini, B.; et al. Next-generation sequencing (NGS) of cell-free circulating tumor DNA and tumor tissue in patients with advanced urothelial cancer: A pilot assessment of concordance. *Ann. Oncol.* **2017**, *28*, 2458–2463. [CrossRef] [PubMed]
51. Soave, A.; Chun, F.K.; Hillebrand, T.; Rink, M.; Weisbach, L.; Steinbach, B.; Fisch, M.; Pantel, K.; Schwarzenbach, H. Copy number variations of circulating, cell-free DNA in urothelial carcinoma of the bladder patients treated with radical cystectomy: A prospective study. *Oncotarget* **2017**, *8*, 56398–56407. [CrossRef] [PubMed]
52. Cheng, M.L.; Shady, M.; Cipolla, C.K.; Funt, S.; Arcila, M.E.; Al-Ahmadie, H.; Rosenberg, J.E.; Bajorin, D.F.; Berger, M.F.; Tsui, D.; et al. Comparison of somatic mutation profiles from cell free DNA (cfDNA) versus tissue in metastatic urothelial carcinoma (MUC). *J. Clin. Oncol.* **2017**, *35*, 4533.
53. National Cancer Institute GDC Data Portal. Available online: https://portal.gdc.cancer.gov/ (accessed on 15 July 2018).
54. Christensen, E.; Nordentoft, I.; Vang, S.; Birkenkamp-Demtröder, K.; Jensen, J.B.; Agerbaek, M.; Pedersen, J.S.; Dyrskjot, L. Optimized targeted sequencing of cell-free plasma DNA from bladder cancer patients. *Sci. Rep.* **2018**, *8*, 1917. [CrossRef] [PubMed]

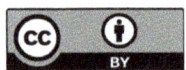

© 2018 by the authors. Licensee MDPI, Basel, Switzerland. This article is an open access article distributed under the terms and conditions of the Creative Commons Attribution (CC BY) license (http://creativecommons.org/licenses/by/4.0/).

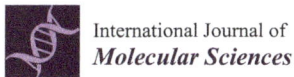

Review

Liquid Biopsy Biomarkers in Bladder Cancer: A Current Need for Patient Diagnosis and Monitoring

Iris Lodewijk [1,2], Marta Dueñas [1,2,3], Carolina Rubio [1,2,3], Ester Munera-Maravilla [1,2], Cristina Segovia [1,2,3], Alejandra Bernardini [1,2,3], Alicia Teijeira [1], Jesús M. Paramio [1,2,3] and Cristian Suárez-Cabrera [1,2,*]

[1] Molecular Oncology Unit, CIEMAT (Centro de Investigaciones Energéticas, Medioambientales y Tecnológicas), Avenida Complutense nº 40, 28040 Madrid, Spain; IrisAdriana.Lodewijk@externos.ciemat.es (I.L.); marta.duenas@ciemat.es (M.D.); carolina.rubio@externos.ciemat.es (C.R.); ester.munera@ciemat.es (E.M.-M.); cristina.segovia@ciemat.es (C.S.); Alejandra.bernardini@externos.ciemat.es (A.B.); aliciateijeira.merced@gmail.com (A.T.); jesusm.paramio@ciemat.es (J.M.P.)
[2] Biomedical Research Institute I+12, University Hospital "12 de Octubre", Av Córdoba s/n, 28041 Madrid, Spain
[3] Centro de Investigación Biomédica en Red de Cáncer (CIBERONC), 28029 Madrid, Spain
* Correspondence: cristian.suarez@externos.ciemat.es; Tel.: +34-91-496-6438

Received: 28 July 2018; Accepted: 21 August 2018; Published: 24 August 2018

Abstract: Bladder Cancer (BC) represents a clinical and social challenge due to its high incidence and recurrence rates, as well as the limited advances in effective disease management. Currently, a combination of cytology and cystoscopy is the routinely used methodology for diagnosis, prognosis and disease surveillance. However, both the poor sensitivity of cytology tests as well as the high invasiveness and big variation in tumour stage and grade interpretation using cystoscopy, emphasizes the urgent need for improvements in BC clinical guidance. Liquid biopsy represents a new non-invasive approach that has been extensively studied over the last decade and holds great promise. Even though its clinical use is still compromised, multiple studies have recently focused on the potential application of biomarkers in liquid biopsies for BC, including circulating tumour cells and DNA, RNAs, proteins and peptides, metabolites and extracellular vesicles. In this review, we summarize the present knowledge on the different types of biomarkers, their potential use in liquid biopsy and clinical applications in BC.

Keywords: bladder cancer; liquid biopsy; biomarkers

---

1. Introduction: Bladder Cancer Issues and Liquid Biopsy

Bladder cancer (BC) is the most common malignancy of the urinary tract, representing a highly prevalent disease which affects primarily elderly people. For both sexes combined, it is the 9th most common cancer diagnosed worldwide and a significant cause of tumour-related death, with an estimated 165,000 deaths per year [1]. BC represents an important health problem with an age-standardized incidence rate (per 100,000 person-years) of 9 in men versus 2.2 in women and an age-standardized mortality rate (per 100,000 person-years) of 3.2 and 0.9, respectively [2–4]. The incidence and mortality rate are stagnant due to the scarcity of newly developed effective treatments and options for prevention [5,6].

BC can be divided in two major classes based on tumour stage, I) non-muscle invasive bladder cancer (NMIBC), which is either confined to the urothelium (carcinoma in situ (CIS)-or stage Ta, 5-year survival rate of 95.4%) or the lamina propia (stage T1, 5-year survival rate of approximately 88%) and II) muscle-invasive bladder cancer (MIBC) (stage T2, T3 and T4, representing 5-year survival rates of 69.4%, 34.9% and 4.8%, respectively) [7,8]. NMIBC represents the most frequent form of BC, presented by approximately 70–80% of patients at diagnosis and is primarily treated by transurethral resection of the bladder tumour (TURBT), which is considered fundamental for the diagnosis and prognosis of the disease [9,10]. Dependent upon certain pathological characteristics (e.g., size and number of implants), TURBT is followed by intravesical instillation with chemotherapeutics, such as mitomycin, or the immunotherapeutic Bacillus Calmette-Guérin (BCG) [11,12]. However, despite TURBT and chemo/immunotherapy as first-line treatment, NMIBC displays a high recurrence incidence (50–70%) with tumour progression towards invasive tumours in at least 10–15% of the cases, due to minimal residual disease (MRD) which remained undetected [9,10]. The extraordinary rates of recurrence and the likelihood to progress require continuous follow-up of NMIBC patients by cystoscopy (every 3–6 months during the next 5 years) and urine cytology, making NMIBC one of the most costly malignancies for the National Health systems of developed countries [11,13]. Accordingly, BC represents the most expensive human cancer from diagnosis to death, with an estimated cost of $187,000 per patient in the United States [14]. In 2010, its total annual cost was estimated at $4 billion, which is expected to rise to approximately $5 billion by 2020 [14,15]. In the European Union, in 2012, the total BC expenditure has been determined at €4.9 billion, with health care accounting for €2.9 billion (59%) [16].

The remaining 20–30% of BC patients presents MIBC at diagnosis. Once tumour progression is observed the prognosis declines [17,18]. Treatment of invasive BC currently consists of radical cystectomy followed by platin-based chemotherapy. Nevertheless, clinical benefit of the addition of neoadjuvant chemotherapy (NAC) (like cisplatin, methotrexate, vinblastine and gemcitabine) has been evaluated by several studies [19–21]. NAC is presumed to diminish the burden of micrometastatic disease and can be used to predict chemosensitivity of the tumour [2]. Despite conflicting results shown by multiple randomized phase III trials (due to differences in for example, chemotherapy used, number of cycles and trial design), a significant survival benefit in favour of NAC has been indicated by various meta-analyses [19,20]. Unfortunately, metastatic spreading remains an important problem in a high fraction of the cases (50–70%), resulting in very low survival rates (5-year survival rate of 4.8%) [2,8,22].

Despite multiple trials, no new effective therapeutic options have been developed throughout the last decades [23], with the exception of immunotherapy based on checkpoint inhibitors. Even though these checkpoint inhibitors have shown promising results in patients with advanced or recurrent BC, only 20–35% of the BC patients benefit from this therapy and overall survival is still limited [24,25].

The typical and most important clinical indication for BC is haematuria. Nowadays, a combination of urine cytology and cystoscopy is still the routinely used methodology by excellence for detection, diagnosis and surveillance of this disease. Cytology remains the gold standard for detection of urothelial carcinoma. BC urinary cytology shows a specificity of approximately 98% and a sensitivity of 38% [26] (Table 1). However, the sensitivity of this test significantly increases with malignancy grade, reaching a reasonable sensitivity of >60% for CIS and high-grade lesions [26,27]. In 1997, in order to improve cytology predictive values, Fradet and Lockhard developed an immunofluorescence test (uCyt+) which was based on detection of three BC antigens (M344, LDQ10 and 19A11) in exfoliated cells [28], improving the sensitivity of cytology to approximately 73% but decreasing the specificity to 66% due to the requirement of a large number of exfoliated cells [29] (Table 1). Cystoscopy is currently the gold standard technique in clinical practice for detection and follow-up of BC, achieving a sensitivity of approximately 85–90% and 65–70% to detect exophytic tumours and CIS, respectively [27,30–33]. Nevertheless, this procedure is highly invasive, showing a big inter-observer and intra-observer variation in the tumour stage and grade interpretation [27,30–33].

Therefore, it is clear that there is an urgent need for improvements in diagnosis, prognosis and follow-up of BC patients. Over the last decades, tumour biopsies have revealed details with regard to the genetic profile of tumours, allowing the prediction of prognosis, tumour progression as well as therapy response and resistance [34]. Recently, the potential use of liquid biopsy as a new non-invasive way to determine the genomic landscape of cancer patients, screen treatment response, quantify MRD and assess therapy resistance is gaining significant attention [34–40]. The term "liquid biopsy" means the sampling and analysis of biological fluids, including blood, plasma, urine, pleural liquid, cerebrospinal fluid and saliva (Figure 1) [36,39]. The analysis is based on different cells and molecules which can be obtained from liquid biopsies: circulating tumour cells (CTCs), circulating cell-free tumour DNA (ctDNA), messenger RNAs (mRNAs), micro-RNAs (miRNAs), long non-coding RNAs (lncRNAs), proteins and peptides, metabolites and vesicles (exosomes and endosomes) (Figure 1). Even though the presence of circulating free DNA and RNA in human blood was first demonstrated in 1948 [41], only a few liquid biopsies are currently approved for clinical use. In recent years, cancer research has been mainly focused on the introduction of suitable biomarkers, indicating the presence, recurrence and progression of a disease, as well as the appropriated treatment for a specific type of cancer. Taken together, biomarkers present in liquid biopsies hold great promise, as they are able to record and monitor the disease stage at real time and predict prognosis, recurrence, therapy response and resistance, without invasive intervention.

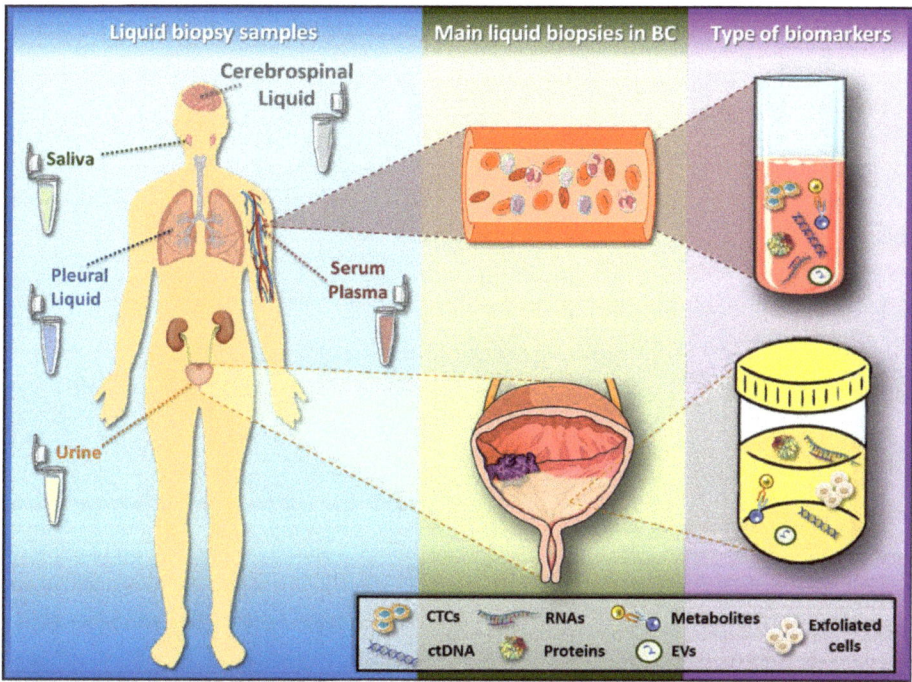

Figure 1. Liquid biopsy samples and biomarkers. Liquid biopsy samples include urine, serum, plasma, saliva, cerebrospinal and pleural fluid, among others. In BC, the liquid biopsies more widely used as detection and surveillance systems are urine (by its intimate contact with the tumour), as well as serum and plasma, which allow the follow-up of advanced disease. These liquid biopsies present several biomarkers, such as circulating tumour cells (CTCs), circulating cell-free tumour DNA (ctDNA), RNAs, proteins, metabolites and extracellular vesicles (EVs). Additionally, exfoliated cells derived from a tumour can be found in urine.

Table 1. Commercial kits to detect and follow-up bladder cancer (BC) using liquid biopsy biomarkers.

Commercial Kits	Biomarker	Assay Type	Sample Type	FDA Approved	Purpose	Predictive Capacity	Source	Refs.
Cytology	Sediment cells	Giemsa and HE staining	Urine	Yes	Diagnostic and surveillance (1)	Sensitivity = 38% Specificity = 98%	-	[26]
uCyt+	Sediment cells	Immunofluorescence	Urine	Yes	Surveillance in adjunct to cystoscopy	Sensitivity = 73% Specificity = 66%	DiagnoCure (2)	[29]
UroVysion	Sediment cells	Multi-target FISH	Urine	Yes	Diagnostic	Sensitivity = 72% Specificity = 83%	Abbott	[42]
UroMark(3)	Sediment cells	Bisulfite-based methylation assay	Urine	No	Diagnostic	Sensitivity = 98% Specificity = 97%	Kelly;Feber	[43]
CellSearch	CTCs	Immunomagnetic enrichment	Plasma/serum	Yes	Surveillance	Sensitivity = 48% Specificity = 98%	Menarini-Silicon Biosystems	[44]
CxBladder	mRNA	RT-qPCR	Urine	No	Diagnostic	Sensitivity = 82% Specificity = 85%	Pacific Edge	[32]
CxBladder Monitor	mRNA	RT-qPCR	Urine	No	Surveillance	Sensitivity = 91% NPV = 96%	Pacific Edge	[45]
Xpert BC Detection	mRNA	RT-qPCR	Urine	No	Diagnostic	Sensitivity = 76% Specificity = 85%	Cepheid	[46]
Xpert BC Monitor	mRNA	RT-qPCR	Urine	No	Surveillance	Sensitivity = 84% Specificity = 91%	Cepheid	[47]
PanC-Dx	mRNA	RT-qPCR	Urine	No	Diagnostic	Sensitivity = 90% Specificity = 83%	Oncocyte	[48]
UROBEST (4)	mRNA	RT-qPCR	Urine	No	Diagnostic and surveillance (5)	Sensitivity = 80% Specificity = 94%	Biofina Diagnostics	-
NMP22	Protein	Sandwich ELISA	Urine	Yes	Surveillance	Sensitivity = 40% Specificity = 99%	Abbott	[49]
NMP22 BladderChek	Protein	Dipstick immunoassay	Urine	Yes	Diagnostic and surveillance (1)	Sensitivity = 68% Specificity = 79%	Abbott	[50]
BTA TRAK	Protein	Sandwich ELISA	Urine	Yes	Diagnostic and surveillance (1)	Sensitivity = 66% Specificity = 65%	Polymedco	[51]
BTA stat	Protein	Dipstick immunoassay	Urine	Yes	Diagnostic and surveillance (1)	Sensitivity = 70% Specificity = 75%	Polymedco	[51]
CYFRA 21.1	Protein	Immunoradiometric assay or ELISA	Urine	No	Diagnostic	Sensitivity = 82% Specificity = 80%	CIS Bio International	[52]
UBC test	Protein	Sandwich ELISA or dipstick immunoassay	Urine	No	Diagnostic	Sensitivity = 64% Specificity = 80%	IDL Biotech	[53]

(1) Although these tests have been proposed for diagnosis and follow-up of BC, predictive values correspond to the detection of primary tumour. (2) DiagnoCure company was dissolved in 2016 and the uCyt+ test is not available at present. (3) The performance of the UroMark test is currently evaluated in Phase III studies. (4) UROBEST is not yet commercially available. (5) Biofina Diagnostics provides these predictive values for diagnostic and surveillance purposes together. NPV = Negative predictive value.

Thus, the potential use of liquid biopsy as a new non-invasive approach to improve BC management is far reaching. Even though their extensive applications are only starting to emerge in clinical practice, multiple studies have indicated the potential use of different biomarkers in liquid biopsies for BC. In this review, we provide an overview of the more important studies regarding the different types of biomarkers in liquid biopsy and their clinical applications in BC.

2. Liquid Biopsy Biomarkers and Their Clinical Applications

2.1. Circulating Tumour Cells (CTCs)

CTCs were first discovered in breast cancer patients in 1869 by Ashworth and colleagues [54]. They are tumour cells of approximately 4 to 50 μm, which are being released from the tumour site into the bloodstream, thereby representing the main mechanism for metastasis [54,55]. CTC detection systems emerged from the need to find new methods to detect early metastatic disease in a less invasive way compared to conventional methods currently available, such as radiological evaluation. In recent years, a wide variety of approaches has been developed for the detection of CTCs, some of which have been implemented in clinical practice. These techniques include immunocytochemistry, reverse-transcriptase polymerase chain reaction, flow cytometry and the CellSearch system, which is the only approach approved by the USA Food and Drug Administration (FDA) [56].

In certain types of solid tumours, such as breast, colorectal cancer and gastric tumours, it has been reported that the presence of CTCs is an indicator of poor prognosis [57–60]. In BC, the presence of CTCs has also been proposed to be associated with a bad prognosis and the amount of CTCs found in blood has been indicated to correlate with short disease-free survival in metastatic BC [61]. However, the relevance for NMIBC is still controversial.

2.1.1. CTC Detection Methods

Since CTCs are very rare and the amount of cells available is around 1 to 10 in 10^6–10^8 white blood cells, their detection, enumeration and molecular characterization is a challenge [62]. Accordingly, an efficient and reliable method for both isolation and characterization of these cells is needed [62,63]. Nowadays, different isolation techniques have been developed, all of which have a first enrichment step before the cells can finally be analysed. Enrichment can be carried out by different methods, including techniques based on physical properties such as size (by microfilters that isolate CTCs regarding to their greater size), density or deformability, as well as on biological properties of CTCs (for example, using immunomagnetic assays) (Figure 2) (reviewed in [64]). Immunomagnetic enrichment can be either negative or positive, both of which are available for in vivo assays, enabling a better sample analysis. Whereas negative enrichment does not rely on the biomarker expression of CTCs but on markers of hematopoietic cells (like CD45, a leukocytic antigen) and allows collection of cells in their intact form (depleting most of the leukocytes and erythrocytes), positive enrichment (using specific CTC biomarkers) has its own advantages including a low false-positive CTC detection rate (Figure 2) (reviewed in [64]).

The CellSearch system (Veridex, LLC, Warren, NJ, USA) is one of those technologies developed and, in this case, approved by the FDA for the isolation of CTCs (Table 1). CellSearch CTC Test is based on immunomagnetic enrichment and, initially, permitted enumeration of CTCs of epithelial origin by targeting only EpCAM for capturing CTCs. However, some studies have pointed out the difficulty in obtaining sufficient EpCAM-expressing CTCs from patients with advanced disease to reach statistically significant conclusions from a study or clinical trial [65]. Therefore, the recent versions of this test also select CTCs by other surface proteins, selecting those cells that are CD45−, EpCAM+ and cytokeratin 8/18+ and/or 19+. Though CellSearch is the most frequently used and still the gold standard today, new ways to detect CTCs have come up recently. CytoTrack is a similar method which allows detection and quantification of CTCs using a scanning fluorescence microscope [66]. For this test, a cocktail of a range of cytokeratins (pan-cytokeratin antibody) and CD45 (to deplete blood cells) is used [66].

Given that CytoTrack relies on a cytokeratin signal to detect cells and CellSearch depends on both EpCAM and cytokeratin expression, these two different approaches could give rise to significantly different results with regard to CTC detection. The advantage of Cytotrack is the possibility of staining with different antibodies which allows identification of new CTC biomarkers [67]. For example, HER2, which is considered a breast cancer biomarker, has also been used as target antigen for this technique [68,69]. By performing a comparative analysis between both systems, CellSearch and Cytotrack, Hillig et al. found that the two CTC technologies have similar recovery of cells spiked into blood (69% vs. 71%, $p = 0.58$, respectively) [67]. However, CellSearch shows a lower variability in the analysis [67]. Another promising method is the Epic CTC Platform, whose detection system is based on the use of cytokeratins as CTC biomarkers and CD45 as hematopoietic marker. Even though this approach is similar to CytoTrack, the Epic CTC platform also integrates downstream capabilities for the evaluation of cell morphology characteristics, protein biomarker expression and genomic analyses (Fluorescence In Situ Hybridization (FISH) and Next-Generation Sequencing (NGS)) [70]. In an analytical validation of the Epic CTC Platform capabilities, Werner et al. assayed the performance, including accuracy, linearity, specificity and intra/inter-assay precision, of CTC enumeration in healthy donor blood samples spiked with varying concentrations of cancer cell line controls [71]. They found a high percentage of nucleated cell recovery for all cancer cell concentrations tested and showed excellent assay linearity ($R^2 = 0.999$). Besides, using a small cohort of metastatic castration-resistant prostate cancer patient samples tested with the Epic CTC Platform, detection of ≥ 1 traditional CTC/mL in 89% of patient samples was shown, whereas 100% of the cancer patient samples had ≥ 1 CTC/mL when additionally considering the cytokeratin negative and apoptotic CTC subpopulations, compared to healthy donor samples (in which zero CTCs were enumerated in all 18 samples) (Figure 2) [70].

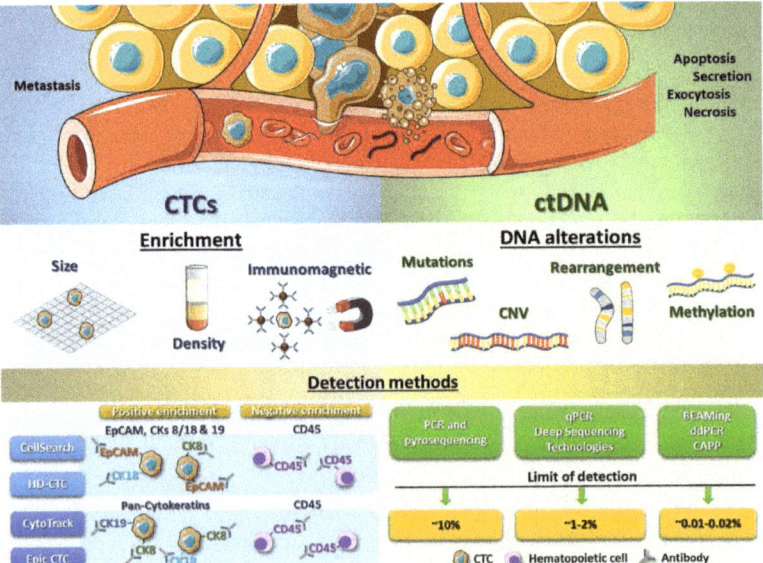

Figure 2. CTC and ctDNA processing methods. Scheme showing some enrichment techniques to isolate CTCs from peripheral blood cells (erythrocytes and leukocytes) and different detection systems based on immunomagnetic assays, using specific antibodies to recognize antigens present in tumour cells (like EpCAM or cytokeratins) as well as to exclude leukocytes (using antibodies against CD45) (left panel). Right panel displays the different DNA alterations (including mutations, copy number variations (CNVs), gene rearrangements or methylation variations) which can be analysed from ctDNA, as well as different detection methods and their correspondent limit of detection.

An improved CellSearch method is HD-CTC (from High Definition CTC; Epic Sciences, Inc., San Diego, CA, USA), which is not only based on EpCAM, cytokeratins and CD45 immunofluorescence staining but also on morphological characterization, size and high throughput counting, allowing the identification of apoptotic cells by DAPI staining and imaging using a high definition scanner (Figure 2). This detection method has been demonstrated to be more sensitive than the original CellSearch [71]. Additional to previously described detection methods, many other approaches have been developed over the last years by multiple commercial laboratories, evidencing the great potential of CTC detection at present and in future clinical procedures (reviewed in [64]).

However, these detection systems usually use small volumes of peripheral blood (<10 mL), showing a yield of 0.1–0.2% with respect to all tumour cells present in whole blood [72]. To overcome this problem in CTC detection and to evaluate large blood volumes, some groups have been exploring the potential of apheresis as CTC isolation method previous to the use of detection systems. In breast and pancreatic cancer patients, apheresis has demonstrated to improve the recovery of CTCs, showing better yield than the CellSearch system [73,74]. Besides, since CTCs probably have representative features of primary tumours, obtaining a sufficient number of CTCs could depict a global view of the tumour alterations and would allow carrying out different genomic analyses in order to define tumour and metastasis features. At present, there is a European Consortium "CTC Therapeutic Apheresis: CTCTrap project" (http://www.utwente.nl/en/tnw/ctctrap/) focused on improving this method in order to characterize all tumour cells circulating in blood and apply it into the clinic in a real-rime liquid biopsy system.

2.1.2. CTCs in Bladder Cancer

CTC detection in BC was first reported in 2000 by Lu et al., when they published a method for CTC detection in peripheral blood of patients with urothelial carcinoma using nested reverse transcription-PCR assay for *UPK2* (Uroplakin II) [75]. Their results were modest, being able to detect 3 out of 29 patients (10.3%) with superficial cancers (pTa-1N0M0), 4 out of 14 patients (28.6%) with MIBC (pT2-4N0M0), 2 out of 5 loco-regional node-positive patients (40.0%) (pN1-2M0) and 6 out of 8 patients (75.0%) with distant metastases [75].

More recently, several studies have evaluated CTCs in BC, mainly using CellSearch Technology, showing an average close to 50% of positive detection for metastatic BC and a low (around 15%) detection level for clinically localized BC [76]. Besides, even though CTC quantification has also been employed for prognosis and patient stratification, the detection of recurrent tumours is approximately 20–44% in patients showing progression upon recurrence. Additionally, Busetto and colleagues found a strong correlation between CTC presence and the time to first recurrence (75%) and they suggested that the time of progression is strongly correlated with CTCs [77].

In 2017, Zhang et al. published a meta-analysis of the impact of CTCs in BC. This study showed that the number of CTCs in peripheral blood is correlated with tumour stage, histological grade, metastasis and regional lymph node metastasis [45]. They also reported that the overall sensitivity and specificity of CTC detection assays are, respectively, 35% (95% CI: 28–43) and 97% (95% CI: 92–99), concluding that the presence of CTCs in peripheral blood is an independent predictive indicator of poor outcomes for urothelial cancer patients [44].

Even though CTC quantitation has to be studied more profoundly, this procedure could be incorporated into risk stratification algorithms and, therefore, aid patient management. In addition, CTC detection may not be accurate to be used as initial screening test but as a method for confirming BC diagnosis, due to the limited diagnostic sensitivity and high overall specificity. With improvements in clinical and laboratory techniques, the detection of CTCs at different time points in the future may allow real-time surveillance of dynamic changes of disease and crucially enhance our understanding of the metastatic cascade, thus facilitating novel targeted therapy approaches.

Regarding BC, the employability of CTCs in diagnosis and prognosis will be determined by the optimal combination of sensitivity, specificity, simplicity and cost of its implementation in the hospital routine. CTC enrichment techniques accompanied by a good cytological characterization may improve the fundamental weakness of cytology in the diagnosis/prognosis of low-grade disease. However, more well-designed, high-quality and large-scale prospective studies, especially including the CTCs and survival, are required to further strengthen current observations and shed more light on the potential of CTCs as a promising biomarker.

2.2. Circulating Cell-Free Tumour DNA (ctDNA)

2.2.1. Detection and Genomic Analysis of ctDNA: First Clinical Approaches

As previously mentioned, the presence of cell-free DNA fragments in human blood was first discovered in 1948 [41]. In 1977, increased total cell-free DNA levels were observed in serum of cancer patients compared to healthy individuals, showing potential for therapeutic evaluation [78]. In blood, fragments of cell-free DNA have a typical size of 160–180 bp and are released from apoptotic as well as necrotic cells and possibly by active secretion, phagocytosis and exocytosis [40,79]. Methylation analysis has been used to trace the tissue of origin of cell-free DNA and showed that the biggest part in plasma is released by blood cells in healthy individuals [80]. At the end of the 1980s, Stroun et al. described that at least part of circulating free DNA in the plasma of cancer patients derived from cancer cells [81]. In 1991, DNA bearing *TP53* mutations were found in urinary sediments from MIBC patients, paving the way for the use of genomics in liquid biopsy [82]. Posteriorly, studies based on mutated *KRAS* sequences in plasma confirmed the tumour origin of mutant cell-free DNA [83]. Mutated genes in plasma were subsequently proposed to represent tumour markers and the term "circulating tumour DNA" was coined. On the other hand, ctDNA levels are very variable between individuals and the presence of metastasis as well as disease burden increase the heterogeneity of ctDNA levels [84]. In fact, the ctDNA fraction in plasma could represent up to 50% of all cell-free DNA in metastatic patients [85], whereas ctDNA may be undetectable in patients with MRD [86].

Despite these findings, poor technological advances have limited progress in this area for decades. For many years, multiple studies have been carried out to improve the detection systems that are used to observe tumour-associated genomic alterations in ctDNA, such as tumour-specific mutations, amplifications, deletions, gene rearrangements or methylation variations (Figure 2). These studies have tried to validate the potential of ctDNA as a diagnostic and prognostic marker in cancer as well as their value in MRD detection and therapeutic monitoring, mainly for patients with advanced malignancies [87–91]. However, the detection and quantification of ctDNA with a sensitivity required for significant clinical practice has not been easy, due to the small number of ctDNA fragments compared to the number of normal circulating DNA fragments.

Initially, allele-specific primers in conventional PCR and Pyrosequencing were used to detect and quantify the percentage of specific mutations in cell-free DNA present in liquid biopsy samples but the restriction to specific mutations as well as a low sensitivity (requiring, at least, a 10% of mutant DNA) has limited the success of these techniques [90,92]. This limitation in detection was improved by using quantitative PCR and different deep sequencing technologies such as NGS, being able to identify a 1–2% of mutations in different types of tumours [92–97]. Nowadays, digital droplet polymerase chain reaction (ddPCR) has improved accuracy and quantification of mutations, enabling more effective extraction and analysis of ctDNA, even in highly diluted cell-free DNA samples [98]. In 2005, Diehl and colleagues described for the first time the quantification of the mutant allele fraction of the *APC* gene in plasma of colorectal cancer patients by means of BEAMing technology, which is an approach based on digital PCR, binding to streptavidin beads, attachment of base pair-specific fluorescent probes and flow cytometry [99,100]. Both ddPCR and BEAMing have allowed the reduction of the detection limit of ctDNA mutations to 0.01–0.02% (Figure 2).

Despite the previously described technological advances, the abovementioned detection systems have some restrictions. Using PCR-based methods, the number of ctDNA alterations detected per assay is limited, only evaluating known and specific mutations. Besides, some techniques (like BEAMing) are laborious processes, keeping off a high productivity. Since the percentage of patients bearing known driver mutations is low, assays based on genome-wide analysis, which detection capacity has increased over the last years, have currently gained much importance. Newman et al. have developed a new system, called "cancer personalized profiling by deep sequencing (CAPP-Seq)" [101]. Here, they designed a multiple panel including somatic alterations from Catalogue Of Somatic Mutations In Cancer (COSMIC) and The Cancer Genome Atlas (TCGA) databases for non-small cell lung cancer, thereby detecting some of these alterations in 100% of high stage patients and in 50% of low stage patients, with a detection limit of approximately 0.02% [101] (Figure 2). Accordingly, these advanced techniques open a wide spectrum of possibilities to increase accuracy of diagnostic and predictive systems in a non-invasive form in cancer patients.

Worthy of note, the exact origin of ctDNA is not completely clear yet. Since ctDNA can be released from apoptotic or necrotic tumour cells which have died, genomic features derived from these cells may not entirely reflect the biology of primary tumours or metastasis at diagnosis, and, consequently, these alterations might not contribute to subsequent tumour progression and/or metastasis. This should also be taken into consideration during the clinical decision-making process.

2.2.2. ctDNA in Bladder Cancer

Regarding ctDNA detection in BC patients, several studies have focused on the detection of different DNA alterations in liquid biopsy samples in order to find predictive biomarkers. In particular, urine has been proposed to be a bona fide liquid biopsy for diagnosis and prognosis of BC, given the proximity of tumours. The presence of ctDNA has been found in urine and plasma of BC patients and multiple studies have shown that high levels of ctDNA could be observed in urine of patients with progressive disease, even if ctDNA was not detected in plasma. These results support the usage of both plasma and urine liquid biopsy to detect BC, as well as to monitor recurrence and progression of the disease (reviewed in [86]).

As previously mentioned, *TP53* mutations in urinary sediments from invasive BC patients were described three decades ago [82]. Ever since, specific mutation hotspots in some genes, such as *PIK3CA*, *TERT*, *FGFR3*, *RAS* and *TP53*, have been targeted to detect mutations in ctDNA from BC patients, which has led to the discovery of associations between the presence of ctDNA mutations in these genes in urine as well as plasma samples and disease recurrence and progression [102–104]. Furthermore, using multiplex ligation-dependent probe amplification and NGS, copy number variations (CNVs) and mutations in tumour-related genes in plasma and urine of non-metastatic BC patients were identified, respectively. In this study, Patel et al. reported that the most common mutated genes were *TP53*, *KRAS*, *PIK3CA*, *BRAF*, *CTNNB1* and *FGFR3* and they found a loss of *CDKN2A* and *CREBBP* and gain of *E2F3*, *SOX4*, *PPARG*, *YWHAZ* and *MYCL1* [102]. The presence of some of these ctDNA mutations in plasma or urine (with a technical threshold of 0.5%) has been associated with early disease recurrence, achieving a sensitivity of 83% and specificity of 100% [102]. In plasma from MIBC patients, who show a high mutation rate, at least one mutation in the *PIK3CA*, *TP53* or *ARDIA1* hotspot regions or promoter region of *TERT* gene has been detected in 90% of the cases, as well as CNVs, observing *TP53* and *RB1* inactivating changes, *MDM2* gain or *CDKN2A* loss [85].

Moreover, loss of heterozygosity (LOH) has been shown by microsatellite-based PCR analysis in serum, plasma and urine of BC patients [69,105,106]. Microsatellite instability and LOH in liquid biopsy samples of BC patients are found relatively frequently using markers to detect alterations on chromosomes 4, 8, 9, 14 and 17 [105,106]. Chromosomal regions 17p and 9p are often affected in BC, disrupting the activity of tumour suppressor genes *TP53* and *CDKN2A*. This LOH seems to be associated with reduced disease-free survival and high risk of disease progression [107,108]. Since mutations and CNVs in ctDNA from plasma and urinary biopsies are detectable in high levels before progression, even in NMIBC patient and especially in urine samples, these biomarkers may be useful for disease monitoring [103]. Besides, some studies have revealed unknown alterations with differential sensitivity to therapeutic agents in metastatic patients, emphasizing the importance of ctDNA analysis as a useful tool for the detection of markers of therapy response and guidance of individualized therapies [86].

On the other hand, epigenetic alterations can be detected in BC patients using methylation -specific PCR (MSP) on ctDNA [69]. The combination of methylation levels of the *POU4F2* and *PCDH17* or *TWIST1* and *NID2* genes in urine samples showed a high capacity to differentiate BC patients from healthy volunteers, with 90% sensitivity and 93–94% specificity in both cases [109,110]. Dulaimi et al. reported the hypermethylation of *APC*, *RASSF1A* or *CDKN2A* (p14ARF) in urine ctDNA from 39 out of 45 BC patients (87% sensitivity and 100% specificity), even detecting 16 cases that showed a negative result in cytology assays [111]. Accordingly, hypermethylated DNA in urine of BC patients seems to be more common than positive cytology [111]. Besides, Hoque and colleagues described the combined methylation analysis of *CDKN2A*, *MGMT* and *GSTP1* using urine, enabling the differentiation between BC patients and control subjects, achieving 69% sensitivity and 100% specificity [112]. Furthermore, promoter methylation of both *CDKN2A* (p14ARF) and *MGMT* has been associated with tumour stage and the addition of *GSTP1* and *TIMP3* promoter methylation allowed to discriminate invasive tumours [112]. In cell-free serum DNA, hypermethylation of *APC*, *GSTP1* or *TIG1* has been shown to allow distinction between BC patients and control subjects with 80% sensitivity and 93% specificity [113]. Thus, the potential importance of methylation markers has been proposed for BC prevention and guidance of individual patient management in unpredictable BCs [114–116].

In addition to the alterations found in ctDNA, some commercial kits are based on DNA modifications present in exfoliated cells of the urine sediment. The UroVysion BC Kit is a multi-target FISH assay using exfoliated cells in urine that identifies aneuploidy of chromosomes 3, 7 and 17, as well as the loss of the 9p21 locus (which harbours tumour suppressor gene *CDKN2A*) [117]. A meta-analysis from 14 studies showed that the UroVysion kit has a diagnostic accuracy of 72% sensitivity and 83% specificity (AUC = 0.87) [42] (Table 1). Furthermore, based on methylation patterns of urine exfoliated cells, the 150 loci UroMark assay allows the detection of primary BC when compared to non-BC urine with a sensitivity of 98% and specificity of 97% (AUC = 0.97) [43] (Table 1).

2.3. Circulating Cell-Free RNAs

The presence of circulating cell-free RNA in liquid biopsy samples of cancer patients was described three decades ago, when alterations in the expression levels of some of them were observed in different types of cancer patients [118–120] and even associations with clinical outcome and disease prognosis were found [121–124]. Ever since, coding (mRNA) and non-coding (miRNA, lncRNA and piwi-interacting RNA) cell-free RNAs have gained much relevance as potential biomarkers in these sample types. Subsequently, principal studies related to each type of cell-free RNA in liquid biopsy in BC are described:

2.3.1. Messenger RNAs

Circulating mRNAs were the first RNA molecules described in liquid biopsy in cancer patients [41]. Due to their intracellular role, cell-free mRNAs could be an important source of information about the status of activated or repressed signalling pathways into the tumour cells. Although a high percentage of these mRNAs are usually degraded by RNases, showing lack of stability and high variability between individuals [125–127], some mRNAs have demonstrated to have potential as biomarkers with diagnostic and predictive capacities.

With respect to total isoforms, the percentage of a full-length splicing variant of the *CA9* gene in urine sediments has shown to have diagnostic value to identify BC patients (AUC = 0.896) and this percentage was further increased in high grade and stage tumours [128]. Expression levels of *UBE2C* and *KRT20* mRNAs were significantly elevated in urine of urothelial cancer patients (sensitivity 82.5% and 85%; specificity 76.2% and 94.3%, respectively), increasing gradually with tumour grade and stage [129,130]. Bacchetti and collaborators observed significant differences in urine *PON2* expression when compared Ta and T1-3 tumours, showing higher expression in tumours confined to the basement membrane than in those invading other histological layers [131].

In order to improve the sensitivity and specificity of diagnostic and prognostic systems based on urine samples, several research groups have investigated different mRNA panels. Urquidi et al. carried out the combination of three different gene signatures [32,132,133] together with 6 other independent genes from different biomarker studies, after which they stablished a new diagnostic gene signature based on detected expression of 18 mRNAs (*ANXA10*, *BIRC5*, *CA9*, *CCL18*, *CDK1*, *CTSE*, *DSC2*, *IGF2*, *KFL9*, *KRT20*, *MDK*, *MMP1*, *MMP9*, *MMP10*, *MMP12*, *RAB1A*, *SEMA3D* and *SNAI2*) in urine samples from BC patients, achieving 85% sensitivity and 88% specificity (AUC = 0.935) [134]. Recently, the CxBladder Monitor and the Xpert Bladder Cancer Monitor (Table 1), two urine-based tests for BC surveillance which measure the expression levels of different sets of five mRNAs (*CDK1*, *CXCR2*, *HOXA13*, *IGFBP5* and *MDK*; and *ABL1*, *ANXA10*, *CRH*, *IGF2* and *UPK1B*, respectively), have been evaluated as follow-up methods for NMIBC patients after TURBT of primary or recurrent tumours. The CxBladder Monitor test was able to predict new recurrences after surgery with a sensitivity of 91% and a negative predictive value (NPV) of 96% (AUC = 0.73) [45,135], whereas the second test achieved a sensitivity of 84% and a specificity of 91% (AUC = 0.872) [47]. Biofina Diagnostics laboratory has developed a test based on ten differentially-expressed genes for the diagnosis and surveillance of BC from urine (UROBEST), achieving 80% sensitivity and 94% specificity (AUC = 0.91). Besides, the commercial laboratory Oncocyte has developed a panel of 43 gene expression biomarkers, PanC-Dx, to distinguish BC from non-cancerous conditions, showing good predictive values from urine samples (AUC = 0.91; sensitivity of 90% with a specificity of 82.5%) (Table 1) [48].

Besides instability and low abundance of circulating mRNAs, another problem associated to the use of mRNAs as biomarkers in liquid biopsy samples is the necessity of appropriate reference genes to compare the expression of target genes. Some studies have evaluated the expression of several potential housekeeping genes in urine samples, such as *PPIA*, *GAPDH*, *UBC*, *PGK1* and *ACTB* [132,136,137]. However, the potential of these and other genes as normalizers in biofluid samples should be studied more profoundly.

2.3.2. microRNAs

Over the last decade, microRNAs have represented a type of biomolecules widely studied as biomarkers in different pathologies, including several types of cancers [138,139]. Moreover, miRNAs expression is very homogeneous among individuals, showing specific expression profiles in different types of tissue [140]. Additionally, miRNAs are protected by a protein complex and they are usually included in exosomes, thereby preserving their integrity and avoiding RNase-mediated degradation [141,142]. Due to these properties, miRNAs are very stable in liquid biopsy samples, such as serum, plasma and urine [137,143], which makes them potential candidates as biomarkers in non-invasive diagnostic and prognostic methods. On the other hand, the new systems designed to perform RT-qPCR from miRNAs allow the study of a wide number of miRNAs from very small amounts of total RNA.

In BC, multiple studies have identified individual miRNAs or panels with predictive features. Some of the most relevant studies of miRNAs in urine samples are discussed next. Downregulation of miR-145 allows to distinguish BC patients from healthy controls (77.8% sensitivity and 61.1% specificity for NMIBC, AUC = 0.729; 84.1% and 61.1% for MIBC, respectively, AUC = 0.790) and shows correlation with tumour grade [144]. Furthermore, miR-106b and miR-146a-5p have shown to be upregulated in BC patients, correlating with tumour stage and with grade and invasion, respectively [145,146]. In addition, high expression of miR-452 and miR-222 (with respect to the miR-16 expression level as normalizer gene) has shown to have diagnostic value (AUC = 0.848 and AUC = 0.718, respectively) [147] and the miR-126: miR-152 ratio has also enabled the detection of BC (AUC = 0.768) [148]. Upregulation of miR-214 has been associated with NMIBC patients but not with tumour grade or stage. Curiously, BC patients with lower levels of miR-214 presented a higher risk of recurrence [149]. Zhang et al.

described that increased expression of miR-155 in urine is associated with tumour grade, stage, recurrence and invasion, allowing the discrimination of NMIBC patients, cystitis patients and healthy controls (80.2% sensitivity and 84.6% specificity) [150]. Besides, urine miR-200a has shown to have predictive properties, observing an association between low expression levels of this miRNA and high risk of recurrence in NMIBC patients [144]. Moreover, upregulation of miR-92a-3p and downregulation of miR-140-5p have been related to progression after recurrence [151].

On the other hand, there are some studies about miRNA expression in serum or plasma samples from BC patients, even though they are less frequent. High expression of miR-210 has been observed in serum of BC patients, correlating with tumour grade and stage and predicting progression (AUC = 0.898) [152]. In the case of plasma, expression of miR-19a is increased in tumour patients and associated with tumour grade [153], miR-200b is upregulated in MIBC, whilst miR-92 and miR-33 present inverse correlation with tumour stage [154].

Moreover, in the last years, several groups have developed multiple panels of miRNA expression, both in urine and in serum samples, to detect and monitor BC. Some of the main miRNA profiles are described in Table 2.

However, appropriate genes for normalization of miRNA expression in biofluids are unclear so far. In tissue samples, miRNA expression is usually normalized using the expression of small nuclear RNAs (snRNAs). Nevertheless, expression and stability of snRNAs is minimized in this type of sample [137], being inadequate as housekeeping genes. Although some authors have suggested some miRNAs, such as miR-16, miR-28-3p and miR-361-3p, as reference genes in urine samples [147,155], additional extensive studies are needed to determine specific housekeeping genes in the different types of liquid biopsies in this pathology. As observed for other tissues and disease conditions, specifically designed studies are required in order to find appropriate miRNAs, which do not show variation among the population to be separated (e.g., patients vs healthy controls, different disease state, metastatic vs non-metastatic disease), in serum and urine. In 2016, Martinez-Fernandez et al. described the use of two miRNAs, miR-193a and miR-448, as normalizers for urine studies [137]. However, these results still have to be validated in a well-designed clinical trial.

2.3.3. Long Non-Coding RNAs

Long non-coding RNAs (lncRNAs) are transcripts longer than 200 nucleotides that are not translated into protein and can modify gene expression at transcriptional, post-transcriptional and epigenetic levels [156]. Although lncRNAs have not been as widely studied as mRNAs or miRNAs, multiple studies have shown that expression of these molecules can be altered in cancer, promoting tumour development, progression and metastasis [157] and, therefore, their use as biomarkers in biofluids is of growing interest.

UCA1 (Urothelial cancer associated 1) is the most studied lncRNA in BC so far. Wang and collaborators determined that high expression of this lncRNA in urine sediments allows detection of high-grade superficial bladder tumours [158]. More recently, a meta-analysis of six studies, including 578 BC patients and 562 healthy controls, confirmed that upregulation of *UCA1* is able to predict BC (sensitivity of 81% and specificity of 86%, AUC = 0.88) [159]. Moreover, blood *UCA1* levels are upregulated in patients with metastatic BC after cisplatin treatment, increasing WNT6 protein expression and activating Wnt signalling, which results in cisplatin resistance [160]. Besides, overexpression of other lncRNAs, such as *HOTAIR*, *HOX-AS-2*, *MALAT1*, *HYMAI*, *LINC00477*, *LOC100506688* and *OTX2-AS1*, has been found in urine exosomes of high-grade MIBC patients [161]. On the other hand, other lncRNAs with biomarker potential are *ABHD11-AS1* and *H19* genes, whose increased expression has been associated with primary BC and early relapse, respectively, in tissue samples [162,163]. Future studies of these molecules in liquid biopsy samples of BC patients could be of great interest.

Table 2. Main miRNA panels for diagnosis, prognosis and recurrence surveillance of BC using liquid biopsy samples.

Studies [References]	Type of Sample	Clinical Application	miRNA Panels	Predictive Capacity
Sapre N. [164]	Urine	Recurrence surveillance	miR16, miR200c, miR205, miR21, miR221 and miR34a	Sensitivity = 88% Specificity = **48%** AUC = **0.74**–0.85
Pardini B. [155]	Urine	Diagnostic and prognosis	NMIBC G1 + G2 *: miR-30a-5p, let-7c-5p, miR-486-5p, miR-205-5p and let-7i-5p	AUC = 0.73
			NMIBC G3 *: miR-30a-5p, let-7c-5p, miR-486-5p, miR-21-5p, miR-106b-3p, miR-151a-3p, miR-200c-3p, miR-183-5p, miR-185-5p, miR-224-5p, miR-30c-2-5p and miR-10b-5p	AUC = 0.95
			MIBC *: miR-30a-5p, let-7c-5p, miR-486-5p, miR-205-5p, miR-451a, miR-25-3p, miR-30a-5p and miR-7-1-5p	AUC = 0.99
Jiang X. [165]	Serum	Diagnostic	miR-152, miR-148b-3p, miR-3187-3p, miR-15b-5p, miR-27a-3p and miR-30a-5p	AUC = 0.899
Jiang X. [166]	Serum	Prognosis	MIBC: miR-422a-3p, miR-486-3p, miR-103a-3p and miR-27a-3p	AUC = **0.880**–0.894
Du L. [167]	Urine	Diagnostic	miR-7-5p, miR-22-3p, miR-29a-3p, miR-126-5p, miR-200a-3p, miR-375 and miR-423-5p	Sensitivity = 82–85% Specificity = 87–96% AUC = **0.916**–0.923
Urquidi V. [168]	Urine	Diagnostic	miR-652, miR-199a-3p, miR-140-5p, miR-93, miR-142-5p, miR-1305, miR-30a, miR-224, miR-96, miR-766, miR-223, miR-99b, miR-140-3p, let-7b, miR-141, miR-191, miR-146b-5p, miR-491-5p, miR-339-3p, miR-200c, miR-106b *, miR-143, miR-429, miR-222 and miR-200a	Sensitivity = 87% Specificity = 100% AUC = 0.982

* Including traditional BC risk factors (age and smoking status). Bold numbers indicate values from validation set.

In addition, expression of different types of cell-free RNAs can be combined to improve the accuracy of individual tests. Accordingly, Eissa and colleagues developed a panel from urine samples which combines the expression of one mRNA (*HYAL1*; Hyaluronoglucosaminidase 1), two miRNAs (miR-210 and miR-96) and one lncRNA (*UCA1*), thereby achieving a sensitivity of 100% and a specificity of 89.5% [169].

2.3.4. Other Non-Coding RNAs and Its Future Potential as Biomarkers

Additionally, other non-coding RNAs, such as piwi-interacting RNAs (piRNAs) and circular RNAs (circRNAs) have been linked to BC. Although these molecules and their roles in cancer have been only recently studied, they could be good candidates as new biomarkers.

piRNAs are short single strands (26–31 nucleotides) of non-coding RNAs which can repress the expression of target genes, mediated by their binding to PIWI proteins (members of Argonaute proteins subfamily) [170]. Recently, several studies have reported that piRNAs can be widely detected in human plasma. Besides, the expression of some piRNAs has been found to be deregulated in patients with colorectal, prostate and pancreatic cancer [171,172]. Downregulation of piRNA DQ594040 has been associated with BC, whereas its overexpression can inhibit cell proliferation and promote cell apoptosis by upregulation of the TNFSF4 protein [173]. However, specific piRNAs have not yet been found in liquid biopsies from patients with BC.

circRNAs are a type of RNA which are covalently closed in a loop at the $3'$ and $5'$ ends. For this reason, these RNAs are more resistant than linear RNAs to degradation mediated by exonucleases and, therefore, show a prolonged half-life [174]. Although intra- and extra-cellular roles of these molecules are still largely unknown, some of them have shown relevance in several cancer types [175,176]. Overexpression of some circRNAs, such as circTCF25, circRNA-MYLK, circRNA-CTDP1 and circRNA-PC, has been observed in BC tissue samples. These circRNAs competitively bind to tumour suppressor miRNAs, acting as RNAs sponge and inhibiting their function [177–179]. Stability and functional properties of circRNAs make them interesting molecules to use as biomarkers in liquid biopsy samples.

2.4. Proteins and Peptides

The presence of proteins in liquid biopsy in cancer patients was first published in 1847 by Dr. Henry Bence Jones (reviewed in Reference [180]). Proteins and peptides (protein mass < 15 kDa) might be great candidates as biomarkers, since they are directly related to the "real-time" dynamic molecular cell phenotype. Nevertheless, the relevance of proteins and peptides as potential biomarkers in liquid biopsies has only been extensively studied over the last decade, due to limited technological advances. In BC, proteomic blood analyses [181,182] are scarce compared to the multiple studies performed with urine [53,132,169,183–201]. Plasma comprises the highly complex human-derived proteome, including the presence of a wide variety of proteins, which results in challenges with regard to detection and analysis systems. On the other hand, the urine proteome has been broadly studied and well-characterized, providing reference standards for data comparison and validation in the discovery of BC diagnostic markers [202].

2.4.1. Peptide Biomarkers

In 2006, Theodorescu and colleagues have reported a diagnostic 22-peptide biomarker panel, using capillary electrophoresis coupled to mass spectrometry, which enables the differentiation between urinary BC patient samples and control samples (from prostate cancer, prostate hyperplasia, renal diseases and urinary tract infection), achieving 100% sensitivity and 73% specificity [195]. However, out of the 22 peptides, only fibrinopeptide A has been identified. Even though this peptide biomarker panel allows a good discrimination between advanced cancer and controls, less advanced tumours could not be correctly classified by this panel. Accordingly, the use of a predictive four polypeptide panel (fragments of membrane-associated progesterone receptor component 1, Collagen α-1 (I), Collagen α-1 (III) and Uromodulin) has been proposed as a relevant approach to distinguish between NMIBC and MIBC, reaching 92% sensitivity and 68% specificity [196]. Recently, the previously mentioned studies have been refined by Frantzi and collaborators, who discriminated two different panels using urine by performing a multi-centre study including 1357 patients. A 116-peptide biomarker panel (including identified Apolipoprotein A (APOA), β2-microglobulin, collagen fragments, fibrinogen A, Haemoglobin A, histidine-rich glycoprotein, insulin and small proline-rich protein 3) has been indicated for BC diagnosis, achieving 91% sensitivity and 68% specificity. The second panel has been proposed to encompass 106 peptide biomarkers (including identified ADAM22, ADAMTS1, Apolipoprotein A-1 (APOA-1), collagen fragments and HSPG2) allowing the detection of BC recurrences with 87% sensitivity and 51% specificity [197].

2.4.2. Protein Biomarkers

Multiple proteomic studies have identified proteins (mass >15 kDa) and modifications with diagnostic and prognostic value in BC. However, a large variability has been observed between individual biomarker studies, reflecting proteomic complexity and the excess of applied proteomic approaches. Additionally, suboptimal experimental design of the individual studies contributes to inter-study inconsistency. Nevertheless, reproducible findings have also been reported in several independent studies. Some of the most relevant analyses are discussed next.

Differential expression of urinary α-1-antitrypsin (A1AT) has been indicated between BC patients and hernia patients (AUC = 0.729) as well as between BC patients and healthy controls (74% sensitivity and 80% specificity, AUC = 0.820) [198,199]. The upregulation of A1AT in patients with BC has subsequently been emphasized in an analysis by Linden and colleagues (66% sensitivity and 85% specificity) [200]. Besides, several studies have shown an increased abundance of apolipoprotein E (APOE) (89% sensitivity and 31% specificity, AUC = 0.745–0.756) and fibrinogen β (AUC = 0.720–0.831) in BC urinary biopsies compared to control patients [200,201]. Additionally, multiple studies have validated the importance of different apoliprotein types, reporting an increased abundance of APOA-1 in urine of BC patients (89–94.6% sensitivity and 85–92% specificity) compared to control patients, as well as an upregulation of APOA-2 (AUC = 0.631–0.864) in BC patients compared to hernia patients [183,198,201]. Besides, the differential expression of urinary carbonic anhydrase I and S100A8 between BC patients and hernia patients (AUC = 0.837 and AUC = 0.836, respectively) has been reported [198]. Moreover, Ebbing and colleagues have performed a study, including 181 samples from BC, prostate and renal cancer patients as well as healthy controls, in order to study the heterodimer S100A8/S100A9, known as calprotectin [184]. They showed a significant increase of calprotectin in BC biopsies (AUC = 0.880, 81% sensitivity and 93% specificity) compared to samples of the above-mentioned other tumour types and healthy controls [184]. In addition, Miyake et al. reported an increased abundance of COL4A1, COL13A1 and the combination of both collagens (COL4A1 + COL13A1) in BC urinary biopsies compared to healthy controls (sensitivity 68.2%, 54.6% and 72.1%; specificity 68.9%, 77.1% and 65.6%, respectively) [203]. Besides, the diagnostic sensitivity of this protein combination has been found to improve with malignancy grade, observing a value of 57.4% for low-grade tumours versus 83.7% for high-grade tumours [203].

The identification of biomarkers related to BC aggressiveness has been described by a limited number of studies. Zoidakis et al. performed a study including 108 BC patient samples and 97 urinary biopsies from control patients with benign disease (for example urolithisasis, benign prostate hyperplasia, infection/inflammation or haematuria) and found a differential expression of myeloblastin, aminopeptidase N and profilin-1 [185]. In addition, Nuclear interacting factor 1/Zinc finger 335 (NIF-1) and histone H2B have been described to be differently abundant in urinary biopsies from MIBC patients, NMIBC patients and benign controls [186].

Additionally, multiple analyses have been performed using protein panels, which might enhance accuracy in BC detection. In 2012, Goodison and colleagues proposed the use of a diagnostic 8-protein biomarker panel (angiogenin (ANG), APOE, CA9, IL8, matrix metallopeptidase 9 (MMP9), MMP10, plasminogen activator inhibitor 1 (PAI-1) and vascular endothelial growth factor A (VEGFA)) to distinguish BC patients and healthy controls in a study encompassing 127 urine biopsies, achieving 92% sensitivity and 97% specificity (AUC = 0.980) [187]. Additionally, Rosser et al. showed that a similar protein biomarker panel, namely the previously described 8-protein biomarker panel without CA9, enables the differentiation between BC patients and patients with different urological disorders (74% sensitivity and 90% specificity) [188]. Besides, Urquidi and collaborators reported a 3-protein biomarker panel (PAI-1, CD44 antigen and C-C motif chemokine 18 (CCL18)) to discriminate BC patients from healthy controls [204]. In 2014, Rosser et al. described the combination of 10 proteins (ANG, APOE, CA9, IL8, MMP9, MMP10, SDC1, Serpin Family A Member 1 (SERPINA1), Serpin Family E Member 1 (SERPINE1) and VEGFA) as a potential biomarker panel to detect recurrent disease in urine (79% sensitivity and 88% specificity) [189]. Two years later, Shimizu and colleagues published a comparable study using a similar protein panel (including PAI-1 and A1AT instead of SERPINA1 and SERPINE1) which allowed the differentiation of BC patients from benign and healthy controls, achieving 85% sensitivity and 81% specificity [190]. Recently, Soukap and collaborators reported the value of a 2-protein biomarker panel (synuclein G and midkine) combined with cytology in BC detection (91.8% sensitivity and 97.5% specificity) and showed that the addition of CEACAM1 and ZAG2 proteins to this panel enables the prediction of BC recurrences, achieving 92.7% sensitivity and 90.2% specificity [191].

As previously mentioned, only a limited number of plasma proteomic studies have currently been reported. Bansal et al. have proposed two differently expressed proteins, S100A8 and S100A9, distinguishing BC patients from healthy controls (AUC = 0.850–0.856 and AUC = 0.902–0.957) [181,182]. Moreover, in pre-operative compared to post-operative BC sera samples, a significantly increased abundance of annexin V was observed as well as a reduction of CA1, S100A4, S100A8 and S100A9 [181]. An upregulation of CA1 has also been observed in BC patients compared to healthy controls (AUC = 0.891–0.908) [181,182].

Overall, the previously described studies emphasize the diagnostic value of protein biomarker panels and individual protein biomarkers. However, their clinical value is still compromised due to suboptimal experimental design including benign or healthy controls (instead of clinically relevant patients) in many of the reported analyses, resulting in over-representation of BC. Nevertheless, some FDA-approved and non-approved diagnostic protein biomarkers are currently commercially available for clinical practice in BC (Table 1) and will be discussed next.

One of the most extensively studied proteins in BC urinary biopsies is Nuclear Matrix Protein 22 (NMP22) and multiple studies have demonstrated the use of this protein as a diagnostic BC biomarker, achieving 75–100% sensitivity and 75.9–91.8% specificity [169,192–194]. Mowatt and colleagues reported a pooled data analysis, encompassing a total of 13885 patients from 41 studies, showing that the performance of biomarker NMP22 exceeds cytology in BC detection with regard to sensitivity of the approach (68% versus 44%), mainly due to an improved detection of low-grade tumours [50,205]. Two assays, NMP22 BC test kit and NMP22 BladderChek Test, are currently in clinical use to detect NMP22 in urine. The NMP22 BC test kit represents the original approach based on a quantitative sandwich enzyme-linked immunosorbent assay (ELISA) test using two antibodies and has been FDA-approved for BC surveillance achieving 40% sensitivity and 99% specificity [49] (Table 1). On the other hand, the NMP22 BladderChek Test relies on a qualitative approach designed as a point of care (POC) analysis. The NMP22 BladderChek Test has been approved by the FDA for both BC surveillance and BC diagnosis (68% sensitivity and 79% specificity) [50] (Table 1). Grossman and collaborators analysed the clinical accuracy of the NMP22 BladderChek Test in two multi-centre studies [206,207], showing an increased sensitivity compared to cytology (56% versus 16%, respectively) in patients with haematuria but it did not reach the level of specificity obtained by cytology (86% versus 99%, respectively) [207]. Additionally, a combination of NMP22 BladderChek Test and cystoscopy has been observed to significantly enhance the detection of BC recurrence (up to 99%) compared to cystoscopy alone (91%) [206].

Next to NMP22, the bladder tumour antigen (BTA) has been approved by the FDA as a diagnostic biomarker in BC [208,209]. A pooled data analysis of 23 studies encompassing a total of 2258 BC patients and 2994 non-cancer individuals has shown that BTA allows for the differentiation of BC patients, achieving a mean sensitivity of 64% and specificity of 76.6% [53]. Two assays, BTA stat and BTA TRAK, have been developed for the detection of BTA in urine. BTA TRAK is an ELISA based approach, which has been approved for BC diagnosis, achieving 66% sensitivity and 65% specificity [51,210] (Table 1). BTA stat represents a qualitative assay for POC analysis, accepted for BC diagnosis with 70% sensitivity and 75% specificity [51,210] (Table 1). Besides, it has to be taken into account that multiple studies excluded patients with benign genitourinary conditions and including these patients would drastically diminish the BTA test specificity [211]. Therefore, this biomarker has currently limited clinical value.

On the other hand, cytokeratin fragment 21.1 (CYFRA 21.1) represents an ELISA test detecting soluble cytokeratin 19 fragments [52]. Multiple studies have reported that CYFRA 21.1 allows differentiation between liquid biopsies of BC patients and patients with non-cancer conditions, achieving 70–90% sensitivity and 73–86% specificity (AUC = 0.87–0.90) [52,53,212]. The specificity of this test dramatically decreases with the inclusion of patients with history of BCG and radiotherapy, excluding current use of the CYFRA 21.1 assay as a BC surveillance test [213,214].

Additionally, bladder cancer rapid test represents an urinary BC (UBC) test based on the detection of soluble fragments of cytokeratin 8 and 18, either using a quantitative ELISA or qualitative POC assay [215]. Multiple reports have shown that the UBC test enables the discrimination of BC patients compared to non-cancer individuals with a mean sensitivity of 64.4% and specificity of 80.3% [53,215]. Subsequently, Babjuk et al. described an increase in sensitivity (79%) as well as a decrease in specificity (49%) for the UBC test, once patients with benign conditions or other urinary tract malignancies were included [216]. In these cases, the BTA tests exceed the UBC rapid test regarding their use in BC detection [216].

2.5. Metabolites

The application of metabolomics in cancer is increasing over the years as this approach has shown importance in the search for candidate biomarkers. Since tumour cells are known to have altered metabolic pathways, metabolites in body fluids could be promising for the assessment of pathology, progression and prognosis of cancer [217]. Moreover, metabolomics has recently proved to be useful in the area of biomarker discovery for cancers in which early diagnostic and prognostic is urgently needed, such as BC. Given that the bladder is in intimate contact with urine, this body fluid has been mined heavily for metabolite biomarkers [218].

The use of metabolomic analysis in BC has been primarily focused on the distinction between normal-appearing urothelium and BC. Zhou et al. found a urinary four-biomarker panel (5-hydroxyvaleric acid, cholesterol, 3-phosphoglyceric acid and glycolic acid) including important metabolic characteristics (e.g., organic acid metabolism, steroid hormone biosynthesis, glycolysis and glyoxylate metabolism) and defined this panel as a combinatorial biomarker for the differentiation between BC patients and healthy controls (AUC = 0.804 with 78.0% sensitivity and 70.3% specificity in the validation set) [219,220]. Besides, Huang and colleagues reported the elevation of component I and decrease of carnitine C9:1 in BC urine samples, compared to healthy controls, as a promising biomarker panel for the identification of BC patients (92.6% sensitivity and 96.9% specificity; AUC = 0.963) [221]. However, the structure and biological function of component I is still unclear and required to be studied as it has not been previously observed in nature. Nevertheless, carnitines are an example of disturbed fatty acid transportation, fatty acid-oxidation, or energy metabolism that is happening in tumour cells [221]. Supporting these findings, Ganti proposed that acylcarnitine appearance in BC patient urine samples varies widely in function of tumour grade, suggesting that consistently lower levels of acylcarnitines are present in the urinary biopsies of BC patients with low grade tumours as compared to both BC patients with high grade tumours as well as healthy controls [222]. These results have raised the possibility that fatty acid abnormalities might be involved in the pathogenesis of the tumour.

Moreover, Sahu and colleagues confirmed unique pathway alterations that differentiate MIBC and NMIBC [223]. MIBC appears to preferentially enhance cyclooxygenase (COX) and lipoxygenase (LOX) signalling (Eicosanoids, prostaglandins and trombaxanes (p-value < 0.004), increase heme catabolism (p = 0.0001) and alter nicotinamide adenine dinucleotide (NAD+) synthesis (kynurenine (p = 0.0212), anthranilate (p = 0.0111) and quinolate (p = 0.0015)) [223] with a possible influence in inflammatory cell regulation, cell proliferation and angiogenesis [224,225]. Supporting these results, Loras and colleagues were recently able to identify metabolites in urine enabling the discrimination of BC patients with a high sensitivity (87.9%) and specificity (100%) and a negative likelihood value of 0.1, as well high negative predictive values for low, low-intermediate and high-intermediate and high-risk patients [226]. Metabolomic analysis revealed altered phenylalanine, arginine, proline and tryptophan intermediate metabolism associated to NMIBC [226]. These studies suggest that different stages/grades of BC might generate distinct metabolic profiles, which might be due to the fact that cancer cells in advanced grades/stages require more energy for survival and continuous growing.

Next to the use of urinary analysis for the identification of metabolites as possible biomarkers, the evaluation of global serum profiles of BC, kidney cancer and non-cancer controls has revealed potential biomarkers for BC, including eicosatrienol (AUC = 0.98), azaprostanoic acid (AUC = 0.977), docosatrienol (AUC = 0.972), retinol (AUC = 0.801) and 14'-apo-beta-carotenal (AUC = 0.767) [227].

Overall, the BC metabolic signature is mainly characterized by alterations in metabolites related to energy metabolic pathways, amino acid and fatty acid metabolism, which are known to be crucial for cell proliferation as well as glutathione metabolism, a determinant in maintaining cellular redox balance [228]. However, the absence of a standard for sample acquisition, use of different platforms to profile metabolites, environmental stress and food intake strongly influence the composition of the metabolome and all these factors have led to a large diversity of metabolomic profiles obtained from different laboratories. These issues need to be considered, since they heavily affect the quality of the results by introducing bias and artefacts. Nevertheless, despite remaining challenges, metabolomics shows great clinical promise. The improved sensitivity, specificity of technics and the development of an in-depth reference metabolome may help to identify good metabolic biomarkers which can eventually be translated into the clinic.

2.6. Extracellular Vesicles

The concept of extracellular vesicles (EVs) has evolved from being considered garbage bags to the demonstration that extracellular vesicles could play very interesting roles and functions in cancer biology by promoting survival and growth of disseminated tumour cells; enhancing invasiveness; promoting angiogenesis, migration, tumour cell viability and inhibiting tumour cell apoptosis [229,230]. EVs include microvesicles, apoptotic bodies and exosomes, with the latter being mostly studied at present. Therefore, in this review, we will mainly focus on the potential of exosomes as cancer biomarkers in BC.

Exosomes are small (30–100 nm) membrane vesicles released into the extracellular environment due to fusion of multivesicular bodies with the plasma membrane. They were first described in 1983 in two different papers, published simultaneously [231,232] and currently tumour-released microvesicles, which are abundant in the body fluids of patients with cancer, are suggested to be involved in tumour progression [233]. Besides, it has been demonstrated that exosomes may help in immune response modulation, presentation of antigens to immune cells and intercellular communication through transfer of proteins, mRNAs and miRNAs, which could be a useful tool for diagnostic, predictive and prognostic purposes in different types of tumours. Regarding this, Valenti and colleagues showed that another kind of EVs, microvesicles, released by human melanoma and colorectal carcinoma cells, can promote the differentiation of monocytes to myeloid-derived suppressor cells, which support tumoral growth and immune escape [234].

Currently, there is an increasing interest in the application of exosomes as non-invasive cancer biomarkers and many studies have demonstrated that molecules, such as the lncRNAs *HOTAIR*, *HOX-AS-2*, among others and proteins, like EDIL3 and periostin, are significantly altered in patients with BC [161]. Therefore, EVs are proposed to be enriched in proteins that can be associated with signalling pathways related to tumorigenesis. In this way, Silvers reported that EVs collected from urine of six BC patients (pT1-pT3) showed, at least, a fifteen fold enrichment in the protein levels of β-Hexosaminidase (HEXB), S100A4 and Staphylococcal nuclease and tumour domain containing 1 (SND1) compared to the urinary protein levels of six healthy volunteers ($p < 0.05$) [235]. However, despite these promising preliminary results, the size of this study population is confined and additional extensive research is required for the validation of these data.

Furthermore, based on their stability in body fluids, especially exosomal miRNAs are discussed to be useful diagnostic and prognostic biomarkers in liquid biopsies. Baumgart and colleagues showed that exosomes from invasive BC cell lines, compared to non-invasive BC cell lines, are characterized by a specific miRNA signature which could play a role in the modification of the tumour microenvironment ($p < 0.05$; FC > 1.5) [236]. These results confirmed the hypothesis that the molecular content of exosomes is, at least in part, similar to that of host cells and reflects their cellular properties. However, Baumgart also analysed urinary exosomes from BC patients and they exhibited only in part the miRNA alterations detected in cell line exosomes [236]. Therefore, further analyses will have to clarify the functional relevance of exosomal miRNAs and their role as molecular markers in liquid biopsies.

Even though EVs are a promising source of cancer biomarkers, few studies have been done and no exosomal biomarkers have been implemented in BC clinical practice so far. In general, the interest in EVs is growing but the introduction as established predictive biomarkers has been hampered by challenges in exosome isolation and characterization, indicating the need for new sensitive platforms which allow more accurate isolation and detection methods. Furthermore, the use of an efficient, rapid and reproducible isolation method is fundamental for analytical reproducibility.

3. Summary and Discussion

Among body fluids, urine and saliva are the most attractive fluids for liquid biopsy due to their accessibility and low invasiveness of collection. As somatic alterations detected in ctDNA are reflective for those present in tumour tissue, the ctDNA profile could be a practical method for obtaining the tumour genome independently of direct tissue sequencing. Additionally, mutations in ctDNA of cancer patients could be detected over one year prior to clinical diagnosis, which emphasizes the great potential of liquid biopsy for the detection of cancer at early stages [98,237,238]. At present, there are several diagnostic kits based on the detection of mutations in liquid biopsy samples using ctDNA or CTCs from the bloodstream. Most of them have been designed for blood/plasma/serum samples using qPCR and NGS techniques. Only the diagnostic kit Trovera (initially designed for the identification of mutations in *BRAF*, *KRAS*, *EGFR* in plasma samples; Trovagene) is marketed for both plasma and urine samples. A diagnostic alternative is based on the detection of both circulating RNA and extracellular vesicles (such as exosomes), for which multiple diagnostic kits are brought on the market in order to detect and monitor prostate (like ExoDx Prostate; IntelliScore) or bladder (like CxBladder; Pacific Edge, among others) cancer in urine samples.

Although it is true that urine can reflect genetic alterations of a large number of solid tumours [239], it will probably be more relevant for the diagnosis and monitoring of tumours of the genitourinary tract. In these cases, the content of nucleic acids from the tumour cells is released directly into the urine, which minimalizes the DNA/RNA contamination background of blood cells as observed in plasma (Figure 3) [240].

As previously mentioned, the high recurrence rate and the need for expensive diagnostic and monitoring methods, such as cystoscopy, make BC the most expensive human cancer from diagnosis to death. For this reason, efforts to develop diagnostic, prognostic and follow-up systems for BC have been enormous in recent years, with various systems published for liquid biopsy samples. Accordingly, several diagnostic laboratories have launched different diagnostic and monitoring systems for BC patients, which are based on the determination of gene expression or protein biomarkers in urine samples (Table 1). Moreover, the identification of metabolites as potential biomarker in BC liquid biopsy has also been explored. Several authors have found specific metabolites that are able to identify patients with BC, even before appearance of the first clinical symptoms of this disease [241]. However, the main concern regarding metabolomics in urine as a diagnostic system is the variability of glomerular filtration, both with medication and dietary habits as the main confounding factors [242,243]. Therefore, large cohort studies and standardization of sample taking and processing procedures will be necessary to finally establish metabolomics as a diagnostic approach.

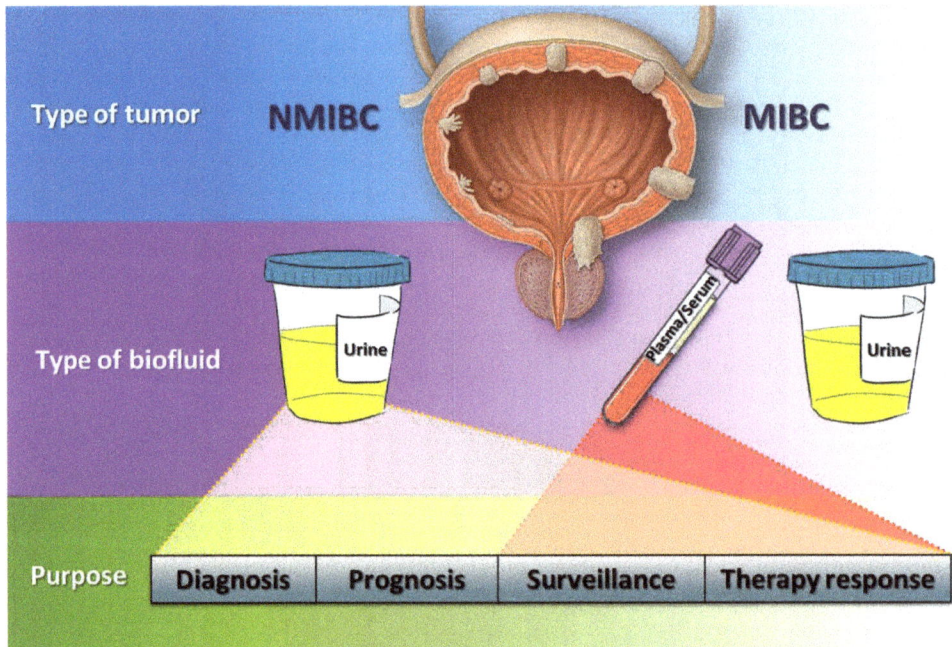

Figure 3. Hypothetical flowchart of liquid biopsies management in BC. In NMIBC patients, urine could be the best type of biofluid for diagnosis, prognosis, surveillance and therapy response due to its intimate contact with the tumour, whilst in MIBC patients, though urine could also be used, plasma and serum acquire more importance to monitor patients.

Regarding MIBC patient follow-up, it should be taken into account that, even though cystectomy is performed in most cases, progression of bladder tumours is produced by metastasis in other tissues and organs. In case of metastatic tumours, blood becomes perhaps the most appropriate fluid for follow-up and to explore possible therapies once progression of the disease is established (Figure 3). Therefore, the determination of mutations or alterations of gene expression patterns has been explored from both ctDNA in plasma/serum and from the isolation of CTCs in the bloodstream (reviewed in [244–246]). However, care must be taken with predictions regarding the future of these new technologies and the studies that support them. Some of the current FDA-approved systems for the diagnosis and monitoring of BC do not meet sensitivity and specificity requirements (e.g., the NMP22 determination), whereas other tests have such high costs that their use in daily health practice is limited (e.g., the UroVysion test). Consequently, there is an urgent need for suitable studies in order to validate biomarkers for early detection. Nevertheless, conventional case-control studies have proven not to be adequate, emphasizing the importance of prospective cohort studies, consisting of serial samples at different time points from a person at-risk, as well as large randomized trials, validating biomarker clinical benefit compared to actual gold standard methods. Additionally, a coherent and comprehensive set of guidelines must be delineated to ensure success once an approach is approved for clinical set-up. For example, Pepe et al. described a prospective randomized open blinded end-point (PROBE) study design which takes into account components related to the clinical context and outcomes, criteria for measuring biomarker performance, the biomarker test itself and the size of the study as a guidance for the design of a biomarker accuracy study [247]. Besides, sample repositories (crucial for the discovery and evaluation of biomarkers with potential use in clinical medicine) should follow this design strategy in order to maximize biomarker values.

4. Concluding Remarks

In general, physicians and researchers agree that liquid biopsy is the most promising strategy for diagnostics, selection of treatments and follow-up in various tumour types. However, it is important that the development of these new diagnostic and follow-up systems come together with the appropriate proposals for changes in the therapeutic procedure, either with a better characterization of the patients or with an adequate proposal of an effective treatment line. On the other hand, the lack of validation of these systems, which are capable of detecting a tumour burden much smaller than the imaging technologies, currently prevents them from clinical practice, since they can generate great anxiety among patients and possibly lead to overtreatment of the patient. Therefore, more studies with long follow-up periods and large cohorts are required to demonstrate that the positive result in a liquid biopsy test is valid as a starting point to initiate or change an oncologic treatment. However, despite the difficulties and current limitations in liquid biopsy technologies and the current lack of robust and confident methodologies that unequivocally allow diagnosis, prognosis or detection of therapy response, with the current accumulation of clinical evidence, we are convinced that it will only be a matter of time until liquid biopsy replaces tissue biopsy in all solid tumours.

Author Contributions: All authors contributed equally to review the current literature and write specific sections. The whole work was coordinated by J.M.P. and C.S.-C. All the authors agreed with the final version.

funding: This study was funded by the following: FEDER cofounded MINECO grant SAF2015-66015-R, grant ISCIII-RETIC RD12/0036/0009, PIE 15/00076 and CB/16/00228 to Jesús M. Paramio.

Conflicts of Interest: The authors declare no conflict of interest.

References

1. Ferlay, J.; Soerjomataram, I.; Dikshit, R.; Eser, S.; Mathers, C.; Rebelo, M.; Parkin, D.M.; Forman, D.; Bray, F. Cancer incidence and mortality worldwide: Sources, methods and major patterns in GLOBOCAN 2012. *Int. J. Cancer* **2015**, *136*, E359–E386. [CrossRef] [PubMed]
2. Witjes, J.A.; Lebret, T.; Compérat, E.M.; Cowan, N.C.; de Santis, M.; Bruins, H.M.; Hernández, V.; Espinós, E.L.; Dunn, J.; Rouanne, M.; et al. Updated 2016 EAU guidelines on guscle-invasive and metastatic bladder cancer. *Eur. Urol.* **2017**, *71*, 462–475. [CrossRef] [PubMed]
3. Babjuk, M.; Böhle, A.; Burger, M.; Capoun, O.; Cohen, D.; Compérat, E.M.; Hernández, V.; Kaasinen, E.; Palou, J.; Rouprêt, M.; et al. EAU guidelines on non-muscle-invasive urothelial carcinoma of the bladder: Update 2016. *Eur. Urol.* **2017**, *71*, 447–461. [CrossRef] [PubMed]
4. Babjuk, M. Trends in bladder cancer incidence and mortality: Success or disappointment? *Eur. Urol.* **2017**, *71*, 109–110. [CrossRef] [PubMed]
5. Robertson, A.G. Comprehensive molecular characterization of muscle-invasive bladder cancer. *Cell* **2017**, *171*, 540–556. [CrossRef] [PubMed]
6. Berdik, C. Unlocking bladder cancer. *Nature* **2017**, *551*, S34–S35. [CrossRef] [PubMed]
7. Humphrey, P.A.; Moch, H.; Cubilla, A.L.; Ulbright, T.M.; Reuter, V.E. The 2016 WHO Classification of tumours of the urinary system and male genital organs—Part B: Prostate and bladder tumours. *Eur. Urol.* **2016**, *70*, 106–119. [CrossRef] [PubMed]

8. Noone, A.; Howlader, N.; Krapcho, M.; Miller, D.; Brest, A.; Yu, M.; Ruhl, J.; Tatalovich, Z.; Mariotto, A.; Lewis, D.; et al. SEER Cancer Statistics Review, 1975–2015. National Cancer Institute: Bethesda, MD. Available online: https://seer.cancer.gov/csr/1975_2015/ (accessed on 12 August 2018).
9. Knowles, M.A.; Hurst, C.D. Molecular biology of bladder cancer: New insights into pathogenesis and clinical diversity. *Nat. Rev. Cancer* **2015**, *15*, 25. [CrossRef] [PubMed]
10. Pietzak, E.J.; Bagrodia, A.; Cha, E.K.; Drill, E.N.; Iyer, G.; Isharwal, S.; Ostrovnaya, I.; Baez, P.; Li, Q.; Berger, M.F.; et al. Next-generation sequencing of nonmuscle invasive bladder cancer reveals potential biomarkers and rational therapeutic targets. *Eur. Urol.* **2017**, *6*, 952–959. [CrossRef] [PubMed]
11. Van Rhijn, B.W.G.; Burger, M.; Lotan, Y.; Solsona, E.; Stief, C.G.; Sylvester, R.J.; Witjes, J.A.; Zlotta, A.R. Recurrence and progression of disease in non-muscle-invasive bladder cancer: From epidemiology to treatment strategy. *Eur. Urol.* **2009**, *56*, 430–442. [CrossRef] [PubMed]
12. Sylvester, R.J.; Oosterlinck, W.; Witjes, J.A. The schedule and duration of intravesical chemotherapy in patients with non-muscle-invasive bladder cancer: A systematic review of the published results of randomized clinical trials. *Eur. Urol.* **2008**, *53*, 709–719. [CrossRef] [PubMed]
13. Shariat, S.F.; Zippe, C.; Lübecke, G.; Boman, H.; Sanchez-Carbayo, M.; Casella, R.; Mian, C.; Friedrich, M.G.; Eissa, S.; Akaza, H.; et al. Nomograms including nuclear matrix protein 22 for prediction of disease recurrence and progression in patients with Ta, T1 or CIS transitional cell carcinoma of the bladder. *J. Urol.* **2005**, *173*, 1518–1525. [CrossRef] [PubMed]
14. Lee, D.J.; Chang, S.S. Cost Considerations in the Management of Bladder Cancer. *Urol. Times*. Available online: http://www.urologytimes.com/modern-medicine-feature-articles/cost-considerations-management-bladder-cancer (accessed on 16 October 2017).
15. Mariotto, A.B.; Yabroff, K.R.; Shao, Y.; Feuer, E.J.; Brown, M.L. Projections of the cost of cancer care in the United States: 2010–2020. *J. Natl. Cancer Inst.* **2011**, *103*, 117–128. [CrossRef] [PubMed]
16. Leal, J.; Luengo-Fernandez, R.; Sullivan, R.; Witjes, J.A. Economic Burden of Bladder Cancer across the European Union. *Eur. Urol.* **2016**, *69*, 438–447. [CrossRef] [PubMed]
17. Wolff, E.M.; Liang, G.; Jones, P.A. Mechanisms of disease: Genetic and epigenetic alterations that drive bladder cancer. *Nat. Clin. Pract. Urol.* **2005**, *2*, 502. [CrossRef] [PubMed]
18. Burger, M.; Catto, J.W.F.; Dalbagni, G.; Grossman, H.B.; Herr, H.; Karakiewicz, P.; Kassouf, W.; Kiemeney, L.A.; La Vecchia, C.; Shariat, S.; et al. Epidemiology and risk factors of urothelial bladder cancer. *Eur. Urol.* **2013**, *63*, 234–241. [CrossRef] [PubMed]
19. Griffiths, G.; Hall, R.; Sylvester, R.; Raghavan, D.; Parmar, M. International phase III trial assessing neoadjuvant cisplatin, methotrexate, and vinblastine chemotherapy for muscle-invasive bladder cancer: Long-term results of the BA06 30894 trial. *J. Clin. Oncol.* **2011**, *29*, 2171–2177. [CrossRef] [PubMed]
20. Advanced Bladder Cancer (ABC) Meta-Analysis Collaboration. Neoadjuvant chemotherapy in invasive bladder cancer: Update of a systematic review and meta-analysis of individual patient data advanced bladder cancer (ABC) meta-analysis collaboration. *Eur. Urol.* **2005**, *48*, 202–205. [CrossRef] [PubMed]
21. Yuh, B.E.; Ruel, N.; Wilson, T.G.; Vogelzang, N.; Pal, S.K. Pooled analysis of clinical outcomes with neoadjuvant cisplatin and gemcitabine chemotherapy for muscle invasive bladder cancer. *J. Urol.* **2013**, *189*, 1682–1686. [CrossRef] [PubMed]
22. Stenzl, A.; Cowan, N.C.; de Santis, M.; Kuczyk, M.A.; Merseburger, A.S.; Ribal, M.J.; Sherif, A.; Witjes, J.A. Treatment of muscle-invasive and metastatic bladder cancer: Update of the EAU guidelines. *Actas Urol. Españolas* **2012**, *36*, 449–460. [CrossRef]
23. Pal, S.K.; Milowsky, M.I.; Plimack, E.R. Optimizing systemic therapy for bladder cancer. *J. Natl. Compr. Cancer Netw.* **2013**, *11*, 793–804. [CrossRef]
24. Bellmunt, J.; de Wit, R.; Vaughn, D.J.; Fradet, Y.; Lee, J.-L.; Fong, L.; Vogelzang, N.J.; Climent, M.A.; Petrylak, D.P.; Choueiri, T.K.; et al. Pembrolizumab as Second-Line Therapy for Advanced Urothelial Carcinoma. *N. Engl. J. Med.* **2017**, *376*, 1015–1026. [CrossRef] [PubMed]
25. Powles, T.; Eder, J.P.; Fine, G.D.; Braiteh, F.S.; Loriot, Y.; Cruz, C.; Bellmunt, J.; Burris, H.A.; Petrylak, D.P.; Teng, S.L.; et al. MPDL3280A (anti-PD-L1) treatment leads to clinical activity in metastatic bladder cancer. *Nature* **2014**, *515*, 558–562. [CrossRef] [PubMed]

26. Blick, C.G.T.; Nazir, S.A.; Mallett, S.; Turney, B.W.; Onwu, N.N.; Roberts, I.S.D.; Crew, J.P.; Cowan, N.C. Evaluation of diagnostic strategies for bladder cancer using computed tomography (CT) urography, flexible cystoscopy and voided urine cytology: Results for 778 patients from a hospital haematuria clinic. *BJU Int.* **2012**, *110*, 84–94. [CrossRef] [PubMed]
27. Van Rhijn, B.W.G.; van der Poel, H.G.; van der Kwast, T.H. Cytology and Urinary Markers for the Diagnosis of Bladder Cancer. *Eur. Urol. Suppl.* **2009**, *8*, 536–541. [CrossRef]
28. Fradet, Y.; Lockhard, C. Performance characteristics of a new monoclonal antibody test for bladder cancer: ImmunoCyt trade mark. *Can. J. Urol.* **1997**, *4*, 400–405. [PubMed]
29. He, H.; Han, C.; Hao, L.; Zang, G. ImmunoCyt test compared to cytology in the diagnosis of bladder cancer: A meta-analysis. *Oncol. Lett.* **2016**, *12*, 83–88. [CrossRef] [PubMed]
30. Glatz, K.; Willi, N.; Glatz, D.; Barascud, A.; Grilli, B.; Herzog, M.; Dalquen, P.; Feichter, G.; Gasser, T.C.; Sulser, T.; et al. An international telecytologic quiz on urinary cytology reveals educational deficits and absence of a commonly used classification system. *Am. J. Clin. Pathol.* **2006**, *126*, 294–301. [CrossRef] [PubMed]
31. Kehinde, E.O.; Al-Mulla, F.; Kapila, K.; Anim, J.T. Comparison of the sensitivity and specificity of urine cytology, urinary nuclear matrix protein-22 and multitarget fluorescence in situ hybridization assay in the detection of bladder cancer. *Scand. J. Urol. Nephrol.* **2011**, *45*, 113–121. [CrossRef] [PubMed]
32. O'Sullivan, P.; Sharples, K.; Dalphin, M.; Davidson, P.; Gilling, P.; Cambridge, L.; Harvey, J.; Toro, T.; Giles, N.; Luxmanan, C.; et al. A Multigene Urine Test for the Detection and Stratification of Bladder Cancer in Patients Presenting with Hematuria. *J. Urol.* **2012**, *188*, 741–747. [CrossRef] [PubMed]
33. Loidl, W.; Schmidbauer, J.; Susani, M.; Marberger, M. Flexible cystoscopy assisted by hexaminolevulinate induced fluorescence: A new approach for bladder cancer detection and surveillance? *Eur. Urol.* **2005**, *47*, 323–326. [CrossRef] [PubMed]
34. Crowley, E.; Di Nicolantonio, F.; Loupakis, F.; Bardelli, A. Liquid biopsy: Monitoring cancer-genetics in the blood. *Nat. Rev. Clin. Oncol.* **2013**, *10*, 472–484. [CrossRef] [PubMed]
35. Bardelli, A.; Pantel, K. Liquid Biopsies, What We Do Not Know (Yet). *Cancer Cell* **2017**, *31*, 172–179. [CrossRef] [PubMed]
36. Di Meo, A.; Bartlett, J.; Cheng, Y.; Pasic, M.D.; Yousef, G.M. Liquid biopsy: A step forward towards precision medicine in urologic malignancies. *Mol. Cancer* **2017**, *16*, 80. [CrossRef] [PubMed]
37. Heitzer, E.; Perakis, S.; Geigl, J.B.; Speicher, M.R. The potential of liquid biopsies for the early detection of cancer. *NPJ Precis. Oncol.* **2017**, *1*, 36. [CrossRef] [PubMed]
38. Khetrapal, P.; Lee, M.W.L.; Tan, W.S.; Dong, L.; de Winter, P.; Feber, A.; Kelly, J.D. The role of circulating tumour cells and nucleic acids in blood for the detection of bladder cancer: A systematic review. *Cancer Treat. Rev.* **2018**, *66*, 56–63. [CrossRef] [PubMed]
39. Siravegna, G.; Marsoni, S.; Siena, S.; Bardelli, A. Integrating liquid biopsies into the management of cancer. *Nat. Rev. Clin. Oncol.* **2017**, *14*, 531–548. [CrossRef] [PubMed]
40. Wan, J.C.M.; Massie, C.; Garcia-Corbacho, J.; Mouliere, F.; Brenton, J.D.; Caldas, C.; Pacey, S.; Baird, R.; Rosenfeld, N. Liquid biopsies come of age: Towards implementation of circulating tumour DNA. *Nat. Rev. Cancer* **2017**, *17*, 223–238. [CrossRef] [PubMed]
41. Mandel, P.; Metais, P. Les acides nucléiques du plasma sanguin chez l'homme. *C. R. Seances Soc. Biol. Fil.* **1948**, *142*, 241–243. [PubMed]
42. Hajdinjak, T. UroVysion FISH test for detecting urothelial cancers: Meta-analysis of diagnostic accuracy and comparison with urinary cytology testing. *Urol. Oncol. Semin. Orig. Investig.* **2008**, *26*, 646–651. [CrossRef] [PubMed]
43. Feber, A.; Dhami, P.; Dong, L.; de Winter, P.; Tan, W.S.; Martínez-Fernández, M.; Paul, D.S.; Hynes-Allen, A.; Rezaee, S.; Gurung, P.; et al. UroMark-a urinary biomarker assay for the detection of bladder cancer. *Clin. Epigenet.* **2017**, *9*, 8. [CrossRef] [PubMed]
44. Zhang, Z.; Fan, W.; Deng, Q.; Tang, S.; Wang, P.; Xu, P.; Wang, J.; Yu, M. The prognostic and diagnostic value of circulating tumor cells in bladder cancer and upper tract urothelial carcinoma: A meta-analysis of 30 published studies. *Oncotarget* **2017**, *8*, 59527. [CrossRef] [PubMed]
45. Lotan, Y.; O'Sullivan, P.; Raman, J.D.; Shariat, S.F.; Kavalieris, L.; Frampton, C.; Guilford, P.; Luxmanan, C.; Suttie, J.; Crist, H.; et al. Clinical comparison of noninvasive urine tests for ruling out recurrent urothelial carcinoma. *Urol. Oncol. Semin. Orig. Investig.* **2017**, *35*, 531. [CrossRef] [PubMed]

46. Valenberg FJP, V. Validation of a mRNA-based urine test for bladder cancer detection in patients with hematuria. *Eur. Urol.* **2017**, *16*, e190–e191. [CrossRef]
47. Pichler, R.; Fritz, J.; Tulchiner, G.; Klinglmair, G.; Soleiman, A.; Horninger, W.; Klocker, H.; Heidegger, I. Increased accuracy of a novel mRNA-based urine test for bladder cancer surveillance. *BJU Int.* **2018**, *121*, 29–37. [CrossRef] [PubMed]
48. Chapman, K. Positive Clinical Results of OncoCyte's PanC-Dx™ Diagnostic Test Demonstrate High Level of Sensitivity and Specificity in Non-Invasive Detection of Bladder Cancer—OncoCyte Corporation. In Proceedings of the American Association for Cancer Research 2015 Annual Meeting, Philadelphia, PA, USA, 19 April 2015.
49. Hatzichristodoulou, G.; Kubler, H.; Schwaibold, H.; Wagenpfeil, S.; Eibauer, C.; Hofer, C.; Gschwend, J.; Treiber, U. Nuclear matrix protein 22 for bladder cancer detection: Comparative analysis of the BladderChek® and ELISA. *Anticancer Res.* **2012**, *32*, 5093–5097. [PubMed]
50. Mowatt, G.; Zhu, S.; Kilonzo, M.; Boachie, C.; Fraser, C.; Griffiths, T.R.L.; N'Dow, J.; Nabi, G.; Cook, J.; Vale, L. Systematic review of the clinical effectiveness and cost-effectiveness of photodynamic diagnosis and urine biomarkers (FISH, ImmunoCyt, NMP22) and cytology for the detection and follow-up of bladder cancer. *Health Technol. Assess.* **2010**, *14*, 1–331. [CrossRef] [PubMed]
51. Glas, A.S.; Roos, D.; Deutekom, M.; Zwinderman, A.H.; Bossuyt, P.M.M.; Kurth, K.H. Tumor Markers in the Diagnosis of Primary Bladder Cancer. A Systematic Review. *J. Urol.* **2003**, *169*, 1975–1982. [CrossRef] [PubMed]
52. Huang, Y.-L.; Chen, J.; Yan, W.; Zang, D.; Qin, Q.; Deng, A.-M. Diagnostic accuracy of cytokeratin-19 fragment (CYFRA 21–21) for bladder cancer: A systematic review and meta-analysis. *Tumor Biol.* **2015**, *36*, 3137–3145. [CrossRef] [PubMed]
53. D'Costa, J.J.; Goldsmith, J.C.; Wilson, J.S.; Bryan, R.T.; Ward, D.G. A Systematic Review of the Diagnostic and Prognostic Value of Urinary Protein Biomarkers in Urothelial Bladder Cancer. *Bladder Cancer* **2016**, *2*, 301–317. [CrossRef] [PubMed]
54. Ashworth, T.R. A case of cancer in which cells similar to those in the tumours were seen in the blood after death. *Aust. Med. J.* **1869**, *14*, 146–147.
55. Stoecklein, N.H.; Fischer, J.C.; Niederacher, D.; Terstappen, L.W. Challenges for CTC-based liquid biopsies: Low CTC frequency and diagnostic leukapheresis as a potential solution. *Expert Rev. Mol. Diagn.* **2016**, *16*, 147–164. [CrossRef] [PubMed]
56. Harouaka, R.; Kang, Z.; Zheng, S.-Y.; Cao, L. Circulating tumor cells: Advances in isolation and analysis, and challenges for clinical applications. *Pharmacol. Ther.* **2014**, *141*, 209–221. [CrossRef] [PubMed]
57. Lv, Q.; Gong, L.; Zhang, T.; Ye, J.; Chai, L.; Ni, C.; Mao, Y. Prognostic value of circulating tumor cells in metastatic breast cancer: A systemic review and meta-analysis. *Clin. Transl. Oncol.* **2016**, *18*, 322–330. [CrossRef] [PubMed]
58. Huang, X.; Gao, P.; Sun, J.; Chen, X.; Song, Y.; Zhao, J.; Xu, H.; Wang, Z. Clinicopathological and prognostic significance of circulating tumor cells in patients with gastric cancer: A meta-analysis. *Int. J. Cancer* **2015**, *136*, 21–33. [CrossRef] [PubMed]
59. Rahbari, N.N.; Aigner, M.; Thorlund, K.; Mollberg, N.; Motschall, E.; Jensen, K.; Diener, M.K.; Büchler, M.W.; Koch, M.; Weitz, J. Meta-analysis Shows That Detection of Circulating Tumor Cells Indicates Poor Prognosis in Patients With Colorectal Cancer. *Gastroenterology* **2010**, *138*, 1714.e13–1726.e13. [CrossRef] [PubMed]
60. Wang, S.; Zheng, G.; Cheng, B.; Chen, F.; Wang, Z.; Chen, Y.; Wang, Y.; Xiong, B. Circulating Tumor Cells (CTCs) Detected by RT-PCR and Its Prognostic Role in Gastric Cancer: A Meta-Analysis of Published Literature. *PLoS ONE* **2014**, *9*, e99259. [CrossRef] [PubMed]
61. Naoe, M.; Ogawa, Y.; Morita, J.; Omori, K.; Takeshita, K.; Shichijyo, T.; Okumura, T.; Igarashi, A.; Yanaihara, A.; Iwamoto, S.; et al. Detection of circulating urothelial cancer cells in the blood using the CellSearch System. *Cancer* **2007**, *109*, 1439–1445. [CrossRef] [PubMed]
62. Neumann, M.H.D.; Bender, S.; Krahn, T.; Schlange, T. ctDNA and CTCs in Liquid Biopsy—Current Status and Where We Need to Progress. *Comput. Struct. Biotechnol. J.* **2018**, *16*, 190–195. [CrossRef] [PubMed]
63. Yoo, C.E.; Park, J.-M.; Moon, H.-S.; Joung, J.-G.; Son, D.-S.; Jeon, H.-J.; Kim, Y.J.; Han, K.-Y.; Sun, J.-M.; Park, K.; et al. Vertical Magnetic Separation of Circulating Tumor Cells for Somatic Genomic-Alteration Analysis in Lung Cancer Patients OPEN. *Nat. Publ. Gr.* **2016**, *6*, 37392. [CrossRef]

64. Yap, T.A.; Lorente, D.; Omlin, A.; Olmos, D.; de Bono, J.S. Circulating tumor cells: A multifunctional biomarker. *Clin. Cancer Res.* **2014**, *20*, 2553–2568. [CrossRef] [PubMed]
65. Wang, L.; Balasubramanian, P.; Chen, A.P.; Kummar, S.; Evrard, Y.A.; Kinders, R.J. Promise and limits of the CellSearch platform for evaluating pharmacodynamics in circulating tumor cells. *Semin. Oncol.* **2016**, *43*, 464–475. [CrossRef] [PubMed]
66. Hillig, T.; Nygaard, A.B.; Nekiunaite, L.; Klingelhöfer, J.; Sölétormos, G. In vitro validation of an ultra-sensitive scanning fluorescence microscope for analysis of circulating tumor cells. *APMIS* **2014**, *122*, 545–551. [CrossRef] [PubMed]
67. Hillig, T.; Horn, P.; Nygaard, A.B.; Haugaard, A.S.; Nejlund, S.; Brandslund, I.; Sölétormos, G. In vitro detection of circulating tumor cells compared by the CytoTrack and CellSearch methods. *Tumor Biol.* **2015**, *36*, 4597–4601. [CrossRef] [PubMed]
68. Frandsen, A.S.; Fabisiewicz, A.; Jagiello-Gruszfeld, A.; Haugaard, A.S.; Petersen, L.M.; Brandt Albrektsen, K.; Nejlund, S.; Smith, J.; Stender, H.; Hillig, T.; Sölétormos, G. Retracing Circulating Tumour Cells for Biomarker Characterization after Enumeration. *J. Circ. Biomark.* **2015**, *4*, 5. [CrossRef] [PubMed]
69. Riethdorf, S.; Soave, A.; Rink, M. The current status and clinical value of circulating tumor cells and circulating cell-free tumor DNA in bladder cancer. *Transl. Androl. Urol.* **2017**, *6*, 1090. [CrossRef] [PubMed]
70. Werner, S.L.; Graf, R.P.; Landers, M.; Valenta, D.T.; Schroeder, M.; Greene, S.B.; Bales, N.; Dittamore, R.; Marrinucci, D. Analytical Validation and Capabilities of the Epic CTC Platform: Enrichment-Free Circulating Tumour Cell Detection and Characterization. *J. Circ. Biomark.* **2015**, *4*, 4. [CrossRef] [PubMed]
71. Marrinucci, D.; Bethel, K.; Kolatkar, A.; Luttgen, M.S.; Malchiodi, M.; Baehring, F.; Voigt, K.; Lazar, D.; Nieva, J.; Bazhenova, L.; et al. Fluid biopsy in patients with metastatic prostate, pancreatic and breast cancers. *Phys. Biol.* **2012**, *9*, 016003. [CrossRef] [PubMed]
72. Greene, B.T.; Hughes, A.D.; King, M.R. Circulating tumor cells: The substrate of personalized medicine? *Front. Oncol.* **2012**, *2*, 69. [CrossRef] [PubMed]
73. Stratmann, A.; Fischer, J.C.; Niederacher, D.; Raba, K.; Schmitz, A.; Kim, P.S.; Singh, S.; Stoecklein, N.H.; Krahn, T. A comprehensive comparison of circulating tumor cell capturing technologies by apheresis of cancer patients. *J. Clin. Oncol.* **2012**, *30*, e21017. [CrossRef]
74. Stoecklein, N.H.; Niederacher, D.; Topp, S.A.; Zacarias Föhrding, L.; Vay, C. Effect of leukapheresis on efficient CTC enrichment for comprehensive molecular characterization and clinical diagnostics. *J. Clin. Oncol.* **2012**, *30*, e21020. [CrossRef]
75. Lu, J.J.; Kakehi, Y.; Takahashi, T.; Wu, X.X.; Yuasa, T.; Yoshiki, T.; Okada, Y.; Terachi, T.; Ogawa, O. Detection of circulating cancer cells by reverse transcription-polymerase chain reaction for uroplakin II in peripheral blood of patients with urothelial cancer. *Clin. Cancer Res.* **2000**, *6*, 3166–3171. [PubMed]
76. Flaig, T.W.; Wilson, S.; van Bokhoven, A.; Varella-Garcia, M.; Wolfe, P.; Maroni, P.; Genova, E.E.; Morales, D.; Lucia, M.S. Detection of circulating tumor cells in metastatic and clinically localized urothelial carcinoma. *Urology* **2011**, *78*, 863–867. [CrossRef] [PubMed]
77. Busetto, G.M.; Ferro, M.; Del Giudice, F.; Antonini, G.; Chung, B.I.; Sperduti, I.; Giannarelli, D.; Lucarelli, G.; Borghesi, M.; Musi, G.; et al. The Prognostic Role of Circulating Tumor Cells (CTC) in High-risk Non–muscle-invasive Bladder Cancer. *Clin. Genitourin. Cancer* **2017**, *15*, e661–e666. [CrossRef] [PubMed]
78. Leon, S.A.; Shapiro, B.; Sklaroff, D.M.; Yaros, M.J. Free DNA in the serum of cancer patients and the effect of therapy. *Cancer Res.* **1977**, *37*, 646–650. [PubMed]
79. Thierry, A.R.; Messaoudi, S.E.; Gahan, P.B.; Anker, P.; Stroun, M. Origins, structures, and functions of circulating DNA in oncology. *Cancer Metastasis Rev.* **2016**, *35*, 347–376. [CrossRef] [PubMed]
80. Sun, K.; Jiang, P.; Chan, K.C.A.; Wong, J.; Cheng, Y.K.Y.; Liang, R.H.S.; Chan, W.; Ma, E.S.K.; Chan, S.L.; Cheng, S.H.; et al. Plasma DNA tissue mapping by genome-wide methylation sequencing for noninvasive prenatal, cancer, and transplantation assessments. *Proc. Natl. Acad. Sci. USA* **2015**, *112*, E5503–E5512. [CrossRef] [PubMed]
81. Stroun, M.; Anker, P.; Maurice, P.; Lyautey, J.; Lederrey, C.; Beljanski, M. Neoplastic Characteristics of the DNA Found in the Plasma of Cancer Patients. *Oncology* **1989**, *46*, 318–322. [CrossRef] [PubMed]
82. Sidransky, D.; Von Eschenbach, A.; Tsai, Y.C.; Jones, P.; Summerhayes, I.; Marshall, F.; Paul, M.; Green, P.; Hamilton, S.R.; Frost, P. Identification of p53 gene mutations in bladder cancers and urine samples. *Science* **1991**, *252*, 706–709. [CrossRef]

83. Sorenson, G.D.; Pribish, D.M.; Valone, F.H.; Memoli, V.A.; Bzik, D.J.; Yao, S.L. Soluble Normal and Mutated Dna-Sequences from Single-Copy Genes in Human Blood. *Cancer Epidemiol. Biomark. Prev.* **1994**, *3*, 67–71.
84. Parkinson, C.A.; Gale, D.; Piskorz, A.M.; Biggs, H.; Hodgkin, C.; Addley, H.; Freeman, S.; Moyle, P.; Sala, E.; Sayal, K.; et al. Exploratory Analysis of TP53 Mutations in Circulating Tumour DNA as Biomarkers of Treatment Response for Patients with Relapsed High-Grade Serous Ovarian Carcinoma: A Retrospective Study. *PLoS Med.* **2016**, *13*, e1002198. [CrossRef] [PubMed]
85. Vandekerkhove, G.; Todenhöfer, T.; Annala, M.; Struss, W.J.; Wong, A.; Beja, K.; Ritch, E.; Brahmbhatt, S.; Volik, S.V.; Hennenlotter, J.; et al. Circulating tumor DNA reveals clinically actionable somatic genome of metastatic bladder cancer. *Clin. Cancer Res.* **2017**, *23*, 6487–6497. [CrossRef] [PubMed]
86. Todenhöfer, T.; Struss, W.J.; Seiler, R.; Wyatt, A.W.; Black, P.C. Liquid Biopsy-Analysis of Circulating Tumor DNA (ctDNA) in Bladder Cancer. *Bladder Cancer* **2018**, *4*, 19–29. [CrossRef] [PubMed]
87. Hegemann, M.; Stenzl, A.; Bedke, J.; Chi, K.N.; Black, P.C.; Todenhöfer, T. Liquid biopsy: Ready to guide therapy in advanced prostate cancer? *BJU Int.* **2016**, *118*, 855–863. [CrossRef] [PubMed]
88. Alix-Panabieres, C.; Pantel, K. Clinical Applications of Circulating Tumor Cells and Circulating Tumor DNA as Liquid Biopsy. *Cancer Discov.* **2016**, *6*, 479–491. [CrossRef] [PubMed]
89. Swisher, E.M.; Wollan, M.; Mahtani, S.M.; Willner, J.B.; Garcia, R.; Goff, B.A.; King, M.-C. Tumor-specific p53 sequences in blood and peritoneal fluid of women with epithelial ovarian cancer. *Am. J. Obstet. Gynecol.* **2005**, *193*, 662–667. [CrossRef] [PubMed]
90. Kimura, H.; Kasahara, K.; Kawaishi, M.; Kunitoh, H.; Tamura, T.; Holloway, B.; Nishio, K. Detection of epidermal growth factor receptor mutations in serum as a predictor of the response to gefitinib in patients with non-small-cell lung cancer. *Clin. Cancer Res.* **2006**, *12*, 3915–3921. [CrossRef] [PubMed]
91. Sozzi, G.; Musso, K.; Ratliffe, C. Detection of microsatellite alterations in plasma DNA of non-small cell lung cancer patients: A prospect for early diagnosis. *Clin. Cancer Res.* **1999**, 2689–2692.
92. Diaz, L.A.; Bardelli, A.; Bardelli, A. Liquid biopsies: Genotyping circulating tumor DNA. *J. Clin. Oncol.* **2014**, *32*, 579–586. [CrossRef] [PubMed]
93. Forshew, T.; Murtaza, M.; Parkinson, C.; Gale, D.; Tsui, D.W.Y.; Kaper, F.; Dawson, S.-J.; Piskorz, A.M.; Jimenez-Linan, M.; Bentley, D.; et al. Noninvasive Identification and Monitoring of Cancer Mutations by Targeted Deep Sequencing of Plasma DNA. *Sci. Transl. Med.* **2012**, *4*, 136ra68. [CrossRef] [PubMed]
94. Leary, R.J.; Sausen, M.; Kinde, I.; Papadopoulos, N.; Carpten, J.D.; Craig, D.; O'shaughnessy, J.; Kinzler, K.W.; Parmigiani, G.; Vogelstein, B.; et al. Detection of Chromosomal Alterations in the Circulation of Cancer Patients with Whole-Genome Sequencing. *Sci. Transl. Med.* **2012**, *28*, 162ra154. [CrossRef] [PubMed]
95. Chan, K.C.A.; Jiang, P.; Zheng, Y.W.L.; Liao, G.J.W.; Sun, H.; Wong, J.; Siu, S.S.N.; Chan, W.C.; Chan, S.L.; Chan, A.T.C.; et al. Cancer genome scanning in plasma: Detection of tumor-associated copy number aberrations, single-nucleotide variants, and tumoral heterogeneity by massively parallel sequencing. *Clin. Chem.* **2013**, *59*, 211–224. [CrossRef] [PubMed]
96. Murtaza, M.; Dawson, S.-J.; Tsui, D.W.Y.; Gale, D.; Forshew, T.; Piskorz, A.M.; Parkinson, C.; Chin, S.-F.; Kingsbury, Z.; Wong, A.S.C.; et al. Non-invasive analysis of acquired resistance to cancer therapy by sequencing of plasma DNA. *Nature* **2013**, *497*, 108–112. [CrossRef] [PubMed]
97. Lebofsky, R.; Decraene, C.; Bernard, V.; Kamal, M.; Blin, A.; Leroy, Q.; Rio Frio, T.; Pierron, G.; Callens, C.; Bieche, I.; et al. Circulating tumor DNA as a non-invasive substitute to metastasis biopsy for tumor genotyping and personalized medicine in a prospective trial across all tumor types. *Mol. Oncol.* **2015**, *9*, 783–790. [CrossRef] [PubMed]
98. Olsson, E.; Winter, C.; George, A.; Chen, Y.; Howlin, J.; Eric Tang, M.-H.; Dahlgren, M.; Schulz, R.; Grabau, D.; van Westen, D.; et al. Serial monitoring of circulating tumor DNA in patients with primary breast cancer for detection of occult metastatic disease. *EMBO Mol. Med.* **2015**, *7*, 1034–1047. [CrossRef] [PubMed]
99. Diehl, F.; Li, M.; Dressman, D.; He, Y.; Shen, D.; Szabo, S.; Diaz, L.A.; Goodman, S.N.; David, K.A.; Juhl, H.; et al. Detection and quantification of mutations in the plasma of patients with colorectal tumors. *Proc. Natl. Acad. Sci. USA* **2005**, *102*, 16368–16373. [CrossRef] [PubMed]
100. Li, M.; Diehl, F.; Dressman, D.; Vogelstein, B.; Kinzler, K.W. BEAMing up for detection and quantification of rare sequence variants. *Nat. Methods* **2006**, *3*, 95–97. [CrossRef] [PubMed]
101. Newman, A.M.; Bratman, S.V.; To, J.; Wynne, J.F.; Eclov, N.C.W.; Modlin, L.A.; Liu, C.L.; Neal, J.W.; Wakelee, H.A.; Merritt, R.E.; et al. An ultrasensitive method for quantitating circulating tumor DNA with broad patient coverage. *Nat. Med.* **2014**, *20*, 548–554. [CrossRef] [PubMed]

102. Patel, K.M.; Van Der Vos, K.E.; Smith, C.G.; Mouliere, F.; Tsui, D.; Morris, J.; Chandrananda, D.; Marass, F.; Van Den Broek, D.; Neal, D.E.; et al. Association of plasma and urinary mutant DNA with clinical outcomes in muscle invasive bladder cancer. *Sci. Rep.* **2017**, *7*. [CrossRef] [PubMed]
103. Christensen, E.; Birkenkamp-Demtröder, K.; Nordentoft, I.; Høyer, S.; van der Keur, K.; van Kessel, K.; Zwarthoff, E.; Agerbæk, M.; Ørntoft, T.F.; Jensen, J.B.; et al. Liquid Biopsy Analysis of FGFR3 and PIK3CA Hotspot Mutations for Disease Surveillance in Bladder Cancer. *Eur. Urol.* **2017**, *71*, 961–969. [CrossRef] [PubMed]
104. Gormally, E.; Vineis, P.; Matullo, G.; Veglia, F.; Caboux, E.; Le Roux, E.; Peluso, M.; Garte, S.; Guarrera, S.; Munnia, A.; et al. *TP53* and *KRAS2* Mutations in Plasma DNA of Healthy Subjects and Subsequent Cancer Occurrence: A Prospective Study. *Cancer Res.* **2006**, *66*, 6871–6876. [CrossRef] [PubMed]
105. Utting, M.; Werner, W.; Dahse, R.; Schubert, J.; Junker, K. Microsatellite analysis of free tumor DNA in urine, serum, and plasma of patients: A minimally invasive method for the detection of bladder cancer. *Clin. Cancer Res.* **2002**, *8*, 35–40. [PubMed]
106. Christensen, M.; Wolf, H.; Orntoft, T.F. Microsatellite alterations in urinary sediments from patients with cystitis and bladder cancer. *Int. J. Cancer* **2000**, *85*, 614–617. [CrossRef]
107. Domínguez, G.; Carballido, J.; Silva, J.; Silva, J.M.; Garcı, J.M.; Mene, J. p14ARF Promoter Hypermethylation in Plasma DNA as an Indicator of Disease Recurrence in Bladder Cancer Patients Advances in Brief p14ARF Promoter Hypermethylation in Plasma DNA as an Indicator of Disease Recurrence in Bladder. *Clin. Cancer Res.* **2002**, *8*, 980–985. [PubMed]
108. Dahse, R.; Utting, M.; Werner, W.; Schimmel, B.; Claussen, U.; Junker, K. TP53 alterations as a potential diagnostic marker in superficial bladder carcinoma and in patients serum, plasma and urine samples. *Int. J. Oncol.* **2002**, *20*, 107–115. [CrossRef] [PubMed]
109. Wang, Y.; Yu, Y.; Ye, R.; Zhang, D.; Li, Q.; An, D.; Fang, L.; Lin, Y.; Hou, Y.; Xu, A.; et al. An epigenetic biomarker combination of PCDH17 and POU4F2 detects bladder cancer accurately by methylation analyses of urine sediment DNA in Han Chinese. *Oncotarget* **2016**, *7*, 2754–2764. [CrossRef] [PubMed]
110. Renard, I.; Joniau, S.; van Cleynenbreugel, B.; Collette, C.; Naômé, C.; Vlassenbroeck, I.; Nicolas, H.; de Leval, J.; Straub, J.; Van Criekinge, W.; et al. Identification and Validation of the Methylated TWIST1 and NID2 Genes through Real-Time Methylation-Specific Polymerase Chain Reaction Assays for the Noninvasive Detection of Primary Bladder Cancer in Urine Samples. *Eur. Urol.* **2010**, *58*, 96–104. [CrossRef] [PubMed]
111. Dulaimi, E.; Uzzo, R.G.; Greenberg, R.E.; Al-Saleem, T.; Cairns, P. Detection of bladder cancer in urine by a tumor suppressor gene hypermethylation panel. *Clin. Cancer Res.* **2004**, *10*, 1887–1893. [CrossRef] [PubMed]
112. Hoque, M.O.; Begum, S.; Topaloglu, O.; Chatterjee, A.; Rosenbaum, E.; Van Criekinge, W.; Westra, W.H.; Schoenberg, M.; Zahurak, M.; Goodman, S.N.; et al. Quantitation of Promoter Methylation of Multiple Genes in Urine DNA and Bladder Cancer Detection. *JNCI J. Natl. Cancer Inst.* **2006**, *98*, 996–1004. [CrossRef] [PubMed]
113. Ellinger, J.; El Kassem, N.; Heukamp, L.C.; Matthews, S.; Cubukluoz, F.; Kahl, P.; Perabo, F.G.; Müller, S.C.; von Ruecker, A.; Bastian, P.J. Hypermethylation of Cell-Free Serum DNA Indicates Worse Outcome in Patients With Bladder Cancer. *J. Urol.* **2008**, *179*, 346–352. [CrossRef] [PubMed]
114. Kim, Y.K.; Kim, W.J. Epigenetic markers as promising prognosticators for bladder cancer. *Int. J. Urol.* **2009**, *16*, 17–22. [CrossRef] [PubMed]
115. Kitchen, M.O.; Bryan, R.T.; Emes, R.D.; Luscombe, C.J.; Cheng, K.; Zeegers, M.P.; James, N.D.; Gommersall, L.M.; Fryer, A.A. HumanMethylation450K Array–Identified Biomarkers Predict Tumour Recurrence/Progression at Initial Diagnosis of High-risk Non-muscle Invasive Bladder Cancer. *Biomark. Cancer* **2018**, *10*. [CrossRef] [PubMed]
116. Phé, V.; Cussenot, O.; Rouprêt, M. Interest of methylated genes as biomarkers in urothelial cell carcinomas of the urinary tract. *BJU Int.* **2009**, *104*, 896–901. [CrossRef] [PubMed]
117. Lotan, Y.; Bensalah, K.; Ruddell, T.; Shariat, S.F.; Sagalowsky, A.I.; Ashfaq, R. Prospective Evaluation of the Clinical Usefulness of Reflex Fluorescence In Situ Hybridization Assay in Patients With Atypical Cytology for the Detection of Urothelial Carcinoma of the Bladder. *J. Urol.* **2008**, *179*, 2164–2169. [CrossRef] [PubMed]
118. Funaki, N.O.; Tanaka, J.; Kasamatsu, T.; Ohshio, G.; Hosotani, R.; Okino, T.; Imamura, M. Identification of carcinoembryonic antigen mRNA in circulating peripheral blood of pancreatic carcinoma and gastric carcinoma patients. *Life Sci.* **1996**, *59*, 2187–2199. [CrossRef]

119. Lo, K.W.; Lo, Y.M.; Leung, S.F.; Tsang, Y.S.; Chan, L.Y.; Johnson, P.J.; Hjelm, N.M.; Lee, J.C.; Huang, D.P. Analysis of cell-free Epstein-Barr virus associated RNA in the plasma of patients with nasopharyngeal carcinoma. *Clin. Chem.* **1999**, *45*, 1292–1294. [PubMed]
120. Kopreski, M.S.; Benko, F.A.; Kwak, L.W.; Gocke, C.D. Detection of tumor messenger RNA in the serum of patients with malignant melanoma. *Clin. Cancer Res.* **1999**, *5*, 1961–1965. [PubMed]
121. Silva, J.; García, V.; García, J.M.; Peña, C.; Domínguez, G.; Díaz, R.; Lorenzo, Y.; Hurtado, A.; Sánchez, A.; Bonilla, F. Circulating *Bmi-1* mRNA as a possible prognostic factor for advanced breast cancer patients. *Breast Cancer Res.* **2007**, *9*, R55. [CrossRef] [PubMed]
122. García, V.; García, J.M.; Peña, C.; Silva, J.; Domínguez, G.; Lorenzo, Y.; Diaz, R.; Espinosa, P.; de Sola, J.G.; Cantos, B.; Bonilla, F. Free circulating mRNA in plasma from breast cancer patients and clinical outcome. *Cancer Lett.* **2008**, *263*, 312–320. [CrossRef] [PubMed]
123. Garcia, V.; Garcia, J.M.; Silva, J.; Martin, P.; Peña, C.; Dominguez, G.; Diaz, R.; Herrera, M.; Maximiano, C.; Sabin, P.; et al. Extracellular Tumor-Related mRNA in Plasma of Lymphoma Patients and Survival Implications. *PLoS ONE* **2009**, *4*, e8173. [CrossRef] [PubMed]
124. March-Villalba, J.A.; Martínez-Jabaloyas, J.M.; Herrero, M.J.; Santamaria, J.; Aliño, S.F.; Dasí, F. Cell-Free Circulating Plasma hTERT mRNA Is a Useful Marker for Prostate Cancer Diagnosis and Is Associated with Poor Prognosis Tumor Characteristics. *PLoS ONE* **2012**, *7*, e43470. [CrossRef] [PubMed]
125. Deligezer, U.; Erten, N.; Akisik, E.E.; Dalay, N. Circulating fragmented nucleosomal DNA and caspase-3 mRNA in patients with lymphoma and myeloma. *Exp. Mol. Pathol.* **2006**, *80*, 72–76. [CrossRef] [PubMed]
126. Reddi, K.K.; Holland, J.F. Elevated serum ribonuclease in patients with pancreatic cancer. *Proc. Natl. Acad. Sci. USA* **1976**, *73*, 2308–2310. [CrossRef] [PubMed]
127. Chomczynski, P.; Wilfinger, W.W.; Eghbalnia, H.R.; Kennedy, A.; Rymaszewski, M.; Mackey, K. Inter-Individual Differences in RNA Levels in Human Peripheral Blood. *PLoS ONE* **2016**, *11*, e0148260. [CrossRef] [PubMed]
128. Malentacchi, F.; Vinci, S.; Della Melina, A.; Kuncova, J.; Villari, D.; Nesi, G.; Selli, C.; Orlando, C.; Pazzagli, M.; Pinzani, P. Urinary carbonic anhydrase IX splicing messenger RNA variants in urogenital cancers. *Urol. Oncol. Semin. Orig. Investig.* **2016**, *34*, 292.e9–292.e16. [CrossRef] [PubMed]
129. Kim, W.T.; Jeong, P.; Yan, C.; Kim, Y.H.; Lee, I.-S.; Kang, H.-W.; Kim, Y.-J.; Lee, S.-C.; Kim, S.J.; Kim, Y.T.; et al. UBE2C cell-free RNA in urine can discriminate between bladder cancer and hematuria. *Oncotarget* **2016**, *7*, 58193–58202. [CrossRef] [PubMed]
130. Guo, B.; Luo, C.; Xun, C.; Xie, J.; Wu, X.; Pu, J. Quantitative detection of cytokeratin 20 mRNA in urine samples as diagnostic tools for bladder cancer by real-time PCR. *Exp. Oncol.* **2009**, *31*, 43–47. [PubMed]
131. Bacchetti, T.; Sartini, D.; Pozzi, V.; Cacciamani, T.; Ferretti, G.; Emanuelli, M. Exploring the role of Paraoxonase-2 in bladder cancer: Analyses performed on tissue samples, urines and cell culturess. *Oncotarget* **2017**, *8*, 28785–28795. [CrossRef] [PubMed]
132. Urquidi, V.; Goodison, S.; Cai, Y.; Sun, Y.; Rosser, C.J. A Candidate Molecular Biomarker Panel for the Detection of Bladder Cancer. *Cancer Epidemiol. Biomark. Prev.* **2012**, *21*, 2149–2158. [CrossRef] [PubMed]
133. Mengual, L.; Burset, M.; Ribal, M.J.; Ars, E.; Marin-Aguilera, M.; Fernandez, M.; Ingelmo-Torres, M.; Villavicencio, H.; Alcaraz, A. Gene Expression Signature in Urine for Diagnosing and Assessing Aggressiveness of Bladder Urothelial Carcinoma. *Clin. Cancer Res.* **2010**, *16*, 2624–2633. [CrossRef] [PubMed]
134. Urquidi, V.; Netherton, M.; Gomes-Giacoia, E.; Serie, D.; Eckel-Passow, J.; Rosser, C.J.; Goodison, S. Urinary mRNA biomarker panel for the detection of urothelial carcinoma. *Oncotarget* **2016**, *7*, 38731–38740. [CrossRef] [PubMed]
135. Kavalieris, L.; O'Sullivan, P.; Frampton, C.; Guilford, P.; Darling, D.; Jacobson, E.; Suttie, J.; Raman, J.D.; Shariat, S.F.; Lotan, Y. Performance Characteristics of a Multigene Urine Biomarker Test for Monitoring for Recurrent Urothelial Carcinoma in a Multicenter Study. *J. Urol.* **2017**, *197*, 1419–1426. [CrossRef] [PubMed]
136. Goodison, S.; Rosser, C.J. Bladder Cancer Detection Composition Kit, and Associated Methods. Google Patents WO2014042763A1, 18 July 2013.
137. Martínez-Fernández, M.; Paramio, J.M.; Dueñas, M. RNA Detection in Urine: From RNA Extraction to Good Normalizer Molecules. *J. Mol. Diagn.* **2016**, *18*, 15–22. [CrossRef] [PubMed]
138. Romero-Cordoba, S.L.; Salido-Guadarrama, I.; Rodriguez-Dorantes, M.; Hidalgo-Miranda, A. miRNA biogenesis: Biological impact in the development of cancer. *Cancer Biol. Ther.* **2014**, *15*, 1444–1455. [CrossRef] [PubMed]

139. Chan, B.; Manley, J.; Lee, J.; Singh, S.R. The emerging roles of microRNAs in cancer metabolism. *Cancer Lett.* **2015**, *356*, 301–308. [CrossRef] [PubMed]
140. Liang, Y.; Ridzon, D.; Wong, L.; Chen, C. Characterization of microRNA expression profiles in normal human tissues. *BMC Genom.* **2007**, *8*, 166. [CrossRef] [PubMed]
141. Ge, Q.; Zhou, Y.; Lu, J.; Bai, Y.; Xie, X.; Lu, Z. miRNA in Plasma Exosome is Stable under Different Storage Conditions. *Molecules* **2014**, *19*, 1568–1575. [CrossRef] [PubMed]
142. Mitchell, P.S.; Parkin, R.K.; Kroh, E.M.; Fritz, B.R.; Wyman, S.K.; Pogosova-Agadjanyan, E.L.; Peterson, A.; Noteboom, J.; O'Briant, K.C.; Allen, A.; et al. Circulating microRNAs as stable blood-based markers for cancer detection. *Proc. Natl. Acad. Sci. USA* **2008**, *105*, 10513–10518. [CrossRef] [PubMed]
143. Weber, J.A.; Baxter, D.H.; Zhang, S.; Huang, D.Y.; How Huang, K.; Jen Lee, M.; Galas, D.J.; Wang, K. The MicroRNA Spectrum in 12 Body Fluids. *Clin. Chem.* **2010**, *56*, 1733–1741. [CrossRef] [PubMed]
144. Yun, S.J.; Jeong, P.; Kim, W.-T.; Kim, T.H.; Lee, Y.-S.; Song, P.H.; Choi, Y.-H.; Kim, I.Y.; Moon, S.-K.; Kim, W.-J.; et al. Cell-free microRNAs in urine as diagnostic and prognostic biomarkers of bladder cancer. *Int. J. Oncol.* **2012**, *41*, 1871–1878. [CrossRef] [PubMed]
145. Zhou, X.; Zhang, X.; Yang, Y.; Li, Z.; Du, L.; Dong, Z.; Qu, A.; Jiang, X.; Li, P.; Wang, C. Urinary cell-free microRNA-106b as a novel biomarker for detection of bladder cancer. *Med. Oncol.* **2014**, *31*, 197. [CrossRef] [PubMed]
146. Sasaki, H.; Yoshiike, M.; Nozawa, S.; Usuba, W.; Katsuoka, Y.; Aida, K.; Kitajima, K.; Kudo, H.; Hoshikawa, M.; Yoshioka, Y.; et al. Expression Level of Urinary MicroRNA-146a-5p Is Increased in Patients With Bladder Cancer and Decreased in Those After Transurethral Resection. *Clin. Genitourin. Cancer* **2016**, *14*, e493–e499. [CrossRef] [PubMed]
147. Puerta-Gil, P.; García-Baquero, R.; Jia, A.Y.; Ocaña, S.; Alvarez-Múgica, M.; Alvarez-Ossorio, J.L.; Cordon-Cardo, C.; Cava, F.; Sánchez-Carbayo, M. miR-143, miR-222, and miR-452 Are Useful as Tumor Stratification and Noninvasive Diagnostic Biomarkers for Bladder Cancer. *Am. J. Pathol.* **2012**, *180*, 1808–1815. [CrossRef] [PubMed]
148. Hanke, M.; Hoefig, K.; Merz, H.; Feller, A.C.; Kausch, I.; Jocham, D.; Warnecke, J.M.; Sczakiel, G. A robust methodology to study urine microRNA as tumor marker: MicroRNA-126 and microRNA-182 are related to urinary bladder cancer. *Urol. Oncol. Semin. Orig. Investig.* **2010**, *28*, 655–661. [CrossRef] [PubMed]
149. Kim, S.M.; Kang, H.W.; Kim, W.T.; Kim, Y.-J.; Yun, S.J.; Lee, S.-C.; Kim, W.-J. Cell-Free microRNA-214 From Urine as a Biomarker for Non-Muscle-Invasive Bladder Cancer. *Korean J. Urol.* **2013**, *54*, 791. [CrossRef] [PubMed]
150. Zhang, X.; Zhang, Y.; Liu, X.; Fang, A.; Wang, J.; Yang, Y.; Wang, L.; Du, L.; Wang, C.; Zhang, X.; et al. Direct quantitative detection for cell-free miR-155 in urine: A potential role in diagnosis and prognosis for non-muscle invasive bladder cancer. *Oncotarget* **2016**, *7*, 3255–3266. [CrossRef] [PubMed]
151. Ingelmo-Torres, M.; Lozano, J.J.; Izquierdo, L.; Carrion, A.; Costa, M.; Gomez, L.; Ribal, M.J.; Alcaraz, A.; Mengual, L. Urinary cell microRNA-based prognostic classifier for non-muscle invasive bladder cancer. *Oncotarget* **2017**, *8*, 18238–18247. [CrossRef] [PubMed]
152. Yang, Y.; Qu, A.; Liu, J.; Wang, R.; Liu, Y.; Li, G.; Duan, W.; Fang, Q.; Jiang, X.; Wang, L.; et al. Serum miR-210 Contributes to Tumor Detection, Stage Prediction and Dynamic Surveillance in Patients with Bladder Cancer. *PLoS ONE* **2015**, *10*, e0135168. [CrossRef] [PubMed]
153. Feng, Y.; Liu, J.; Kang, Y.; He, Y.; Liang, B.; Yang, P.; Yu, Z. miR-19a acts as an oncogenic microRNA and is up-regulated in bladder cancer. *J. Exp. Clin. Cancer Res.* **2014**, *33*, 67. [CrossRef] [PubMed]
154. Adam, L.; Wszolek, M.F.; Liu, C.-G.; Jing, W.; Diao, L.; Zien, A.; Zhang, J.D.; Jackson, D.; Dinney, C.P.N. Plasma microRNA profiles for bladder cancer detection. *Urol. Oncol. Semin. Orig. Investig.* **2013**, *31*, 1701–1708. [CrossRef] [PubMed]
155. Pardini, B.; Cordero, F.; Naccarati, A.; Viberti, C.; Birolo, G.; Oderda, M.; Di Gaetano, C.; Arigoni, M.; Martina, F.; Calogero, R.A.; et al. microRNA profiles in urine by next-generation sequencing can stratify bladder cancer subtypes. *Oncotarget* **2018**, *9*, 20658–20669. [CrossRef] [PubMed]
156. Wang, K.C.; Chang, H.Y. Molecular mechanisms of long noncoding RNAs. *Mol. Cell* **2011**, *43*, 904–914. [CrossRef] [PubMed]
157. Schmitt, A.M.; Chang, H.Y. Long Noncoding RNAs in Cancer Pathways. *Cancer Cell* **2016**, *29*, 452–463. [CrossRef] [PubMed]

158. Wang, X.-S.; Zhang, Z.; Wang, H.-C.; Cai, J.-L.; Xu, Q.-W.; Li, M.-Q.; Chen, Y.-C.; Qian, X.-P.; Lu, T.-J.; Yu, L.-Z.; et al. Rapid Identification of UCA1 as a Very Sensitive and Specific Unique Marker for Human Bladder Carcinoma. *Clin. Cancer Res.* **2006**, *12*, 4851–4858. [CrossRef] [PubMed]
159. Cui, X.; Jing, X.; Long, C.; Yi, Q.; Tian, J.; Zhu, J. Accuracy of the urine UCA1 for diagnosis of bladder cancer: A meta-analysis. *Oncotarget* **2017**, *8*, 35222–35233. [CrossRef] [PubMed]
160. Fan, Y.; Shen, B.; Tan, M.; Mu, X.; Qin, Y.; Zhang, F.; Liu, Y. Long non-coding RNA UCA1 increases chemoresistance of bladder cancer cells by regulating Wnt signaling. *FEBS J.* **2014**, *281*, 1750–1758. [CrossRef] [PubMed]
161. Berrondo, C.; Flax, J.; Kucherov, V.; Siebert, A.; Osinski, T.; Rosenberg, A.; Fucile, C.; Richheimer, S.; Beckham, C.J. Expression of the Long Non-Coding RNA HOTAIR Correlates with Disease Progression in Bladder Cancer and Is Contained in Bladder Cancer Patient Urinary Exosomes. *PLoS ONE* **2016**, *11*, e0147236. [CrossRef] [PubMed]
162. Chen, M.; Li, J.; Zhuang, C.; Cai, Z. Increased lncRNA ABHD11-AS1 represses the malignant phenotypes of bladder cancer. *Oncotarget* **2017**, *8*, 28176–28186. [CrossRef] [PubMed]
163. Ariel, I.; Sughayer, M.; Fellig, Y.; Pizov, G.; Ayesh, S.; Podeh, D.; Libdeh, B.A.; Levy, C.; Birman, T.; Tykocinski, M.L.; et al. The imprinted *H19* gene is a marker of early recurrence in human bladder carcinoma. *Mol. Pathol.* **2000**, *53*, 320–323. [CrossRef] [PubMed]
164. Sapre, N.; Macintyre, G.; Clarkson, M.; Naeem, H.; Cmero, M.; Kowalczyk, A.; Anderson, P.D.; Costello, A.J.; Corcoran, N.M.; Hovens, C.M. A urinary microRNA signature can predict the presence of bladder urothelial carcinoma in patients undergoing surveillance. *Br. J. Cancer* **2016**, *114*, 454–462. [CrossRef] [PubMed]
165. Jiang, X.; Du, L.; Wang, L.; Li, J.; Liu, Y.; Zheng, G.; Qu, A.; Zhang, X.; Pan, H.; Yang, Y.; et al. Serum microRNA expression signatures identified from genome-wide microRNA profiling serve as novel noninvasive biomarkers for diagnosis and recurrence of bladder cancer. *Int. J. Cancer* **2015**, *136*, 854–862. [CrossRef] [PubMed]
166. Jiang, X.; Du, L.; Duan, W.; Wang, R.; Yan, K.; Wang, L.; Li, J.; Zheng, G.; Zhang, X.; Yang, Y.; et al. Serum microRNA expression signatures as novel noninvasive biomarkers for prediction and prognosis of muscle-invasive bladder cancer. *Oncotarget* **2016**, *7*, 36733–36742. [CrossRef] [PubMed]
167. Du, L.; Jiang, X.; Duan, W.; Wang, R.; Wang, L.; Zheng, G.; Yan, K.; Wang, L.; Li, J.; Zhang, X.; et al. Cell-free microRNA expression signatures in urine serve as novel noninvasive biomarkers for diagnosis and recurrence prediction of bladder cancer. *Oncotarget* **2017**, *8*, 40832–40842. [CrossRef] [PubMed]
168. Urquidi, V.; Netherton, M.; Gomes-Giacoia, E.; Serie, D.J.; Eckel-Passow, J.; Rosser, C.J.; Goodison, S. A microRNA biomarker panel for the non-invasive detection of bladder cancer. *Oncotarget* **2016**, *7*, 86290–86299. [CrossRef] [PubMed]
169. Eissa, S.; Matboli, M.; Essawy, N.O.E.; Kotb, Y.M. Integrative functional genetic-epigenetic approach for selecting genes as urine biomarkers for bladder cancer diagnosis. *Tumor Biol.* **2015**, *36*, 9545–9552. [CrossRef] [PubMed]
170. Siomi, M.C.; Sato, K.; Pezic, D.; Aravin, A.A. PIWI-interacting small RNAs: The vanguard of genome defence. *Nat. Rev. Mol. Cell Biol.* **2011**, *12*, 246–258. [CrossRef] [PubMed]
171. Yuan, T.; Huang, X.; Woodcock, M.; Du, M.; Dittmar, R.; Wang, Y.; Tsai, S.; Kohli, M.; Boardman, L.; Patel, T.; et al. Plasma extracellular RNA profiles in healthy and cancer patients. *Sci. Rep.* **2016**, *6*, 19413. [CrossRef] [PubMed]
172. Freedman, J.E.; Gerstein, M.; Mick, E.; Rozowsky, J.; Levy, D.; Kitchen, R.; Das, S.; Shah, R.; Danielson, K.; Beaulieu, L.; et al. Diverse human extracellular RNAs are widely detected in human plasma. *Nat. Commun.* **2016**, *7*, 11106. [CrossRef] [PubMed]
173. Chu, H.; Hui, G.; Yuan, L.; Shi, D.; Wang, Y.; Du, M.; Zhong, D.; Ma, L.; Tong, N.; Qin, C.; et al. Identification of novel piRNAs in bladder cancer. *Cancer Lett.* **2015**, *356*, 561–567. [CrossRef] [PubMed]
174. Jeck, W.R.; Sharpless, N.E. Detecting and characterizing circular RNAs. *Nat. Biotechnol.* **2014**, *32*, 453–461. [CrossRef] [PubMed]
175. Kristensen, L.S.; Hansen, T.B.; Venø, M.T.; Kjems, J. Circular RNAs in cancer: Opportunities and challenges in the field. *Oncogene* **2018**, *37*, 555–565. [CrossRef] [PubMed]
176. Zhang, Y.; Liang, W.; Zhang, P.; Chen, J.; Qian, H.; Zhang, X.; Xu, W. Circular RNAs: Emerging cancer biomarkers and targets. *J. Exp. Clin. Cancer Res.* **2017**, *36*, 152. [CrossRef] [PubMed]

177. Zhong, Z.; Lv, M.; Chen, J. Screening differential circular RNA expression profiles reveals the regulatory role of circTCF25-miR-103a-3p/miR-107-CDK6 pathway in bladder carcinoma. *Sci. Rep.* **2016**, *6*, 30919. [CrossRef] [PubMed]

178. Zhong, Z.; Huang, M.; Lv, M.; He, Y.; Duan, C.; Zhang, L.; Chen, J. Circular RNA MYLK as a competing endogenous RNA promotes bladder cancer progression through modulating VEGFA/VEGFR2 signaling pathway. *Cancer Lett.* **2017**, *403*, 305–317. [CrossRef] [PubMed]

179. Huang, M.; Zhong, Z.; Lv, M.; Shu, J.; Tian, Q.; Chen, J. Comprehensive analysis of differentially expressed profiles of lncRNAs and circRNAs with associated co-expression and ceRNA networks in bladder carcinoma. *Oncotarget* **2016**, *7*, 47186–47200. [CrossRef] [PubMed]

180. Chander, Y.; Subramanya, H. Serological tumor markers—Their role. *Med. J. Armed Forces India* **2000**, *56*, 279–281. [CrossRef]

181. Bansal, N.; Gupta, A.K.; Gupta, A.; Sankhwar, S.N.; Mahdi, A.A. Serum-based protein biomarkers of bladder cancer: A pre- and post-operative evaluation. *J. Pharm. Biomed. Anal.* **2016**, *124*, 22–25. [CrossRef] [PubMed]

182. Bansal, N.; Gupta, A.; Sankhwar, S.N.; Mahdi, A.A. Low- and high-grade bladder cancer appraisal via serum-based proteomics approach. *Clin. Chim. Acta* **2014**, *436*, 97–103. [CrossRef] [PubMed]

183. Chen, Y.T.; Chen, C.L.; Chen, H.W.; Chung, T.; Wu, C.C.; Chen, C.D.; Hsu, C.W.; Chen, M.C.; Tsui, K.H.; Chang, P.L.; Chang, Y.S.; Yu, J.S. Discovery of novel bladder cancer biomarkers by comparative urine proteomics using iTRAQ technology. *J. Proteome Res.* **2010**, *11*, 5803–5815. [CrossRef] [PubMed]

184. Ebbing, J.; Mathia, S.; Seibert, F.S.; Pagonas, N.; Bauer, F.; Erber, B.; Günzel, K.; Kilic, E.; Kempkensteffen, C.; Miller, K.; et al. Urinary calprotectin: A new diagnostic marker in urothelial carcinoma of the bladder. *World J. Urol.* **2014**, *32*, 1485–1492. [CrossRef] [PubMed]

185. Zoidakis, J.; Makridakis, M.; Zerefos, P.G.; Bitsika, V.; Esteban, S.; Frantzi, M.; Stravodimos, K.; Anagnou, N.P.; Roubelakis, M.G.; Sanchez-Carbayo, M.; et al. Profilin 1 is a Potential Biomarker for Bladder Cancer Aggressiveness. *Mol. Cell. Proteom.* **2012**, *11*, M111.009449. [CrossRef] [PubMed]

186. Frantzi, M.; Zoidakis, J.; Papadopoulos, T.; Zürbig, P.; Katafigiotis, I.; Stravodimos, K.; Lazaris, A.; Giannopoulou, I.; Ploumidis, A.; Mischak, H.; et al. IMAC fractionation in combination with LC-MS reveals H2B and NIF-1 peptides as potential bladder cancer biomarkers. *J. Proteome Res.* **2013**, *12*, 3969–3979. [CrossRef] [PubMed]

187. Goodison, S.; Chang, M.; Dai, Y.; Urquidi, V.; Rosser, C.J. A Multi-Analyte Assay for the Non-Invasive Detection of Bladder Cancer. *PLoS ONE* **2012**, *7*, e47469. [CrossRef] [PubMed]

188. Rosser, C.J.; Ross, S.; Chang, M.; Dai, Y.; Mengual, L.; Zhang, G.; Kim, J.; Urquidi, V.; Alcaraz, A.; Goodison, S. Multiplex protein signature for the detection of bladder cancer in voided urine samples. *J. Urol.* **2013**, *190*, 2257–2262. [CrossRef] [PubMed]

189. Rosser, C.J.; Chang, M.; Dai, Y.; Ross, S.; Mengual, L.; Alcaraz, A.; Goodison, S. Urinary Protein Biomarker Panel for the Detection of Recurrent Bladder Cancer. *Cancer Epidemiol. Biomark. Prev.* **2014**, *23*, 247–253. [CrossRef] [PubMed]

190. Shimizu, Y.; Furuya, H.; Bryant Greenwood, P.; Chan, O.; Dai, Y.; Thornquist, M.D.; Goodison, S.; Rosser, C.J. A multiplex immunoassay for the non-invasive detection of bladder cancer. *J. Transl. Med.* **2016**, *14*, 31. [CrossRef] [PubMed]

191. Soukup, V.; Kalousová, M.; Capoun, O.; Sobotka, R.; Breyl, Z.; Pešl, M.; Zima, T.; Hanuš, T. Panel of Urinary Diagnostic Markers for Non-Invasive Detection of Primary and Recurrent Urothelial Urinary Bladder Carcinoma. *Urol. Int.* **2015**, *95*, 56–64. [CrossRef] [PubMed]

192. Jamshidian, H.; Kor, K.; Djalali, M. Urine concentration of nuclear matrix protein 22 for diagnosis of transitional cell carcinoma of bladder. *Urol. J.* **2008**, *5*, 243–247. [PubMed]

193. Soloway, M.S.; Briggman, V.; Carpinito, G.A.; Chodak, G.W.; Church, P.A.; Lamm, D.L.; Lange, P.; Messing, E.; Pasciak, R.M.; Reservitz, G.B.; et al. Use of a new tumor marker, urinary NMP22, in the detection of occult or rapidly recurring transitional cell carcinoma of the urinary tract following surgical treatment. *J. Urol.* **1996**, *156*, 363–367. [CrossRef]

194. Zippe, C.; Pandrangi, L.; Agarwal, A. NMP22 Is a Sensitive, Cost-Effective Test in Patients At Risk for Bladder Cancer. *J. Urol.* **1999**, *161*, 62–65. [CrossRef]

195. Theodorescu, D.; Wittke, S.; Ross, M.M.; Walden, M.; Conaway, M.; Just, I.; Mischak, H.; Frierson, H.F. Discovery and validation of new protein biomarkers for urothelial cancer: A prospective analysis. *Lancet Oncol.* **2006**, *7*, 230–240. [CrossRef]

196. Schiffer, E.; Vlahou, A.; Petrolekas, A.; Stravodimos, K.; Tauber, R.; Geschwend, J.E.; Neuhaus, J.; Stolzenburg, J.U.; Conaway, M.R.; Mischak, H.; et al. Prediction of muscle-invasive bladder cancer using urinary proteomics. *Clin. Cancer Res.* **2009**, *15*, 4935–4943. [CrossRef] [PubMed]
197. Frantzi, M.; Van Kessel, K.E.; Zwarthoff, E.C.; Marquez, M.; Rava, M.; Malats, N.; Merseburger, A.S.; Katafigiotis, I.; Stravodimos, K.; Mullen, W.; et al. Development and validation of urine-based peptide biomarker panels for detecting bladder cancer in a multi-center study. *Clin. Cancer Res.* **2016**, *22*, 4077–4086. [CrossRef] [PubMed]
198. Chen, C.L.; Lai, Y.F.; Tang, P.; Chien, K.Y.; Yu, J.S.; Tsai, C.H.; Chen, H.W.; Wu, C.C.; Chung, T.; Hsu, C.W.; et al. Comparative and targeted proteomic analyses of urinary microparticles from bladder cancer and hernia patients. *J. Proteome Res.* **2012**, *11*, 5611–5629. [CrossRef] [PubMed]
199. Yang, N.; Feng, S.; Shedden, K.; Xie, X.; Liu, Y.; Rosser, C.J.; Lubman, D.M.; Goodison, S. Urinary Glycoprotein Biomarker Discovery for Bladder Cancer Detection using LC-MS/MS and Label-free Quantification. *Clin. Cancer Res.* **2011**, *17*, 247–253. [CrossRef] [PubMed]
200. Lindén, M.; Lind, S.B.; Mayrhofer, C.; Segersten, U.; Wester, K.; Lyutvinskiy, Y.; Zubarev, R.; Malmström, P.U.; Pettersson, U. Proteomic analysis of urinary biomarker candidates for nonmuscle invasive bladder cancer. *Proteomics* **2012**, *12*, 135–144. [CrossRef] [PubMed]
201. Chen, C.L.; Lin, T.S.; Tsai, C.H.; Wu, C.C.; Chung, T.; Chien, K.Y.; Wu, M.; Chang, Y.S.; Yu, J.S.; Chen, Y.T. Identification of potential bladder cancer markers in urine by abundant-protein depletion coupled with quantitative proteomics. *J. Proteom.* **2013**, *85*, 28–43. [CrossRef] [PubMed]
202. Mischak, H.; Kolch, W.; Aivaliotis, M.; Bouyssié, D.; Dihazi, H.; Dihazi, G.H.; Franke, J.; Garin, J.; Gonzalez, A.; Peredo, D.; et al. Comprehensive human urine standards for comparability and standardization in clinical proteome analysis. *Proteom. Clin. Appl.* **2010**, *4*, 464–478. [CrossRef] [PubMed]
203. Miyake, M.; Morizawa, Y.; Hori, S.; Tatsumi, Y.; Onishi, S.; Owari, T.; Iida, K.; Onishi, K.; Gotoh, D.; Nakai, Y.; et al. Diagnostic and prognostic role of urinary collagens in primary human bladder cancer. *Cancer Sci.* **2017**, *108*, 2221–2228. [CrossRef] [PubMed]
204. Urquidi, V.; Kim, J.; Chang, M.; Dai, Y.; Rosser, C.J.; Goodison, S. CCL18 in a multiplex urine-based assay for the detection of bladder cancer. *PLoS ONE* **2012**, *7*, e37797. [CrossRef] [PubMed]
205. Hwang, E.C.; Choi, H.S.; Jung, S., II; Kwon, D.D.; Park, K.; Ryu, S.B. Use of the NMP22 BladderChek test in the diagnosis and follow-up of urothelial cancer: A cross-sectional study. *Urology* **2011**, *77*, 154–159. [CrossRef] [PubMed]
206. Barton Grossman, H.; Soloway, M.; Messing, E.; Katz, G.; Stein, B.; Kassabian, V.; Shen, Y. Surveillance for recurrent bladder cancer using a point-of-care proteomic assay. *J. Am. Med. Assoc.* **2006**, *295*, 299–305. [CrossRef] [PubMed]
207. Grossman, H. Detection of bladder cancer using a proteomic assay. *JAMA* **2005**, *293*, 2467. [CrossRef] [PubMed]
208. Kinders, R.; Jones, T.; Root, R.; Bruce, C.; Murchison, H.; Corey, M.; Williams, L.; Enfield, D.; Hass, G.M. Complement factor H or a related protein is a marker for transitional cell cancer of the bladder. *Clin. Cancer Res.* **1998**, *4*, 2511–2520. [PubMed]
209. Malkowicz, S.B. The application of human complement factor H-related protein (BTA TRAK) in monitoring patients with bladder cancer. *Urol. Clin. N. Am.* **2000**, *27*, 63–73. [CrossRef]
210. Guo, A.; Wang, X.; Gao, L.; Shi, J.; Sun, C.; Wan, Z. Bladder tumour antigen (BTA stat) test compared to the urine cytology in the diagnosis of bladder cancer: A meta-analysis. *J. Can. Urol. Assoc.* **2014**, *8*, E347. [CrossRef] [PubMed]
211. Raitanen, M. The role of BTA stat test in follow-up of patients with bladder cancer: Results from Finn Bladder studies. *World J. Urol.* **2008**, *26*, 45–50. [CrossRef] [PubMed]
212. Jeong, S.; Park, Y.; Cho, Y.; Kim, Y.R.; Kim, H.S. Diagnostic values of urine CYFRA21-1, NMP22, UBC, and FDP for the detection of bladder cancer. *Clin. Chim. Acta* **1970**, *414*, 93–100. [CrossRef] [PubMed]
213. Nisman, B.; Yutkin, V.; Peretz, T.; Shapiro, A.; Barak, V.; Pode, D. The follow-up of patients with non-muscle-invasive bladder cancer by urine cytology, abdominal ultrasound and urine CYFRA 21-1: A pilot study. *Anticancer Res.* **2009**, *29*, 4281–4285. [PubMed]

214. Fernandez-Gomez, J.; Rodríguez-Martínez, J.J.; Barmadah, S.E.; García Rodríguez, J.; Allende, D.M.; Jalon, A.; Gonzalez, R.; Álvarez-Múgica, M. Urinary CYFRA 21.1 Is Not a Useful Marker for the Detection of Recurrences in the Follow-Up of Superficial Bladder Cancer. *Eur. Urol.* **2007**, *51*, 1267–1274. [CrossRef] [PubMed]
215. Hakenberg, O.W.; Fuessel, S.; Richter, K.; Froehner, M.; Oehlschlaeger, S.; Rathert, P.; Meye, A.; Wirth, M.P. Qualitative and quantitative assessment of urinary cytokeratin 8 and 18 fragments compared with voided urine cytology in diagnosis of bladder carcinoma. *Urology* **2004**, *64*, 1121–1126. [CrossRef] [PubMed]
216. Babjuk, M.; Koštířová, M.; Mudra, K.; Pecher, S.; Smolová, H.; Pecen, L.; Ibrahim, Z.; Dvořáček, J.; Jarolím, L.; Novák, J.; Zima, T. Qualitative and quantitative detection of urinary human complement factor H-related protein (BTA stat and BTA TRAK) and fragments of cytokeratins 8, 18 (UBC rapid and UBC IRMA) as markers for transitional cell carcinoma of the bladder. *Eur. Urol.* **2002**, *41*, 34–39. [CrossRef]
217. Cheng, Y.; Yang, X.; Deng, X.; Zhang, X.; Li, P.; Tao, J.; Qin, C.; Wei, J.; Lu, Q. Metabolomics in bladder cancer: A systematic review. *Int. J. Clin. Exp. Med.* **2015**, *8*, 11052–11063. [PubMed]
218. Bauça, J.M.; Martínez-Morillo, E.; Diamandis, E.P. Peptidomics of urine and other biofluids for cancer diagnostics. *Clin. Chem.* **2014**, *60*, 1052–1061. [CrossRef] [PubMed]
219. Jin, X.; Yun, S.J.; Jeong, P.; Kim, I.Y.; Kim, W.-J.; Park, S. Diagnosis of bladder cancer and prediction of survival by urinary metabolomics. *Oncotarget* **2014**, *5*, 1635–1645. [CrossRef] [PubMed]
220. Zhou, Y.; Song, R.; Ma, C.; Zhou, L.; Liu, X.; Yin, P.; Zhang, Z.; Sun, Y.; Xu, C.; Lu, X.; et al. Discovery and validation of potential urinary biomarkers for bladder cancer diagnosis using a pseudotargeted GC-MS metabolomics method. *Oncotarget* **2017**, *8*, 20719–20728. [CrossRef] [PubMed]
221. Huang, Z.; Lin, L.; Gao, Y.; Chen, Y.; Yan, X.; Xing, J.; Hang, W. Bladder Cancer Determination Via Two Urinary Metabolites: A Biomarker Pattern Approach. *Mol. Cell. Proteom.* **2011**, *10*, mcp.M111.007922. [CrossRef] [PubMed]
222. Ganti, S.; Taylor, S.L.; Kim, K.; Hoppel, C.L.; Guo, L.; Yang, J.; Evans, C.; Weiss, R.H. Urinary acylcarnitines are altered in human kidney cancer. *Int. J. Cancer* **2012**, *130*, 2791–2800. [CrossRef] [PubMed]
223. Sahu, D.; Lotan, Y.; Wittmann, B.; Neri, B.; Hansel, D.E. Metabolomics analysis reveals distinct profiles of nonmuscle-invasive and muscle-invasive bladder cancer. *Cancer Med.* **2017**, *6*, 2106–2120. [CrossRef] [PubMed]
224. Madka, V.; Mohammed, A.; Li, Q.; Zhang, Y.; Patlolla, J.M.R.; Biddick, L.; Lightfoot, S.; Wu, X.R.; Steele, V.; Kopelovich, L.; et al. Chemoprevention of urothelial cell carcinoma growth and invasion by the dual COX-LOX inhibitor licofelone in UPII-SV40T transgenic mice. *Cancer Prev. Res.* **2014**, *7*, 708–716. [CrossRef] [PubMed]
225. Miyata, Y.; Kanda, S.; Mitsunari, K.; Asai, A.; Sakai, H. Heme oxygenase-1 expression is associated with tumor aggressiveness and outcomes in patients with bladder cancer: A correlation with smoking intensity. *Transl. Res.* **2014**, *164*, 468–476. [CrossRef] [PubMed]
226. Loras, A.; Trassierra, M.; Castell, J.V. Bladder cancer recurrence surveillance by urine metabolomics analysis. *Sci. Rep.* **2018**, *8*, 9172. [CrossRef] [PubMed]
227. Lin, L.; Huang, Z.; Gao, Y.; Chen, Y.; Hang, W.; Xing, J.; Yan, X. LC-MS-based serum metabolic profiling for genitourinary cancer classification and cancer type-specific biomarker discovery. *Proteomics* **2012**, *12*, 2238–2246. [CrossRef] [PubMed]
228. Rodrigues, D.; Jerónimo, C.; Henrique, R.; Belo, L.; de Lourdes Bastos, M.; de Pinho, P.G.; Carvalho, M. Biomarkers in bladder cancer: A metabolomic approach using in vitro and ex vivo model systems. *Int. J. Cancer* **2016**, *139*, 256–268. [CrossRef] [PubMed]
229. Franzen, C.A.; Blackwell, R.H.; Todorovic, V.; Greco, K.A.; Foreman, K.E.; Flanigan, R.C.; Kuo, P.C.; Gupta, G.N. Urothelial cells undergo epithelial-to-mesenchymal transition after exposure to muscle invasive bladder cancer exosomes. *Oncogenesis* **2015**, *4*, e163-10. [CrossRef] [PubMed]
230. Reclusa, P.; Taverna, S.; Pucci, M.; Durendez, E.; Calabuig, S.; Manca, P.; Serrano, M.J.; Sober, L.; Pauwels, P.; Russo, A.; et al. Exosomes as diagnostic and predictive biomarkers in lung cancer. *J. Thorac. Dis.* **2017**, *9*, S1373–S1382. [CrossRef] [PubMed]
231. Johnstone, R.M.; Adam, M.; Pan, B.T. The fate of the transferrin receptor during maturation of sheep reticulocytes in vitro. *Can. J. Biochem. Cell Biol.* **1984**, *62*, 1246–1254. [CrossRef] [PubMed]
232. Harding, C.; Heuser, J.; Stahl, P. Receptor-mediated endocytosis of transferrin and recycling of the transferrin receptor in rat reticulocytes. *J. Cell Biol.* **1983**, *97*, 329–339. [CrossRef] [PubMed]

233. Iero, M.; Valenti, R.; Huber, V.; Filipazzi, P.; Parmiani, G.; Fais, S.; Rivoltini, L. Tumour-released exosomes and their implications in cancer immunity. *Cell Death Differ.* **2008**, *15*, 80–88. [CrossRef] [PubMed]
234. Valenti, R.; Huber, V.; Iero, M.; Filipazzi, P.; Parmiani, G.; Rivoltini, L. Tumor-released microvesicles as vehicles of immunosuppression. *Cancer Res.* **2007**, *67*, 2912–2915. [CrossRef] [PubMed]
235. Silvers, C.R.; Miyamoto, H.; Messing, E.M.; Netto, G.J.; Lee, Y.-F. Characterization of urinary extracellular vesicle proteins in muscle-invasive bladder cancer. *Oncotarget* **2017**, *8*, 91199–91208. [CrossRef] [PubMed]
236. Baumgart, S.; Hölters, S.; Ohlmann, C.-H.; Bohle, R.; Stöckle, M.; Ostenfeld, M.S.; Dyrskjøt, L.; Junker, K.; Heinzelmann, J. Exosomes of invasive urothelial carcinoma cells are characterized by a specific miRNA expression signature. *Oncotarget* **2017**, *8*, 58278–58291. [CrossRef] [PubMed]
237. Mao, L.; Hruban, R.H.; Boyle, J.O.; Tockman, M.; Sidransky, D. Detection of Oncogene Mutations in Sputum Precedes Diagnosis of Lung Cancer Advances in Brief Detection of Oncogene Mutations in Sputum Precedes Diagnosis of Lung Cancer1. *Cancer* **1994**, *54*, 1634–1637.
238. Wyatt, A.W.; Annala, M.; Aggarwal, R.; Beja, K.; Feng, F.; Youngren, J.; Foye, A.; Lloyd, P.; Nykter, M.; Beer, T.M.; et al. Concordance of Circulating Tumor DNA and Matched Metastatic Tissue Biopsy in Prostate Cancer. *J. Natl. Cancer Inst.* **2017**, *109*, 78–86. [CrossRef] [PubMed]
239. Su, Y.-H.; Wang, M.; Brenner, D.E.; Ng, A.; Melkonyan, H.; Umansky, S.; Syngal, S.; Block, T.M. Human urine contains small, 150 to 250 nucleotide-sized, soluble DNA derived from the circulation and may be useful in the detection of colorectal cancer. *J. Mol. Diagn.* **2004**, *6*, 101–107. [CrossRef]
240. Peng, M.; Chen, C.; Hulbert, A.; Brock, M.V.; Yu, F. Non-blood circulating tumor DNA detection in cancer. *Oncotarget* **2017**, *8*, 69162–69173. [CrossRef] [PubMed]
241. Shao, C.-H.; Chen, C.-L.; Lin, J.-Y.; Chen, C.-J.; Fu, S.-H.; Chen, Y.-T.; Chang, Y.-S.; Yu, J.-S.; Tsui, K.-H.; Juo, C.-G.; et al. Metabolite marker discovery for the detection of bladder cancer by comparative metabolomics. *Oncotarget* **2017**, *8*, 38802–38810. [CrossRef] [PubMed]
242. Maher, A.D.; Zirah, S.F.M.; Holmes, E.; Nicholson, J.K. Experimental and Analytical Variation in Human Urine in ^{1}H NMR Spectroscopy-Based Metabolic Phenotyping Studies. *Anal. Chem.* **2007**, *79*, 5204–5211. [CrossRef] [PubMed]
243. Walsh, M.C.; Brennan, L.; Pujos-Guillot, E.; Sébédio, J.-L.; Scalbert, A.; Fagan, A.; Higgins, D.G.; Gibney, M.J. Influence of acute phytochemical intake on human urinary metabolomic profiles. *Am. J. Clin. Nutr.* **2007**, *86*, 1687–1693. [CrossRef] [PubMed]
244. Thoma, C. Bladder cancer: The promise of liquid biopsy ctDNA analysis. *Nat. Rev. Urol.* **2017**, *14*, 580–581. [CrossRef] [PubMed]
245. Yang, Y.; Miller, C.R.; Lopez-Beltran, A.; Montironi, R.; Cheng, M.; Zhang, S.; Koch, M.O.; Kaimakliotis, H.Z.; Cheng, L. Liquid Biopsies in the Management of Bladder Cancer: Next-Generation Biomarkers for Diagnosis, Surveillance, and Treatment-Response Prediction. *Crit. Rev. Oncog.* **2017**, *22*, 389–401. [CrossRef] [PubMed]
246. Chalfin, H.J.; Kates, M.; van der Toom, E.E.; Glavaris, S.; Verdone, J.E.; Hahn, N.M.; Pienta, K.J.; Bivalacqua, T.J.; Gorin, M.A. Characterization of Urothelial Cancer Circulating Tumor Cells with a Novel Selection-Free Method. *Urology* **2018**, *115*, 82–86. [CrossRef] [PubMed]
247. Pepe, M.S.; Etzioni, R.; Feng, Z.; Potter, J.D.; Thompson, M.L.; Thornquist, M.; Winget, M.; Yasui, Y. Phases of biomarker development for early detection of cancer. *J. Natl. Cancer Inst.* **2001**, *93*, 1054–1061. [CrossRef] [PubMed]

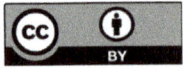

© 2018 by the authors. Licensee MDPI, Basel, Switzerland. This article is an open access article distributed under the terms and conditions of the Creative Commons Attribution (CC BY) license (http://creativecommons.org/licenses/by/4.0/).

MDPI
St. Alban-Anlage 66
4052 Basel
Switzerland
Tel. +41 61 683 77 34
Fax +41 61 302 89 18
www.mdpi.com

International Journal of Molecular Sciences Editorial Office
E-mail: ijms@mdpi.com
www.mdpi.com/journal/ijms

www.ingramcontent.com/pod-product-compliance
Lightning Source LLC
LaVergne TN
LVHW071947080526
838202LV00064B/6695